Technology and Adolescent Mental Health

Megan A. Moreno • Ana Radovic
Editors

Technology and Adolescent Mental Health

Springer

Editors
Megan A. Moreno
Department of Pediatrics
University of Wisconsin-Madison
Madison
Wisconsin
USA

Ana Radovic
Department of Pediatrics
University of Pittsburgh
Children's Hospital of Pittsburgh of UPMC
Pittsburgh
Pennsylvania
USA

ISBN 978-3-319-69637-9 ISBN 978-3-319-69638-6 (eBook)
https://doi.org/10.1007/978-3-319-69638-6

Library of Congress Control Number: 2018932556

Printed on acid-free paper

This Springer imprint is published by the registered company Springer International Publishing AG part of Springer Nature
The registered company address is: Gewerbestrasse 11, 6330 Cham, Switzerland

Preface

In today's world, healthcare providers who see adolescent patients will undoubtedly encounter patients with mental health concerns. Anxiety and depression are common among adolescents and may present with physical, cognitive, or emotional symptoms. Providers who care for adolescents will also experience the encroachment of technology into their patient's lives and health, be it the patient who is distracted and texting during a clinical visit, the patient who asks questions about health information found via a common search engine like Google, or the patient who discloses that he is posting about depression on a popular blogging social media site like Tumblr. Given the overlap in mental health and technology for today's adolescents, this book seeks to inform and empower healthcare providers to take on the challenges and opportunities presented by the intersection of mental health and technology.

With this book's focus on adolescent mental health and technology, our goal was to provide salient information to a range of healthcare providers who may encounter these issues among their adolescent patients. These providers may include primary care providers such as pediatricians, family physicians, or internal medicine providers and specialists including in adolescent medicine and psychiatry. Adolescents also seek care from nurses, social workers, therapists, and counselors, in school-based as well as community-based settings. Providers such as nurse practitioners, physician assistants, and psychologists also provide care to adolescents across these clinical settings. These valuable providers may all be called upon to address mental health concerns among adolescent patients, and we hope this book will provide both familiar and new information to enhance clinical practice.

This book is organized using a public health framework. Thus, the early chapters focus on the epidemiology of mental health and on technology use by teens in health-related ways. Dr. Berman's chapter on adolescent mental health provides an overview of the key mental health conditions, including diagnosis and treatment, among adolescents. Dr. Colditz et al.'s chapter describes current trends and rationale for how and why adolescents use online sources of information for health. Dr. Evans describes ways in which patients with mental health concerns use technology such as the Internet differently compared with peers without mental health concerns.

In the second part of the book, authors dive into associations between the offline and online worlds that affect mental health, presenting both positive and negative outcomes. Dr. Ahrens and Allison Schimmel-Bristow illustrate key aspects of special populations to consider in the relationship between mental health and technology use, including foster youth, disabled youth, and other teens at risk. Dr. Charmaraman et al. describe associations between mental health symptoms, social media use, and self-reported mental health, while Dr. Radovic et al. go into greater detail about social media use and display of depressive symptoms online. Drs. Selkie and Kota describe the phenomenon of cyberbullying and its impact on mental health. Dr. Cheever et al.'s chapter focused on multitasking illustrates how this approach to technology use can affect mental health, as well as other health and academic outcomes. This part also includes two chapters on technology-driven illnesses, including a chapter by Dr. Gentile et al. describing Internet Gaming Disorder, and one by Dr. Cheever et al. describing Problematic Internet Use.

The third part of the book focuses on technology use for the purposes of diagnosis or screening for, intervention, and treatment of mental health conditions. This includes Dr. Doryab's chapter on using technology to identify symptoms of mental illness and Dr. Adrian and Aaron Lyon's chapter discussing new approaches using machine learning to identify risk of suicide. In this part, we also highlight promising approaches to using technology to improve intervention and treatment for mental health concerns and illnesses. Dr. Myers and Jennifer McWilliams provide updates on telemental health. Dr. Santesteban-Echarri et al. describe social media interventions for improving mental health. Dr. Ranney illustrates the emerging role of texting in mental health interventions. Dr. Khan et al. describe promising online intervention approaches for mental health conditions. Drs. DeRosier and Thomas provide a delightful overview of games for mental health, and Dr. Lindheim and Harris describe innovations in mobile applications for mental health. And finally, we conclude with a chapter by Dr. Cash et al. describing organizations that have developed multi-tech approaches including online pages, social media platforms, and other components to present comprehensive programs using technology.

Throughout this book, we aim to provide the most recent, evidence-based approaches that are applicable to clinical practice. To maintain our focus on the application of the information in this book to clinical practice, each chapter includes a patient case illustrating key components of the chapter contents. While we recognize that technology moves quickly, it is our goal that the key approaches and adolescent health considerations described in this book will remain salient even as new platforms and websites emerge. Thus, providers can apply lessons from this read to future tech advances to understand their clinical implications.

Pittsburgh, PA Ana Radovic
Madison, WI Megan Moreno

Contents

Part III Use of Technology for Diagnosis, Intervention, and Treatment

Contributors

Molly Adrian Department of Psychiatry and Behavioral Sciences, University of Washington, Seattle, WA, USA

Kym R. Ahrens Division of Adolescent Medicine, Department of Pediatrics, Center for Child Health Behavior and Development, Seattle Children's Hospital and Research Institute, Seattle, WA, USA

Mario Álvarez-Jiménez Orygen, The National Centre of Excellence in Youth Mental Health, Melbourne, VIC, Australia

Centre for Youth Mental Health, The University of Melbourne, Melbourne, VIC, Australia

Henry Berman University of Washington School of Medicine, Seattle, WA, USA

Karen Bernstein Division of Adolescent Medicine, University of Illinois Hospital, Chicago, Chicago, IL, USA

Jorge A. Blanco-Herrera Iowa State University, Ames, IA, USA

Scottye J. Cash The Ohio State University, Columbus, OH, USA

Linda Charmaraman Wellesley Centers for Women, Wellesley College, Wellesley, MA, USA

Nancy A. Cheever Department of Communications, California State University, Dominguez Hills, Carson, CA, USA

Lauren S. Chernick Pediatric Emergency Department, New York-Presbyterian Children's Hospital, New York, NY, USA

Jason B. Colditz Center for Research on Media, Technology, and Health, University of Pittsburgh School of Medicine, Pittsburgh, PA, USA

Melissa E. DeRosier 3C Institute, Durham, NC, USA

Afsaneh Doryab Carnegie Mellon University, Pittsburgh, PA, USA

Yolanda N. Evans Seattle Children's Hospital, University of Washington, Seattle Children's Hospital, Seattle, WA, USA

Manuela E. Faulhaber Iowa State University, Ames, IA, USA

Douglas A. Gentile Iowa State University, Ames, IA, USA

Tracy Gladstone Wellesley Centers for Women, Wellesley College Wellesley, MA, USA

John Gleeson School of Psychology, Australian Catholic University, Melbourne, VIC, Australia

Jordan L. Harris University of Pittsburgh Medical Center, Pittsburgh, PA, USA

Huma Ali Khan University of Illinois Hospital, Chicago; John H. Stroger, Jr. Hospital of Cook County, , Chicago, IL, USA

Rajitha Kota University of Wisconsin School of Medicine and Public Health, Madison, WI, USA

Oliver Lindhiem Department of Psychiatry, University of Pittsburgh, Pittsburgh, PA, USA

Aaron R. Lyon Department of Psychiatry and Behavioral Sciences, University of Washington, Seattle, WA, USA

Jennifer McWilliams Department of Behavioral Health, Children's Hospital & Medical Center, Omaha, NE, USA

Megan A. Moreno Department of Pediatrics, University of Wisconsin-Madison, Madison, WI, USA

Kathleen Myers Department of Psychiatry and Behavioral Sciences, University of Washington, Seattle, WA, USA

Department of Psychiatry and Behavioral Medicine, Seattle Children's Hospital, Seattle, WA, USA

Kristin Peviani Department of Psychology, Virginia Tech, Blacksburg, VA, USA

Anthony R. Pisani Department of Psychiatry (Psychology) and Pediatrics, University of Rochester Medical Center, Rochester, NY, USA

Brian A. Primack Center for Research on Media, Technology, and Health, University of Pittsburgh School of Medicine, Pittsburgh, PA, USA

Ana Radovic University of Pittsburgh School of Medicine, Children's Hospital of Pittsburgh of UPMC, Pittsburgh, PA, USA

Megan L. Ranney Emergency Digital Health Innovation Program, Department of Emergency Medicine, Alpert Medical School, Brown University, Providence, RI, USA

Simon M. Rice Orygen, The National Centre of Excellence in Youth Mental Health, Melbourne, VIC, Australia

Centre for Youth Mental Health, The University of Melbourne, Melbourne, VIC, Australia

Amanda Richer Wellesley Centers for Women, Wellesley College, Wellesley, MA, USA

Jeffrey N. Rokkum Iowa State University, Ames, IA, USA

Larry D. Rosen Department of Psychology, California State University, Dominguez Hills, Carson, CA, USA

Stephanie Craig Rushing Northwest Portland Area Indian Health Board, Portland, OR, USA

Olga Santesteban-Echarri Orygen, The National Centre of Excellence in Youth Mental Health, Melbourne, VIC, Australia

Centre for Youth Mental Health, The University of Melbourne, Melbourne, VIC, Australia

Department of Psychology, Universitat Rovira i Virgili, Tarragona, Spain

Allison Schimmel-Bristow Department of Counseling, Education Psychology, and Research, The University of Memphis, Memphis, TN, USA

Ellen Selkie Division of Adolescent Medicine, Department of Pediatrics, University of Michigan, Ann Arbor, MI, USA

David Stephens Northwest Portland Area Indian Health Board, Portland, OR, USA

James M. Thomas 3C Institute, Durham, NC, USA

Benjamin Van Voorhees Department of Pediatrics, University of Illinois Hospital, Chicago, Chicago, IL, USA

Michelle S. Woods Center for Research on Media, Technology, and Health, University of Pittsburgh School of Medicine, Pittsburgh, PA, USA

Part I

Epidemiology of Mental Health and Technology

1 An Overview of Adolescent Mental Health

Henry Berman

Overview

You arrive at your office one morning and see that your first patient is Danny, a 15-year-old boy, brought in by his mother.

> *Danny was referred by his pediatrician because of her concerns about changes in his behavior over the past several months. Danny had been a good student, but his grades are deteriorating, and he has recently been truant. He seems withdrawn to his parents and friends, and last week he quit the soccer team, which he had always enjoyed, after a fight with the coach.*

There are a number of diagnoses or conditions that could explain Danny's behavior, including anxiety, depression, ADHD, a history of abuse (domestic violence, sexual, bullying, etc.), disruptions at home, *or* Sex, Drugs, and Rock 'n' Roll, a phrase specialists in adolescent medicine often use to describe normal adolescent behavior. There are seldom hints from a physical examination or a blood test that point to a diagnosis in patients with this kind of presentation. Danny's clinician will need to gather most of the information he needs by interviewing him.

Interviewing Teens

It is not uncommon for teens to show up without an established diagnosis. Before clinicians begin to ask about onset, symptoms, previous history, family history, etc., they need to understand the world of that teen. The established approach to learning about that is the HEADSS interview.[1] HEADSS is the acronym for home, education, activities, drugs, sexual activities/issues, and suicidal ideation or behaviors/depression (see [1, 2] for information about the HEADSS interview and its usefulness).

There are three goals for the HEADSS interview. In order of importance, they are:

1. To establish a relationship with a patient. Teens do not expect an adult to take an interest in their lives and experiences. Just by asking such questions, and listening without judgment, a clinician can gain trust quickly. Trust is the essence of adolescent medicine—teens who trust their medical provider will answer questions honestly, and are more likely to adhere to recommended treatments [3].

H. Berman, M.D.
University of Washington School of Medicine, Seattle, WA, USA
e-mail: henry.berman@seattlechildrens.org

[1] The author of this chapter created the HEADS system as a way to obtain a "social history." Several years later, S for suicidal ideation and behaviors/depression was added, thus converting the approach to a psychosocial history.

M.A. Moreno, A. Radovic (eds.), *Technology and Adolescent Mental Health*,
https://doi.org/10.1007/978-3-319-69638-6_1

The HEADSS interview uses the same approach as a "cognitive interview," created to interview witnesses and victims. A succinct explanation for this approach is: "Rapport is essential and the interviewer, therefore, needs to be socially skilled in order to put the interviewee at their ease and give them license to tell their story in detail. The interviewer needs to be very attentive to what the interviewee is saying. This attentiveness and freedom from interruption seems to encourage interviewees to provide copious detail, apparently serving as affirmation that they are being taken seriously (in our research, incidents lasting minutes were recalled in interviews exceeding an hour)" [4].

2. To assess how well a teen is progressing in managing the journey from the end of childhood to beginning of adulthood, discussed in the last section of this chapter.
3. To identify risk factors and/or risky behaviors.

(With teens, one never knows what a simple question will elicit. Simon Clarke, an Australian specialist in adolescent medicine, had the following experience: "One nice youngster, who was 14, with severe learning difficulties, had a reading age of 7. He had spent 3 years in first class, 2 years in second and 2 years in third. When I asked, 'Did you burn your school down?' he replied, 'yes,' much to the surprise of his jailors") [5].

In addition, a complete HEADSS interview may yield a diagnosis that would not have been considered using a standard medical workup.

Case

JH is a 15-year-old boy who had been taken to the emergency department by ambulance several times because of seizures. The ED staff had not been able to determine the cause, so they referred JH to the pediatrics clinic for a comprehensive workup. The resident who assessed the patient could not find any condition that may have caused the seizures, so he asked for help from the clinic attending. HEADSS had been developed by then but had not been disseminated. The resident had not been taught the HEADSS interview; the attending, however, was familiar with that approach to interviewing.

Even though there did not seem to be any purpose in asking HEADSS questions of a patient with a seizure disorder, the attending physician felt this was the one thing he could do that the resident had not. To the question, "What grade are you in?" the patient responded "eighth grade." (A 15-year-old would generally be in ninth grade.) The most common reason for a student to be held back was poor attendance, so the physician asked, "How many days of school did you miss last year?" The patient replied, "I haven't been to school for a year." To the follow-up question "Why is that?" the patient answered "I am afraid to leave my apartment."

It was a small step for the physician to come to the conclusion that JH suffered from extreme anxiety and would have had severe panic attacks which, in turn, had caused hyperventilation, which lowers carbon dioxide (CO_2). Very low CO_2 can cause carpopedal spasms, which *appear* to be a seizure. By the time an ambulance brought JH to the ED, he had been breathing normally for long enough that all of his blood tests were normal. The correct diagnosis was made only because the question "What grade are you in?" is part of the HEADSS interview.

To determine the underlying cause or causes of behavior changes, clinicians need to understand not only the adolescent but also adolescence. They need to be able to sort out "normal" behaviors for this age group from concerns caused by life situations and also from problems that have a diagnosis and need further evaluation. This chapter discusses the likely causes of worrisome behaviors and provides information on each, including prevalence and the most effective treatments.

Common Mental Health Concerns in Adolescents

Anxiety Disorders

Background on Anxiety Disorders

These are among the most common of mental illnesses in teens; the NIH estimates a 25% lifetime prevalence in 13- to 18-year-olds. However, an NIMH study found that only 18% of adolescents with clinical anxiety ever receive treatment [6]. Identifying and managing adolescent anxiety can be challenging. Symptoms and the focus of anxiety are varied and are often misidentified in primary care as somatic complaints due to "normal" teenage stress. They frequently become manifest in early adolescence and can be incapacitating.

Diagnosing an Anxiety Disorder

The DSM-5 criteria for generalized anxiety disorder (GAD) state that the diagnosis requires the presence of excessive anxiety and worry about a variety of topics, events, or activities; in addition, worry occurs more often than not for at least 6 months and is clearly excessive.

Many individuals with GAD experience symptoms such as sweating, nausea, or diarrhea.

- The anxiety, worry, or associated symptoms make it hard to carry out day-to-day activities and responsibilities. They may cause problems in relationships, at school or at work, or in other important areas.
- These symptoms are unrelated to any other medical conditions and cannot be explained by the effect of substances, including a prescription medication, alcohol, or recreational drugs.
- These symptoms are not better explained by a different mental disorder.

The first two questions of the GAD-7 [44] (Generalized Anxiety Disorder, seven questions) serve as a screening for general anxiety. If the answers to the first two questions add up to three or more, then all seven questions should be asked. GAD-7 [44] is Chart 1.1 in Appendix.

A second validated tool for diagnosing anxiety in subjects 8 to 18 is Screening Children for Anxiety-Related Emotional Disorders (SCARED). Chart 1.2 in the Appendix includes a brief version, the SCARED-5, and the URL for the full SCARED. One advantage of the SCARED tool is that it provides a score for each of the five types of anxiety.

Why Would We Consider Anxiety as the Cause of Danny's Behaviors?

- He may have difficulty concentrating in class because he is afraid something awful might happen, leading to a falloff in his school performance.
- Perhaps he has begun to miss school because he has social anxiety. He is afraid that his teacher will call on him and he won't know the right answer, so the other students will make fun of him.
- Perhaps the coach criticized him for letting an opponent score, and he was so humiliated he quit the team.

Treating an Anxiety Disorder

Mild anxiety disorders that do not appear to be causing serious problems can be managed with support from a clinician, along with nonmedication interventions. These include breathing exercises, muscle relaxation, therapeutic imaging, journaling, exercise, and involvement in art or music. Today, some of these modalities may be taught using technology. Websites and apps exist to support teaching breathing exercises and muscle relaxation. Journaling can happen both offline and online, and art and music are accessed in both tactile and virtual worlds. Another modality of treatment is biofeedback. Biofeedback harnesses the power of technology to visually show vital signs such as breathing and heart rate. Then, as a patient learns to relax, he or she can visualize the change in these vital signs in real time. A review of the literature found that "biofeedback of various modalities is effective for anxiety reduction" [7].

For patients who have moderate anxiety that is causing them some, but not severe, problems, cognitive behavioral therapy (CBT) is the best choice. For patients who are resistant to therapy, medication is *helpful*, while for patients with moderate-to-severe anxiety, medication is *necessary*. One study that included 488 children and adolescents found that medication alone was more effective than CBT alone; the two together had an excellent success rate of 81% [8].

Patients who need medication are treated with an SSRI (selective serotonin reuptake inhibitor). (The FDA has approved sertraline (Zoloft) for the treatment of anxiety in teens. If it is not effective, or there are too many side effects, then clinicians generally "cross-taper" to a different SSRI.)

The DSM-5 describes five kinds of anxiety: general anxiety, separation anxiety, social anxiety, panic disorder, and phobias. Several of these—phobias in particular—respond well to desensitization. Other forms of anxiety are well treated by encouraging the teen to "avoid the avoidance," since avoiding the situation that causes anxiety makes it worse. Sometimes the level of fear or anxiety is reduced by pervasive avoidance behaviors. Panic attacks feature prominently within the anxiety disorders as a particular type of fear response. They are not limited to anxiety disorders and can be seen in other mental disorders as well.

School Refusal Behaviors

Case

WG, a senior in high school, was referred to the adolescent clinic by the gastroenterology clinic where he had been evaluated for nausea and vomiting that had caused him to miss school for the past month. Their doctors had done a series of tests, all of which were normal, and had sent him to the adolescent clinic in the hope that they could determine the cause of his symptoms. WG was asked to describe his experience; it was noteworthy that the symptoms occurred only on school days.

When asked when his symptoms had started, he replied "early July." And when asked had any particular event occurred before he had become sick, he said, "My father came home from work one day and beat up my mother so severely she was afraid she was going to die." His father subsequently spent some time in jail and was released with the requirement that he stay away from the house for several months and take a course in anger management.

His father returned to the home at the beginning of September, and WG said everything was fine now. But, no surprise, his mother was not fine. She worked evenings and slept at home during the day. Subconsciously, WG knew she was still in danger—and if he was home, she would be safe.

"School refusal behaviors" (previously called "school phobia" or "school avoidance") refer to a child-motivated refusal to attend school and/or difficulty remaining in classes for an entire day. Although it is not classified as one of the anxiety disorders, it is caused by the interaction of several of them, so is discussed here. The problem may manifest as lengthy absences from school, skipping classes during the day, being late to school, or misbehaving in the morning in an attempt to miss school. Some youths manage to attend school but do so with great dread and distress.

Extended school refusal behaviors can lead to serious short-term and long-term consequences if left unaddressed. These consequences include academic problems, social alienation, family conflict and stress, school dropout, delinquency, and occupational and marital problems in adulthood. School refusal is extraordinarily difficult to treat. Teens who suffer from both separation anxiety (making it difficult for them to *leave* for school) and social anxiety (making it difficult for them to *be* in school) are particularly difficult to help. Also, any of the other anxiety disorders or any combination can potentiate school refusal.

Common symptoms include anxiety, depression, withdrawal, fatigue, crying, and physical complaints such as stomachaches and headaches. More disruptive symptoms may include tantrums, dawdling, noncompliance, arguing, refusing to move, running away from school or home, and aggression [9].

Barriers: Anxiety is the stepchild of behavioral medicine. For example, the psychiatry department of a highly regarded children's hospital opened a program in the rural part of the state in order to provide care to the children who had no access to mental health services. The announcement of the program described which children would be eligible to receive care: those who have a diagnosis of mild-to-moderate depression or disruptive behavior [e.g., hyperactive/impulsive ADHD and/or an oppositional behavior disorder]. There was no mention of anxiety.

Why are teens with anxiety underserved? Perhaps it is because teens with depression look and act depressed, whereas those with anxiety may show no outward signs of their disorder. In addition, there are five different kinds of anxiety, each presenting in a different way. For the most part, clinicians receive little training in understanding this complex diagnosis.

Depression

Major Depressive Episode (from the DSM-5) condensed

To qualify for "major depressive disorder" (MDD), patients need to have been experiencing symptoms almost every day for at least 2 weeks that are more intense than the normal fluctuations in mood that all of us experience in our daily lives. They need to have at least five of nine symptoms to qualify; one of these five has to be either depressed mood or loss of interest or pleasure in activities. The NIH estimates that 12.5% of the US population aged 12 to 17 has had depression. The prevalence of depression is much higher in females (19.5%) than males (5.8%). As for age, the prevalence in 12-year-olds is 5.4%, rising to 16.1% at age 15. And depression is more common in Whites (13.4%) and Hispanics (12.6%) than in Asians (9.7% and Blacks (9.0%). It is highest in teens with two of more races (15.6%) [10].

What About His Behaviors Would Lead Us to the Conclusion That Danny May Have Depression?

A. Symptoms

1. *Depressed mood most of the day*, almost every day, indicated by subjective report or *by the report of others*. This mood might be characterized by sadness, emptiness, or *hopelessness*.
2. *Markedly diminished interest or pleasure in all or almost all activities* most of the day.
3. Significant weight loss or weight gain when not dieting.
4. Inability to sleep or oversleeping.
5. Psychomotor agitation or retardation.
6. Fatigue or loss of energy.
7. Feelings of worthlessness or excessive or inappropriate guilt.
8. *Diminished ability to think or concentrate*, or indecisiveness.
9. Recurrent thoughts of death (not just fear of dying), recurrent suicidal ideation without a specific plan, or a suicide attempt or a specific plan for killing themselves.

People who die from suicide usually had exhibited one or more warning signs through what they said or what they did, including talking about suicide or having no reason to live, withdrawing from activities, visiting or calling people to say goodbye, or giving away prized possessions. They also may have had mood changes such as depression, loss of interest, anxiety, and irritability. One study found that patients with a previous suicide attempt were 38 times more likely to eventually die from suicide than those with no past attempts [11].

B. Symptoms cause clinically significant distress or *impairment in social, occupational, or other important areas of functioning*.
C. The episode is not due to the effects of a substance or to a medical condition.

Depression can cause low energy and concentration difficulties. *At school, this may lead to poor attendance, a drop in grades, or frustration with schoolwork in a formerly good student.*

The American Academy of Pediatrics recommends that all adolescents 11–21 be screened for depression with the PHQ-2 (Patient Health Questionnaire, two questions); if the answer to either question is "yes," then the full PHQ-9 is administered (Chart 1.3, PHQ-A, Appendix).

In the past 2 weeks, have you been bothered by:

	0	1	2	3
	Not at all	Several days	More than half the days	Nearly every day
1. Little interest or pleasure in doing things?				
2. Feeling down, depressed, irritable, or hopeless?				

Treating Depression

Mild depression that does not appear to be causing problems can be managed with support from a clinician along with non-medication interventions. These include breathing exercises, muscle relaxation, therapeutic imaging, journaling, exercise, and involvement in art or music.

For patients who have mild-to-moderate depression that is causing them some, but not severe, distress, cognitive behavioral therapy may be helpful. Moderately severe depression is treated by medication, therapy, or both, and severe depression is treated with both. A review article published in 2006 found that treating depressed teens with medication alone was more effective than therapy alone; the combination was the most effective [12].

Fluoxetine (Prozac) is the only SSRI approved by the FDA for treating children and adolescents for depression. However, if it is not effective, or causes persistent side effects, other medications in the same family are used.

Persistent Depressive Disorder: PDD (Dysthymia)

Dysthymia is a chronic condition characterized by depressive symptoms that occur for most of the day, more days than not, for at least 1 year (2 years in adults). This disorder is often associated with impaired school performance and poor social interactions, plus irritability and crankiness. Adolescents with this condition also have low self-esteem and are pessimistic and are at high risk to develop major depression. The symptoms must have been present for at least 1 year. During this period, any symptom-free interval cannot have lasted longer than 2 months. Treatment includes both medication and talk therapy.

Bipolar Disorder

The phrase "bipolar disorder" is used to describe a set of "mood swing" conditions, the most severe of which, in the past, was called "manic depression." These patients suffer recurrent episodes of high or elevated moods (mania or hypomania) and depression. Most experience both the highs and the lows. Occasionally people can experience a mixture of both highs and lows at the same time, or switch during the day, giving a "mixed" picture of symptoms. A very small percentage of sufferers of bipolar disorder only experience the "highs." People with bipolar disorder experience normal moods in between their mood swings [13].

A clinician concerned about these behaviors should refer such a patient to a psychiatrist, requesting an urgent assessment due to greater severity and more complicated medication management.

Barriers to receiving care for all of these depressive disorders include a severe shortage of child and adolescent psychiatrists.

ADHD

What Is ADHD (Attention-Deficit/Hyperactivity Disorder)?

The DSM-5 defines ADHD as a persistent pattern of inattention and/or hyperactivity-impulsivity that interferes with functioning or development, has symptoms presenting in two or more settings (e.g., at home, school, or work; with friends or relatives; in other activities), and negatively impacts directly on social, academic, or occupational functioning. Several symptoms must have been present before age 12. A patient may have hyperactivity/impulsivity alone, inattention alone, (labeled ADHD without hyperactivity/impulsivity), or the "combined type." The NIH estimates a prevalence of 11% [14].

It is difficult to come to any definitive conclusions about the epidemiology of ADHD. Most studies are based on patients of different gender or of different ethnic backgrounds or different socioeconomic status. Results can be distorted by the source of the subjects (e.g., if based on patients seen in clinical settings, it will exclude teens who were not seen by a provider and who may be of a different age or gender). Or the variable may be how concerned parents are about school grades; the more important grades are to parents, the more likely they will bring their children to a clinician's office for an evaluation, and the more likely it will be that ADHD is found.

A comprehensive analysis by the National Committee on Health Statistics found that 13.3% of boys and 5.6% of girls aged 4–17 had ever been diagnosed with ADHD. Prevalence was highest among non-Hispanic white children and lowest among Hispanic children. And prevalence was higher for children with family income less than 200% of the federal poverty threshold than for children with family income at 200% or more of the poverty threshold. Most experts believe that girls are more apt to have inattentive ADHD than the hyperactive version. Since being inattentive is less obvious than being hyperactive/impulsive, that might be the basis for some of the difference in gender frequency [15].

What Is the Cause of ADHD?

Our present understanding is that ADHD is caused by a deficit in the circulation of several neurotransmitters, primarily dopamine. The frontal lobes, basal ganglia, corpus callosum, and cerebellum have emerged as the primary areas of the brain showing deficits. These areas are interconnected by a network of neurons. Together, they regulate attention, thoughts, emotions, behavior, and actions. Studies in ADHD patients have showed slower maturation or reduced activity in these areas of the brain. The activity between these areas is maintained by neurotransmitters, in particular dopamine, with involvement of the frontal lobes, basal ganglia, corpus callosum, and cerebellum [16].

A deficit in the amount of dopamine leads to a delay in the development of "executive functions." Executive functions are a set of cognitive processes—including attentional control, inhibitory control, working memory, cognitive flexibility, and planning—that are necessary for the cognitive control of behavior [17].

There is a strong genetic factor. A twin study with 1938 pairs found there was heritability of 0.75–0.91, robust across familial relationships (twin, sibling, and twin sibling) and across definitions of ADHD [18]. It is not unusual for parents to say that there is no family history of ADHD. But a query about behaviors, as opposed to a diagnosis, may lead to a discussion of a father who never graduated from high school or a mother who is always late, often loses her keys, cannot hold down a job, etc. And, as the clinician asks parents about their teen, they may suddenly come to the realization that they themselves may have undiagnosed ADHD.

What About His Behaviors Would Lead Us to the Conclusion That Danny May Have ADHD?

His grades are deteriorating. Many teens with ADHD have above-average intelligence. They do well in lower grades where most of their classes are with one teacher in one room. That teacher knows that Danny needs reminders to pay attention, and she is happy to do that, since he is very receptive to her reminders. Once these teens are in a school situation where each class is in a different room, with a different teacher, their problems with being organized move from the background to the foreground. These problems are exacerbated by the increasing complexity of the course work and in the importance of homework. Danny may be discouraged by his poor grades, so he skips school to play video games. (Video games are characterized by continuous action and are, therefore, particularly attractive to teens with ADHD with their very short attention spans.)

Difficulty in sustaining attention can show up in problems in certain sports. Soccer is a particular problem for teen athletes at the high school level. There are 20 players scattered over a field that measures about 70 *yards* in width and 100 *yards* in length. Who is supposed to do what, when, and where? With experience, teens learn, but it takes more concentration than a sport like basketball, where everyone is moving all the time; there are only ten players, and the court is 94 by 50 *feet*. The problem is even more likely to occur at practice—when only a few players are involved in practicing a particular aspect of the game.

Teens with ADHD are *less likely to have friends*. Acting without thinking, blurting out comments, and not paying attention to conversations—all of these behaviors can interfere with their ability to make and keep friends.

Diagnosing ADHD

The diagnosis is made based on answers by parents, teachers, and the teen to a structured questionnaire (Chart 1.4, Teen Behavior Checklist, Appendix).

DSM-5 lists the 18 questions that determine the likelihood of the diagnosis. If the score for *either* "inattention" or "hyperactive/impulsive" is ≥6, and the behaviors cause problems in more than one setting, the clinician can make tentative diagnosis of ADHD. (For subjects 18 or older, only five need to be positive.) For children, it is important to ask teachers to answer the same questions; however, that is seldom useful with teens. They can have up to six teachers, each with 30 students per class, making it difficult for a given teacher to notice behaviors of any one student. And whereas they can't miss noticing a hyperactive student, they are not likely to pay as much attention to one who is only inattentive.

Is It a "Real Diagnosis?"

No blood test or radiological procedure is useful in diagnosing ADHD. That contributes to the confusion surrounding the disorder. In addition, pronouncements about ADHD from celebrities, the media, neighbors, and grandparents create additional barriers. Fortunately, the medications act very quickly, so clinicians can determine easily if they are effective. The patient can stop at any time without risks or side effects. At times the improvement is so quick and so substantial that the parent is amazed, calling it "a magic pill."

Is ADHD Overdiagnosed?

The section on ADHD in the CDC site states that "less than 1 in 3 children with ADHD received both medication treatment and behavior therapy, the preferred treatment approach for children ages 6 and older" [19].

Treatment of ADHD

Case

JS is a 13-year-old boy brought in by his mother because of poor grades, despite his high intelligence. Two years earlier he had been diagnosed with ADHD, and his clinician had recommended medication. His mother believed that his symptoms could be treated with vitamins and diet, but there was no improvement. She still had doubts about giving her son medication, but after a discussion about the risks and side effects, she agreed to do a trial. After 2 weeks there was some improvement. The dose was increased, and at the next visit, when his clinician asked how he was doing, JS answered "good." When asked what he meant by "good," he answered "I can read boring stuff." [Anyone reading this book has had to "read boring stuff."]

ADHD is best treated by a combination of medication and modification of the behaviors of the teen and the parents. Studies have shown that medication alone can be effective—especially in highly structured home settings—but behavioral modification without the use of medication is not an effective treatment [20].

Medication

There are scores of medications with various chemical compositions, different ways of affecting the brain, different doses, and different durations of actions (see References for a very useful guide for ADHD meds [21]).

The Risks of Not Treating a Teen with Medication

There is a substantial body of literature that demonstrates the effectiveness of medication to reduce a number of problems frequently caused by teens with ADHD. These include:

The reduction of driving risks and impairments associated with ADHD. Teens with ADHD are nearly four times more likely to have had an accident, while they were the driver of a vehicle [22].

A decrease in legal troubles. The estimated probability of *not* being convicted of a crime during a 4-year treatment period was 0.49 for men and 0.75 for women. The same probability during the nontreatment period was 0.37 for men and 0.69 for women [23].

Teens with ADHD who are not on medication are 2.7 times more likely to drop out before high school graduation [24].

Stimulant treatment of children with ADHD was associated with improved reading achievement, decreased school absenteeism, and a modest improvement in grades [25].

Teens with ADHD also experience a greater risk for developing oppositional and defiant behavior (≥50%), conduct problems and antisocial difficulties (25–45%), learning disabilities (25–40%), low self-esteem, and depression (25%) [26].

Three Outcomes of Treatment with Medication:

- There may be dramatic improvement in all aspects of concern immediately or after adjusting medication.
- School performance may improve, but the teen still forgets to hand in homework, and grades suffer.
- There may be minimal improvement in home situations.

If problems persist, it is critical that parents work closely with their teen on behavior management.

Behavior Modification

The first step in modifying the behaviors of the teen and the parents is to "demystify" the cause of the problems. A discussion of the effects of the neurotransmitters on executive functions, as listed above, makes it clear that teens' behaviors are not their "fault," thereby reducing some of the parent-teen conflicts. The next step is "contingency management."

Contingency management, derived from the theory of Operant Conditioning by B.F. Skinner [27], is based on the idea that parents or caregivers provide privileges or preferred activities only when the teen completes a given task. The theory proposes that the requested behavior will increase the frequency of successful completion when desired activities or privileges are allowed, but only after requested behaviors have been completed by the teen. The corollary of this is that when reinforcing events are not contingent upon a given behavior, the behavior will decrease in strength [28].

Because teens with ADHD often have deficits in "active working memory," their ability to remember can be remarkably short. Discussing that one characteristic of ADHD with parents is particularly important. Parents often focus on their teen's forgetting to do chores or saying they will do something soon and then never doing it at all. Once they understand that they are not being ignored, or lied to, they can learn that they need to ask for simple tasks, like taking out the garbage, to be done "now." For tasks that are more complex, and can be postponed, like folding the laundry, the teen must enter a reminder into their iPhone—and do that immediately (before they forget). That way they will remember to do it later, without their parents having to remind them. A few weeks of parents being persistent in these efforts will lead to their teen remembering, with only occasional lapses.

Technology and ADHD

It appears that the use of technology can be a blessing or a curse for teens with ADHD. One study shows that working memory (WM) can be improved by training in children with ADHD by computerized, systematic practice of WM tasks. This training also improved response inhibition and reasoning and resulted in a reduction of the parent-rated inattentive symptoms of ADHD" [29]. Another found that gaming had negative effects on boys—and, in particular, those with ADHD. Boys had more than eight times the probability, odds ratio (OR), of having problematic gaming. Symptoms of ADHD, depression, and anxiety were associated with ORs of 2.43, 2.47, and 2.06, respectively, in relation to coexisting problematic gaming [30]. And a third found that children with ADHD had higher scores on the Internet Addiction Test (IAT), used the internet for longer hours, and went to sleep late than those without ADHD [31].

Summary

It is not uncommon for primary care clinicians to miss the diagnosis of inattentive ADHD. In addition, the short- and long-term consequences are often not appreciated. Also, few clinicians have been taught about the importance of going beyond medication and adding the kinds of structure discussed above.

Twenty years ago, the American Medical Association established a council for the following purpose: to deal with public and professional concern regarding possible overprescription of ADHD medications, particularly methylphenidate, by reviewing issues related to the diagnosis, optimal treatment, and actual care of patients with ADHD, and of evidence of patient misuse of ADHD medications. Among their conclusions were the following:

> "ADHD is one of the best-researched disorders in medicine, and the overall data on its validity are far more compelling than for most mental disorders and even for many medical conditions."

> "ADHD is associated with significant potential comorbidity and functional impairment, and its presence at any age increases the risk of behavioral and emotional problems at subsequent stages of life. It is thus a chronic illness with persistence common into adolescence and beyond."

> "Optimal treatment of ADHD involves an individualized plan based on any comorbidity as well as child and family preferences. This treatment generally will include pharmacotherapy (usually with stimulant medication) along with adjunctive psychoeducation, behavioral therapy, environmental changes, and, at times, supportive psychotherapy of the child, the family, or both"[2] [32].

This summary describes most of the barriers to the diagnosis and treatment of ADHD in teens. Additional barriers include the shortage of professionals to implement the AMA's "optimal treatment," as well as the cost of the stimulants needed for effective treatment.

Understanding Adolescent Mental Health in Context of Life and Stress

Behavioral Problems Related to Stress

The American Psychological Society found that in a survey of over 1000 teens, they reported that their stress level during the school year far exceeded what they believe to be healthy (5.8 on a 10-point scale). Note: their assessment even in the summer, with no school, was a level of 4.6. Teens also reported feeling overwhelmed (31%) and depressed or sad (30 percent) as a result of stress. More than one-third of teens reported fatigue or feeling tired (36%), and nearly one-quarter (23%) reported skipping a meal due to stress [33].

The best way to determine if a teen's symptoms are primarily due to stress is to use the HEADSS system (discussed in the introduction to the chapter), listening for the possibility of a stressful situation. The following are examples of questions that can elicit useful information.

Home

Who is in Peter's household? Perhaps his mother remarried several months ago—there is now a stepfather and some stepsiblings too. Suppose his father died recently after a long illness—how is

[2] Russell Barkley, PhD, has written a number of books and articles about ADHD—for both clinicians and for parents. *Taking Charge of ADHD—the Complete Authoritative Guide for Parents*, the Guilford Press, 2013, is particularly helpful. The book includes tips for changing behavior.

affecting him? How does he get along with those he shares a house with? Does his father abuse him physically—perhaps even sexually? Does he have an older brother who bullies him? If his parents are divorced, are there issues around custody? If so, does one parent insist on seeing him every other weekend even when he does not want to be with that parent? Did his family move recently? And being in a new school—the year had already started—has it been difficult to become included in any group?

Education

What grade is Madison in? Perhaps she is 15 and in 11th grade—she had skipped a grade in elementary school and could do the work for several years but is now over her head. How many days of school has she missed this year? Perhaps she has had 15 absences in the first 3 months; she often has severe abdominal pain upon awakening—likely to be secondary to anxiety.

What are Madison's grades, "and how does she feel about them? Does she have a 3.3 grade-point average, but her parents are pushing her to get her grades up to 3.6? Or does she have a 2.3 average, and her parents are worried that she won't get any financial aid for college to supplement their low earnings? Does she want to attend an elite school, but several months ago got her PSAT scores and they were only 1010? (An example from a recent adolescent medicine listserv: "The patient has an older sister who goes to a prestigious college but is upset she did not get into an even more prestigious place. The parents talk about how crazy other parents in the area are in terms of unreasonable expectations for their children, yet one of the issues the patient has with her father is that he is 'helicopter parenting.'").

If her grades are lower than they were in the past, is she getting enough sleep? If not, is it because the work is so difficult that she stays up past midnight to finish it? Or does she complete it by 11:00 but texts her friends until 1 a.m.? Is there a television set in her bedroom?

Activities

How does Omar like to spend his time? Perhaps he liked soccer, but his performance did not live up to his older brother's, so he managed to have a fight with his coach, is now off the team, and no longer has the burden of equaling his brother. Does he have close friends—what are they like? Are they all A students and he feels inadequate with his 3.3 GPA? Or is *he* the A student and his friends appreciate his help in preparing for exams? And what does he mean by "friends?" Does he see them only in school, or does he spend a lot of time with them after school and on weekends? Are they face-to-face friends, or are they Facebook "friends?"

Does he attend a house of worship regularly and enjoy it, or does he feel it is a burden—his parents won't let him miss a service? Does Omar have a part-time job—Saturdays only—and can he use the money? Or is money tight and he has to work 3 hours each night and falls behind in his homework or has no spare time to spend with friends?

Drugs

Does Mateo smoke cigarettes or use alcohol or smoke marijuana and drive while high or ride in his best friend's car while his friend is driving after smoking marijuana? Does he use oxycodone—if so, where does he get it, and where does he get the money to purchase it? Does he have friends who use fentanyl and urge him to try it because the high is mind-blowing? Has he ever gotten into trouble when he is high?

Sexual Experiences/Concerns

Does Aisha have a dating relationship? If so, what attracts her to that person (be sure to be gender neutral until the patient describes the friend)? Has she had a sexual experience? If so, ask about it. Was it entirely consensual? How old is that partner? More than 2 years older increases the possibility of less-than-consensual sex. It also raises the possibility of being illegal. (Clinicians should know the law in their state about what is a crime in these situations.) Has she been involved with "sexting?" If so, does she understand what problems that might cause for her? (A 13-year-old girl was brought in by her mother who was concerned about some of her behaviors, including sending her "boyfriend" a picture of herself from the waist up. The girl was outraged: "I had my bra on!")

Is she attracted to the same sex, the opposite sex, both, or neither? If she has had sexual intercourse, was a condom used? Plus, another method of contraception? And did Aisha's partner use a condom *every time* they had intercourse? Has she ever had a sexual experience against her will? Does she have any questions about sex?

Summary

The answers to these questions may identify the underlying problem. There is often a cascade effect—parents get divorced, and the custodial parent can't afford their house and so moves to a less expensive part of town. It is too far for the patient to see their friends regularly and their new friends smoke marijuana. They get busted, or they develop amotivational syndrome and their grades drop.

Do they have a "disorder" or have there been too many stressful situations in their life? The "treatment" is likely to be an adult who they trust. Perhaps a grandparent, or the mother of one of their good friends. Or a teacher/school counselor. Or a clinician who has earned their trust by listening, not judging, and by being available.

Sex, Drugs, and Rock 'n' Roll

Understanding Normal Teenage Behavior

Adolescence begins at the end of childhood and ends at the beginning of adulthood. In order to appreciate just how overwhelming this may seem to 12-year-olds facing that journey, look at it from their point of view:

If they want to become autonomous adults, they must:

- Find out who they are.
- Convince their parents they can take care of themselves responsibly.
- Develop a set of ethical guidelines.
- Learn how to live with rules that help them get along in the world, neither accepting nor rejecting them blindly.
- Learn how to have close relationships.
- Learn how to deal with people in a practical way.
- Learn how to deal with their sexuality, both physically and emotionally.
- Explore what they want to do with their lives.
- Begin to acquire the skills they will need to be self-supporting.
- Learn to view their parents realistically, and limit their battles with them to a necessary minimum.
- Develop realistic aspirations and find role models that embody them [34].

Certain behavioral features common among adolescents may have evolved to promote attainment of the necessary skills for independence. These age-related behaviors, such as an adolescent-associated increase in risk-taking, have often been attributed to increases in pubertal hormones. However, it appears that the primary cause is developmental events occurring in the brain during adolescence.

Giedd et al. (1999) published a landmark study on brain development during childhood and adolescence. The prior assumption about the adolescent brain had been that there was growth and change up to about the age of 12 and after that there were no significant changes in brain structure. The article reported that pediatric neuroimaging studies confirmed linear increases in white matter but demonstrated "nonlinear changes in cortical gray matter, with a preadolescent increase followed by a post-adolescent decrease" [35].

Spear (2000) noted "We provide evidence from recent brain imaging and animal studies that there is a heightened responsiveness to incentives and socioemotional contexts during this time, when impulse control is still relatively immature. These findings suggest differential development of bottoms-up limbic systems, implicated in the incentive and emotional processing, to top-down control systems during adolescence prone to emotional reactivity, increasing the likelihood of poor outcomes" [36].

More recently, Casey, Jones, and Hare (2008) wrote "Adolescents knowingly engage in risky behavior, and this is often due to influences of feelings, emotions, and peers .... Our model suggests that the adolescent is capable of making rational decisions, but in emotionally charged situations the more mature limbic system will win over the prefrontal control system." Adolescents show adult levels of intellectual capability but do not yet have full capacity to override impulses in emotionally charged situations that require decisions in the heat of the moment [37].

It is important for clinicians to pay attention to aspects of adolescent brain development other than risk-taking, as articulated in an article by Guyer et al. (2009). "This general model of adolescent brain development has been extended beyond the study of risk-taking in several ways… Adolescence is also a time of important changes in the processing of social and emotional information, much of which is subserved by the same regions and systems that undergird the motivational and self-regulatory changes described by writers who have focused on risk-taking. For instance, there is evidence that adolescents are highly responsive to the social rewards afforded by positive peer evaluation and that *such rewards activate the same brain regions as non-social rewards.*" [Italics added by author] [38].

The critical role that peers play in the life of teens is also emphasized by the following observation: "We also have evidence that the presence of peers leads adolescents to more steeply discount delayed rewards, leading to increased preference for immediate, although smaller, ones" [39].

Of particular interest for readers of this book, a recent study found that in adolescents, "symptoms of video game addiction depend not only on video game play but also on concurrent levels of online communication. Those who are very socially active online report fewer symptoms of game addiction" [40].

Knowledge of key elements in the development of the adolescent brain can enable clinicians to counsel their teen patients more effectively. For example:

- Understanding that, despite their intellectual level, adolescents are susceptible to making poor decisions "in the heat of the moment," clinicians realize that they need to urge their female patients who are sexually active to consider long-acting, reversible, contraception (LARC).
- Being knowledgeable about the critical importance of peer relationships gives clinicians insight into the puzzling behavior of teens who, even at their own detriment, refuse to "rat" on their friends.
- Knowing the propensity of teens to take more risks in the presence of their peers, clinicians might want to warn their patients about the extreme risks of drinking heavily at a party because they want to fit in.

It appears that an increased emphasis on reducing risky behaviors of "normal teenagers" is worth the effort of law-makers, parents, clinicians, and perhaps the media, as can be seen in the chart below:

Behavior	Earlier rate	Year	New rate	Year
Teen birth rate[a]	61.8 per 1000 adolescent females	1991	24.2 per 1000 adolescent females	2014
Use of marijuana in past month for 8th graders[b]	6.5%	2015	5.4%	2016
Of those, daily use	1.1%	2015	0.7%	2016
Cigarette use (≥½ pack a day) by high school students	10.7%	1991	1.8%	2016
12th graders being drunk over past year	53.2%	2001	37.3%	2016

[a]HHS Office of Adolescent Health 2014

[b]This and the remaining behaviors are from the Monitoring the Future annual survey by the National Institute on Drug Abuse of the NIH; it surveys students in 8th, 10th and, 12th grades

This chapter is about teens with difficulties—ranging from severe problems to normal adolescence. It is important for clinicians to remind themselves that, for the most part, they see teens who are healthy only occasionally—for exams for sports or camp—but see those who have a problem often. Most teens are doing well—the most recent CDC data show that close to 83% of teens are in excellent or very good health and another 15% are in good health [41].

And they are not only healthy, but most are also happy. Psychiatrist Daniel Offer was a pioneer in the study of adolescents; he challenged prevailing beliefs that adolescence is inherently a time of storm and stress. In 1963, Offer received 8 years of federal grants to study the psychological development of normal adolescents. In the first phase of the study, 73 boys were selected from two suburban Chicago area high schools and followed for 8 years. The major finding for the high school phase was that stability and not turmoil was the overriding characteristic of normal adolescents. This finding contradicted the then current notion of normal development. At that time, it was believed that all adolescents go through major turmoil as they move through the high school years. In 1981, Offer and two colleagues published a book based on the Offer Longitudinal Study that concluded that "eighty-five percent of the adolescents they tested reported being happy most of the time" [42].

Offer's study is considered the "gold standard" for research about *normal* adolescents. The author could not identify any other longitudinal study of healthy teens. However, in 2010, the NIMH published *Lifetime Prevalence of Mental Disorders in U.S. Adolescents* [43]. The study concluded that approximately one in every four to five youth in the USA will meet criteria for a mental disorder with severe impairment across their lifetime. We can infer from that that 75–80% of youth will *not* experience such a disorder in their lifetime.

Resources

Society for Adolescent Health and Medicine website:
www.adolescenthealth.org/

Appendix

Chart 1.1 GAD-7

Over the last 2 weeks, how often have you been bothered by the following problems?	Not at all	Several days	More than half the days	Nearly every day
1. Feeling nervous, anxious, or on edge	0	1	2	3
2. Not being able to stop or control worrying	0	1	2	3
3. Worrying too much about different things	0	1	2	3
4. Having trouble relaxing	0	1	2	3
5. Being so restless that it is hard to sit still	0	1	2	3
6. Becoming easily annoyed or irritable	0	1	2	3
7. Feeling afraid as if something awful might happen	0	1	2	3
Add columns Total score ____	___	___	___	___

If you checked off problems, how difficult have they made it for you to do your schoolwork, take care of things at home, or get along with other people?
Not difficult at all ___ Somewhat difficult ___ Very difficult ___ Extremely difficult___
Scoring: A total score of ≥10 means the patient is likely to have an anxiety disorder
Spitzer RL, et al. A brief measure for assessing generalized anxiety disorder. Arch Intern Med. 2006;166:1092–97

Chart 1.2 SCARED. Screening for Childhood Anxiety-Related Disorders (SCARED). Below is the **SCARED-5**. If the score for this assessment is ≥3, use the full SCARED questionnaire: ww.psychiatry.pitt.edu/sites/default/files/Documents/assessments/SCARED%20Child.pdf

During the past 3 months are the following statements "not true or hardly ever true," "somewhat true or sometimes true," or "very true or often true?" (scored 0 to 2)	People tell me that I worry too much 0 1 2
I get frightened for no reason at all 0 1 2	I am scared to go to school 0 1 2
I am afraid to be alone in the house 0 1 2	I am shy 0 1 2
Total points for SCARED 5:	*Scoring: ≥ 3 separates anxiety from non-anxiety*

Chart 1.3 PHQ-9 modified for adolescents (PHQ-A)

	0	1	2	3
	Not at all	Several days	More than half the days	Nearly every day
1. Little interest or pleasure in doing things?				
2. Feeling down, depressed, irritable, or hopeless?				
3. Trouble falling asleep or staying asleep or sleeping too much?				
4. Feeling tired or having little energy?				
5. Poor appetite or overeating?				
6. Feeling bad about yourself—Or that you are a failure or let yourself or your family down?				
7. Trouble concentrating on things, such as reading the newspaper, doing homework, or watching television?				
8. Moving or speaking so slowly that other people could have noticed. Or the opposite—Being so fidgety or restless that you have been moving around a lot more than usual?				
9. Thoughts that you would be better off dead or of hurting yourself in some way?				
Total each column				

Total: ________

If you said yes to *any* problems, how *difficult* have these problems made it for you to do your work, take care of things at home, or get along with other people?

Not difficult at all ___ Somewhat ____ Very ____Extremely ___

Scoring:

0–4 No depression symptoms
5–9 Mild depression symptoms
10–14 Moderate depression symptoms (therapy)
15–19 Moderate to severe depression symptoms (therapy and/or meds)
20 or more severe depression symptoms (therapy and meds)

If the patient responds "yes" to question 9, the risk of suicide needs to be determined and a plan developed

Chart 1.4 Teen behavior checklist (updated as per DSM-5)

Name of Person Being Rated ______________________

Name of Rater, if not Patient ______________________ Date__________________

Inattentive Behaviors

Check the column that best describes the teen's behavior *over the past 6 months*

	Never or rarely	Sometimes	Often	Very often
1. Fails to give close attention to details or makes careless mistakes in school work, at work, or during other activities (e.g., overlooks or misses details, work is inaccurate)				
2. Has difficulty sustaining attention to tasks or activities (e.g., has difficulty remaining focused during lectures, conversations, or lengthy reading)				
3. Does not seem to listen when spoken to directly (e.g.., mind seems elsewhere, even in the absence of any obvious distraction)				
4. Does not follow through on instructions and fails to finish school work, chores, or duties in the workplace (e.g., starts tasks but quickly loses focus and is easily distracted)				
5. Has difficulty organizing tasks and activities (e.g., difficulty managing sequential tasks, difficulty keeping materials and belongings in order, has poor time management, fails to meet deadlines)				
6. Avoids, dislikes, or is reluctant to engage in tasks that require **sustained** mental effort (e.g., schoolwork or homework; for older adolescents and adults, preparing reports, completing forms, reviewing lengthy papers)				
7. Loses things necessary for tasks or activities (e.g., school materials, pencils, books, tools, wallets, keys, paperwork, eyeglasses, phones). Sometimes loses **completed** homework				
8. Is easily distracted by extraneous stimuli (for older adolescents, may include unrelated thoughts)				
9. Is forgetful in daily activities (e.g., doing chores, running errands; for older adolescents and adults, returning calls paying bills)				
Total				

Hyperactive/Impulsive Behaviors

	Never or rarely	Sometimes	Often	Very often
10. Fidgets with hands or feet or squirms in seat				
11. Leaves seat in classroom or in other situations in which remaining seated is expected (e.g., leaves his or her place in the classroom, in the office or other workplace, or in other situations that require remaining in place)				
12. Frequently feels restlessness				

	Never or rarely	Sometimes	Often	Very often
13. Has difficulty engaging in leisure activities or doing fun things **quietly**				
14. Is "on the go" or acts as if "driven by a motor" (e.g., is unable to be or uncomfortable being still for an extended time, as in restaurants, meetings; may be experienced by others as being restless or difficult to keep up with)				
15. Talks excessively [**ends *hyperactivity***]				
16. Blurts out an answer before questions have been completed (e.g., completes people's sentences, cannot wait for turn in conversation)				
17. Has difficulty awaiting turn (e.g., while waiting in line)				
18. Interrupts or intrudes on others (e.g., butts into conversations, games, or activities; may start using other people's things without asking or receiving permission; may intrude into or take over what others are doing) [**ends *impulsivity***]				
Total				

Do these behaviors cause significant difficulties?
Home: yes ___ no___ School: yes ___ no ___
Scoring: Add each of the columns in the Inattentive ADHD set. Combine totals for "Often" and "Very Often." Do the same for the hyperactive/impulsive behaviors. See article for next step
[Content from DSM-5. Structure created by author]

References

1. Katzenellenbogen R. HEADSS: The "Review of Systems" for adolescents. Virtual Mentor. AMA J Ethics. 2005;7(3):Clinical Pearl.
2. Goldenring JM, Rosen D. Getting into adolescent heads: an essential update. Contemp Pediatr. 2004;21(64):1–19.
3. Litt IF, Cuskey WR. Compliance with medical regimens during adolescence. Pediatr Clin N Am. 1980; 27(1):3–15.
4. Waddington PAJ, Bull R. Cognitive interviewing as a research technique. Social Res Update. 2007;50:Summer.
5. Berman HS, Dashefsky HS. Teens and their doctors. The story of the development of adolescent medicine. Sagamore Beach, MA: Science History. p. 65.
6. https://www.nimh.nih.gov/health/statistics/prevalence/any-anxiety-disorder-among-children.shtml.
7. Yucha CB, Montgomery D. Evidence-based practice in biofeedback and neurofeedback. A faculty publication by the University of Nevada, Las Vegas. 2009. http://digitalcommons.library.unlv.edu/nursing_fac_articles/1.
8. Walkup, et al. Cognitive behavioral therapy, sertraline, or a combination in childhood anxiety. N Engl J Med. 2008;359:2753–66.
9. Berman HS. Teens who don't go to school. J Child Adolesc Behav. 2015;3:3.
10. NIH. A complicated picture. https://www.nimh.nih.gov/about/directors/thomas-insel/blog/2011/antidepressants-a-complicated-picture.shtml.
11. Harris EC, Barraclough B. Suicide as an outcome for mental disorders: a meta-analysis. Br J Psychiatry. 1997;170:205–28.
12. Ruple SJ, Blecke DM, Renfrow M. Cognitive therapy for depression. Am Fam Physician. 2006;73:83–6.
13. NIDA. January Bipolar disorder. 2014. https://www.nimh.nih.gov/health/topics/bipolar-disorder/index.shtml.
14. CDC. https://www.cdc.gov/ncbddd/adhd/data.html.
15. NCHS Association between diagnosed ADHD and selected characteristics among children aged 4–17 years: United States, 2011–2013. NCHS Data Brief No. 201, May 2015.
16. Giedd JN, et al. Brain imaging of attention deficit/hyperactivity disorder. Ann N Y Acad Sci. 2001; 931:33–49.
17. https://en.wikipedia.org/wiki/Executive_functions.
18. Levy F, et al. Attention-deficit hyperactivity disorder: a category or a continuum? Genetic analysis of a large-scale twin study. J Am Acad Child Adolesc Psychiatry. 1997;36:737–44.
19. CDC ADHD. https://www.cdc.gov/ncbddd/adhd/data.html.
20. The MTA Cooperative Group. A 14-month randomized clinical trial of treatment strategies for attention deficit/hyperactivity disorder. Arch Gen Psychiatry. 1999;50:1073–86.
21. Googling "North Shore LIJ ADHD" and selecting "medication guide" will open a remarkable chart that has a photo of every one of these medications, in each dose, in full color. The chart can be obtained free of charge.

22. Fischer M, et al. Hyperactive children as young adults: driving abilities, safe driving behavior, and adverse driving outcomes. Accid Anal Prev. 2007;39: 94–105.
23. Lichtenstein P, et al. Medication for attention deficit–hyperactivity disorder and criminality. N Engl J Med. 2012;367:2006–14.
24. Barbaresi WJ, et al. Modifiers of long-term school outcomes for children with attention-deficit/hyperactivity disorder: does treatment with stimulant medication make a difference? Results from a population-based study. J Dev Behav Pediatr. 2007;28(4): 274–87.
25. Robyn L, et al. Stimulant treatment in children with attention-deficit/hyperactivity disorder moderates adolescent academic outcome. J Child Adolesc Psychopharmacol. 2008;18(5):449–59.
26. Adapted from Barkley RA, Murphy KR. Attention deficit hyperactivity disorder: a clinical workbook. 3rd ed. New York: Guilford; 2006.
27. Skinner BF. Science and human behavior. New York, London: The Free Press, Collier-Macmillan; 1953.
28. Graziano AM, editor. Behavior therapy with children II. Aldine Transaction; 2008.
29. Klingberg T, et al. Computerized training of working memory in children with ADHD—a randomized, controlled trial. J Am Acad Child Adolesc Psychiatry. 2005;44:177–86.
30. Vadlin S, et al. Associations between problematic gaming and psychiatric symptoms among adolescents in two samples. Addict Behav. 2016;61:8.
31. Weinstein A, et al. Internet addiction and attention deficit hyperactivity disorder among schoolchildren. Isr Med Assoc J. 2015;17(12):731–4.
32. Slanetz PJ, et al. For the council on scientific affairs. Diagnosis and treatment of attention-deficit/hyperactivity disorder in children and adolescents. JAMA. 1998;279:1107–0.
33. American Psychological Association survey shows teen stress rivals that of adults. 2014. http://www.apa.org/news/press/releases/2014/02/teen-stress.aspx.
34. Williams LH, Berman HS, Rose LM. The too precious child. The perils of being a super-parent and how to avoid them. New York: Atheneum Macmillan; 1987. pp. 229–30.
35. Giedd JN, et al. Brain development during childhood and adolescence: a longitudinal MRI study. Nat Neurosci. 1999;2:861–3.
36. Spear LP. The adolescent brain and age-related behavioral manifestations. Neurosci Biobehav Rev. 2000;24:417–63. [Abstract].
37. Casey BJ, Jones RM, Hare TA. The adolescent brain. Ann N Y Acad Sci 2008;1124:111–26.
38. Guyer A, et al. Probing the neural correlates of anticipated peer evaluation in adolescence. Child Dev. 2009;80:1000–15.
39. O'Brien L, Steinberg L. Impact of peers on delay discounting. Presented at the biennial meeting of the Society for Research on Adolescence, Philadelphia; 2010.
40. Carras MC, et al. Video gaming in a hyperconnected world: a cross-sectional study of heavy gaming, problematic gaming symptoms, and online socializing in adolescents. Comput Hum Behav. 2017;68:472–79.
41. CDC. https://ftp.cdc.gov/pub/Health_Statistics/NCHS/NHIS/SHS/2014_SHS_Table_C-5.pdf.
42. Offer D, Ostrov E, Howard HI. The adolescent, a psychological self-portrait. New York: Basic Books; 1981.
43. Merikangas KS, et al. Lifetime prevalence of mental disorders in U.S. adolescents: results from the National Comorbidity Survey Replication–Adolescent Supplement (NCS-A). J Am Acad Child Adolesc Psychiatry. 2010;49(10):980–9.
44. Spitzer RL, et al. A brief measure for assessing generalized anxiety disorder. Arch Intern Med. 2006;166:1092–7.

2 Adolescents Seeking Online Health Information: Topics, Approaches, and Challenges

Jason B. Colditz, Michelle S. Woods, and Brian A. Primack

Background

Adolescence is a developmental stage characterized by curiosity and uncertainty [1]. By virtue of their physical development within complex social environments, adolescents encounter new experiences that demand external insights and reassurances. This includes health-related questions about whether personal experiences are "normal" and how new experiences should be handled. Traditionally, adolescents have relied on trusted adults (e.g., parents, physicians, teachers), peers, and traditional print or audiovisual media for answers to health questions.

While traditional media resources remain important sources of health information for adolescents, online resources are increasingly available and utilized. As of 2015, 84% of adolescents in the USA report having ever received health information from the Internet, and one-quarter report getting "a lot" of Internet health information [2]. In a sense, the Internet has democratized access to useful health information. However, online resources also incorporate novel biases that can affect health knowledge and beliefs.

There are known biases in the way that adolescents seek out, understand, and utilize online health information. Some of these biases are a function of health literacy and information-seeking approaches. Others are germane to the online environment and how information is presented. For example, informational websites offer authoritative answers to myriad health questions. However, conflicting information may be presented across multiple sites. Additionally, the quality and comprehensiveness of information varies among sources. For example, many sites are commercial and present information that supports particular health products or practices. Social media sites also provide substantial information to most adolescents [3]. These sites can also incorporate compelling video clips from interactive audiovisual platforms, such as YouTube. These technologies offer opportunities for answering old health questions in new, compelling, and interactive ways. The ways that adolescents seek out online health information will continue to adapt with the availability of novel information resources.

An Evolving Online Ecosystem

Many webpages and search platforms present easily navigated static information, but they do not offer opportunities for dialogue. The rise of technology—such as webpage comment interfaces and

J.B. Colditz, M.Ed. (✉) • M.S. Woods, B.A
B.A. Primack, M.D., Ph.D.
Center for Research on Media, Technology, and Health, University of Pittsburgh School of Medicine, Pittsburgh, PA, USA
e-mail: colditzjb@pitt.edu

M.A. Moreno, A. Radovic (eds.), *Technology and Adolescent Mental Health*,
https://doi.org/10.1007/978-3-319-69638-6_2

dedicated social networking sites—has changed the dynamic of online interaction. Myspace, which was the most popular social networking site among adolescents in the early 2000s, faced sharp declines in participation as adolescents gravitated toward newer platforms [4]. Facebook, which is now highly popular among adolescents, has been predicted to face a similar decline [5]. In addition to changes among platforms, the functions and features within them have evolved over the years. For example, as smartphones became popular, so did the sharing of images and videos via social media platforms such as Snapchat and Instagram. As the online landscape continues to evolve toward interconnectivity and artificially intelligent platforms, adolescents' online behavior is likely to adapt in turn.

Nearly all adolescents in developed countries have access to diverse online resources at home, at school, and/or via mobile devices [6]. Adolescents are sometimes referred to as "digital natives" because they cannot remember a time before Internet communication technologies [7]. The technological landscape will continue to change around these digital natives. While they may obtain health information through new technological channels, the types of health questions and concerns associated with adolescence are largely unchanged.

Overview of Adolescents' Online Health Information Seeking

Results from a recent survey conducted by the Center on Media and Human Development at Northwestern University help to frame how adolescents utilize online resources to seek health information. The authors conducted a nationally representative survey of 1156 US adolescents, aged 13–18, in English- and Spanish-speaking households in 2014–2015 [8]. The survey detailed what types of health information adolescents seek and what online sources they consult. A summary of descriptive results are publicly available via a comprehensive online report [2].

Health Topics [2]

With 95% of adolescents rating their health as good or excellent, it makes sense that the health topics they personally consider "very important" are primarily related to general well-being. However, nearly one-third of adolescents identified topics related to sexual health and mental or behavioral health as very important. Figure 2.1 presents the top five health topics of importance within each of these groupings and the extent to which corresponding information is sought online. Across general well-being, sexual health, and mental/behavioral health, there are incongruities between a topic's importance and whether or not adolescents search for it. For example, although nearly 50% of adolescents rate "personal hygiene" as very important, just over 10% searched for hygiene information online. However, roughly equal proportions of adolescents rate exercise important (45%) and report having searched about it online (42%). Such incongruity may indicate that some information is adequately covered via other sources such as trusted adults [9]. Identifying health topics that are rated as both important and commonly searched for could help to prioritize health education interventions for adolescents.

There is also discordance around what adolescents identify as being personally important versus what they believe is important among other adolescents their age. For example, 59% of adolescents identify drug/alcohol abuse as very important among their peer group, whereas 32% rate it as comparably important to themselves. Similarly, with respect to sexually transmitted infections, 57% consider this topic to be very important among peers, as compared to 32% who find it personally important. When searching for health information online, adolescents more frequently investigate topics with which they personally identify, rather than those that they attribute to being important among peers. This may indicate that adolescents' online health information seeking is personally motivated, rather than an expression of topical curiosity.

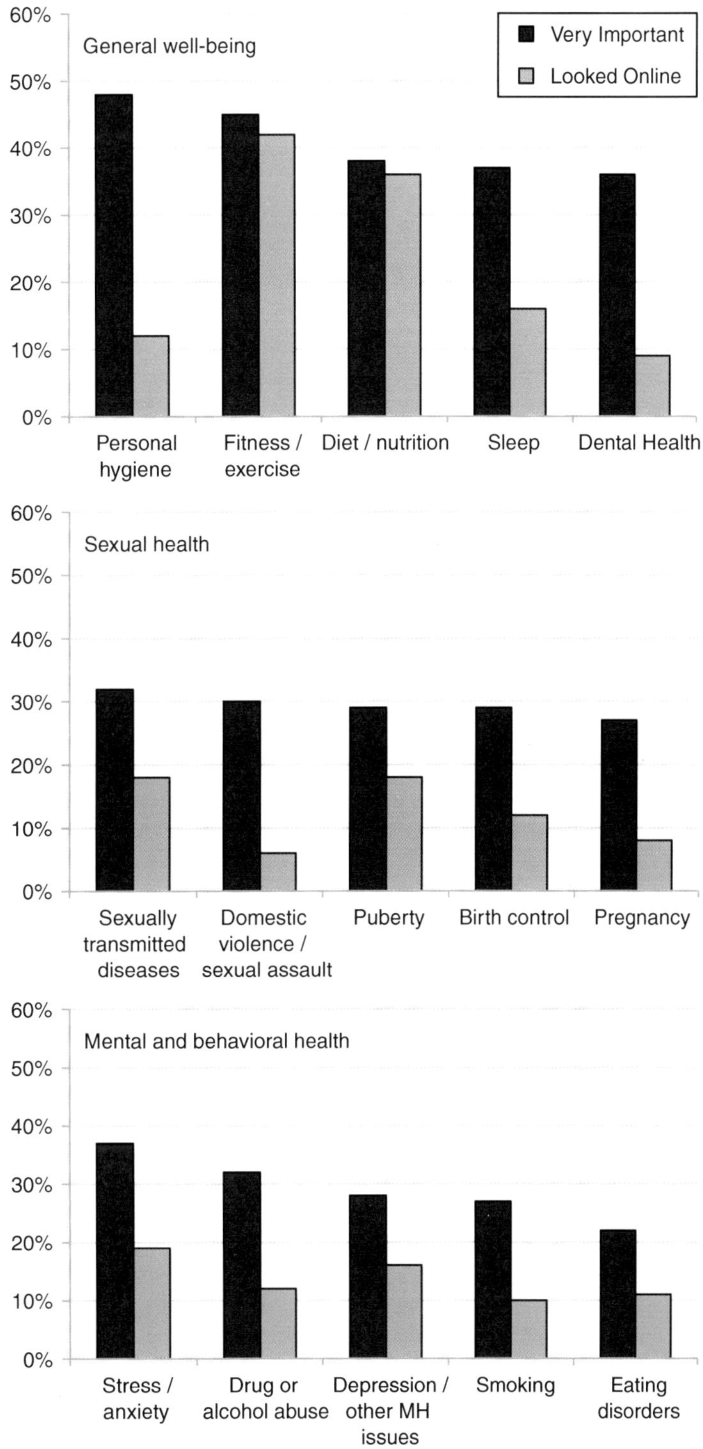

Fig. 2.1 Proportion of adolescents endorsing a health topic as very important and looking for health information online [2]

Of the 84% of adolescents in the USA who report having ever received health information online, 45% report that they had done so to learn better self-care habits, 33% to check symptoms, 24% to treat a personal health condition, and 12% to obtain medication information. Of adolescents who report seeking online health information, 34% report that they changed their behavior as a result. Such behavior change is more likely to happen in circumstances in which an intrinsic desire to change motivates health information seeking [9].

Health Information Sources [2]

An adolescent's choice of information source is influenced by the health topic. For information about serious health conditions (e.g., cancer, heart attacks), adolescents favor parental advice. For sensitive health topics such as birth control or depression, adolescents tend to look up the information online. In both situations, adolescents generally indicate that they are somewhat less likely to consult a doctor and not at all likely to talk to someone on a hotline. Overall, 11% of adolescents indicate that they have gone online for information on a health topic that could be uncomfortable to discuss with parents.

Despite the popularity of Internet use among adolescents, they continue to get a large amount of information from trusted adults. For example, adolescents indicate that they get "a lot" of information from their parents (55%), school health classes (32%), and doctors or nurses (29%). Additionally, adolescents report that they are more satisfied with information obtained from trusted adults compared with information from other sources. About 75% of adolescents report getting very little or no information from traditional media such as newspapers, magazines, or radio. Adolescents rely on peers, television, and books to a slightly larger extent. One-quarter of adolescents indicate that they get "a lot" of health information from the Internet. A greater percentage of adolescents get at least some health information online (61%) compared with getting information from friends (49%). Adolescents are also more satisfied with online health information than they are with information obtained from friends.

While four out of five adolescents are at least "somewhat" satisfied with information obtained from the Internet, there are many reasons they report being dissatisfied. Primarily, dissatisfied adolescents reported being faced with information that was conflicting (42%), unreliable (40%), or not relevant to their situation (35%). Other reasons for dissatisfaction included taking too long to navigate information, encountering vague information, and/or being unable to find an answer (26–29%).

Among adolescents who reported seeking out health advice online, the top four methods ever used included the Google search platform (58%), medical websites (37%), Wikipedia (26%), and YouTube (24%). Despite the popularity of social media platforms, they do not appear to be popular for seeking out health information among adolescents. Among adolescents who do seek health information on social media platforms, the most commonly used platforms are Facebook (11%) and online health blogs (9%). Fewer than 5% of adolescents report following any health-related groups on social networking sites.

In summary, adolescents continue to rely on trusted adults to provide health information, and they are largely satisfied with information that they receive. Beyond that, adolescents tend to favor online sources, particularly for sensitive health topics. Adolescents seeking online health information rely primarily on Google searches.

Google Is a Verb

A 2003 observational study of online search strategies identified Google as the most popular search engine for a dolescents seeking health information [10]. At that time, it was used roughly as much as the next four most popular search engines combined. Since "google" was added to mainstream dictionaries as a verb in 2006 [11, 12], "googling" has become synonymous with seeking online knowledge in a general sense. However, because 89% of adolescents who seek health information online report that they sometimes or often do so by "googling it" [2], it is likely that they literally mean using the Google search engine.

Adolescents report managing the many results returned when searching for a common health term challenging [2, 13]. It is perhaps because of this overload of information that adolescents tend to focus on only the first page of search results. In fact, half of adolescents who search for health information trust that the first result "is usually the best one" and rarely explore search results beyond that [2].

Google provides results linking to Wikipedia, medical websites, and YouTube, which are also popular sites for adolescents seeking health information. Since around 2012, some Google searches have begun to return "featured snippets" that summarize likely answers to questions based on popular search results. Some adolescents may perceive these snippets as providing concise, authoritative answers to health queries. Additionally, advertisements are commonly featured near the top of Google search results, which makes commercially oriented results more likely to be seen. Results from search platforms may also be different depending on search history, location, and what device or web browser is used. Additionally, the underlying search algorithms may occasionally change, and results may reflect more popular or timely search trends among other platform users.

For the examples of Google search results presented later in this chapter, we relied on a desktop computer with a web browser set to "private" or "incognito" and without any "safe search" restrictions in place (e.g., parental controls). While this allows for more generalizable search results, adolescents may encounter different results based on when and how they connect to the Google platform.

Table 2.1 Selected online health information resources for adolescents

Organization and website	Overview
"TeensHealth" of the Nemours Foundation **teenshealth.org**	Educational content that covers a variety of topics including general well-being, sexual health, mental health, substance use, school and jobs, motor vehicle safety, and other areas of adolescent development
"Young Women's Health" of Boston Children's Hospital **youngwomenshealth.org**	Educational content about general well-being, sexual health, mental health, and other health concerns as they relate to young women
"Young Men's Health" of Boston Children's Hospital **youngmenshealthsite.org**	Educational content about general well-being, sexual health, mental health, and other health concerns as they relate to young men
"Go Ask Alice!" of Columbia University **goaskalice.columbia.edu**	An interactive question and answer site that provides individualized feedback from a team of health promotion specialists and healthcare providers

Information Seeking Across Specific Health Domains

Adolescents seek online information about a variety of health topics, and several reputable organizations provide relevant health resources to this end (e.g., Table 2.1). However, adolescents face challenges that inhibit their abilities to retrieve information based on what health information is popular or most easily accessible. Other challenges relate to how adolescents understand, interpret, and engage with online health information. Adolescents encounter these challenges when searching across a variety of health topics, including general well-being, sexual health, and mental/behavioral health.

General Well-Being

General well-being issues were commonly endorsed as "very important" by adolescents (Fig. 2.1). The pattern in Fig. 2.1 also suggests that more complex topics are more commonly sought online. For example, while dental care is fairly straightforward (e.g., brush, rinse, floss), topics such as weight loss can elicit a wide breadth of complex and conflicting information [14].

Information-Seeking Shortcuts

When evaluating complex topics around general well-being, adolescents may incorporate "shortcuts" to simplify the task. For example, online health information can be filtered through cognitive heuristics such as *lay reasoning* and *attribution to others* [15]. Lay reasoning integrates simple information from non-expert sources (e.g., peer influence, popular culture, political viewpoints) or common platitudes (e.g., "an apple a day keeps the doctor away") as precedent to more complex information communicated by reputable health resources. For example, a celebrity plainly endorsing "eating meat is animal cruelty" is more readily interpretable than lengthy dietary guidelines that weigh social and health considerations surrounding particular meat products. Attribution to others can serve to dismiss conflicting health perspectives as overly dramatic, scaremongering, and/or disproportionately oppositional. This may occur around particularly contentious topics such as vaccination, where individuals of opposing viewpoints might be attributed stereotypical labels (e.g., "vaxxers" versus "anti-vaxxers") and their conflicting perspectives more conveniently dismissed. Another mental shortcut that can influence online health information seeking is *positive hypothesis testing* in which adolescents may selectively seek information that confirms preexisting health beliefs [16]. For example, an adolescent may google the name of a particular health regimen of interest and focus attention toward results that provide positive affirmation of its practices and virtues, regardless of the veracity of information provided. These information-seeking shortcuts reduce the cognitive demand of evaluating complex and conflicting information. They may also reduce the potential for cognitive dissonance experienced when health-driven behaviors are based in weak or counterfactual evidence [17].

Pop-Health Beliefs

Within the realm of diet and nutrition in particular, some health topics can be classified as popularized health, or *pop-health*. For example, the Paleolithic "Paleo" diet has risen to recent popularity through celebrity endorsements, branded merchandise, cross-promotion with popularized exercise programs, and conference tours [18]. Scientific evidence supporting the efficacy of this diet continues to be debated within the nutrition field [19, 20]. While some of the lay public remains skeptical, others are less critical and several books focusing on this diet have become bestsellers [18, 21]. This particular diet is one of many examples of fad diets, juice cleanses, and get-fit-quick exercise regimens touted by celebrities [22]. Often these health practices are based in weak or circumstantial evidence. Adolescents who haven't been instructed on critical appraisal of information skills may be vulnerable to popular and pseudoscientific health claims [23]. In particular, pop-health trends may be compelling because adolescents face developmental concerns about body image and social pressure to conform with peers who actively engage in novel health practices.

Sexual Health

Adolescents tend to be concerned about parents and health providers being judgmental about sexual health topics [24]. Concerns about stigma and privacy drive many adolescents to seek out sexual health information online. Even when using online resources, anonymity is a particular concern among adolescents. For example, adolescents prefer sites that do not require providing personally identifying information and sites that have an existing answer section in case their particular health question has already been asked [24]. As the credibility of online health information is also a concern, adolescents tend to prefer resources that list authors' qualifying health credentials [24].

Adolescents seeking sexual health information online are most likely to search for information about sexually transmitted infections and puberty (Fig. 2.1). However, as was the case for topics of general well-being, perceived importance and degree of online searching does not always match. For example, while domestic violence and sexual assault are highly important sexual health topics among adolescents, these are infrequently searched for online. When adolescents turn to online sources for information, certain search strategy challenges arise for topics such as sexual health.

Search Strategies

Googling the word "sex" provides over three billion results. The first page of results might include online editorials from popular *Women's Health* or *Men's Health* magazines that provide guidance on how to "please your partner" or "last longer in bed." Other top search results might include links to graphic narratives, images, or videos. Reputable and developmentally appropriate health resources are scarce among these top results. Searching for "sex" is an example of an overly simplistic strategy for which search results provide the most popular online content. These top results may offer very little age-appropriate content to answer the sexual health questions adolescents find most important.

A more targeted search for "sexual health" first elicits a featured definition from the World Health Organization and then several top results from reputable organizations that are directly relevant to developmentally appropriate topics such as puberty, sexually transmitted infections, and understanding healthy relationship boundaries. For health practitioners, it might seem obvious to google "sexual health." However, this is unlikely to be an initial search approach among adolescents without such conceptual insights or who do not use formal health terminology to frame sexual practices.

Adolescents seek online answers to particular sexual health questions that are not covered in sexual health curricula or topics that are too uncomfortable to discuss with an adult [25]. Thus, adolescents may use online searches to supplement rather than replace current sexual health knowledge. An examination of information seeking in this realm categorized adolescents' search objectives as *definitional*, *functional*, *normative*, *experiential*, *relational*, and *factual* [25]. For example, a query such as "How do I know if I am pregnant?" would be considered factual, while a query such as "How do I know if a girl likes me?" would belong in the relational category [25]. Adolescents are also likely to seek additional online information about what constitutes "normal" sexual development and behavior. Such information seeking is less about understanding statistical norms in a public health sense and more about self-evaluating whether individual life experiences are considered physically or socially appropriate [26].

Search Results

Taking into account search ranks and top results, health-related search results can be biased in ways that favor personal experiences and editorialized narratives over evidence-based recommendations. For example, an assessment of Google search results related to human papillomavirus vaccines revealed significantly higher search rankings for pages that were critical of vaccination, offered less biographical information about authors, and included more unsubstantiated testimonials [27]. Similarly, in the results of a systematic search about adolescent birth control, information about long-acting reversible contraception was often omitted or ran counter to widely accepted clinical guidelines [28].

Without advanced conceptual insights or grasp of clinical terminology, adolescents are apt to discount relevant information that they do not understand. For example, as adolescents search for information about STIs (sexually transmitted infections), they may dismiss information related to STDs (sexually transmitted diseases) as "completely different" [29]. In general, adolescents may not understand sexual health terminology in a way that leads to engagement with age-appropriate and evidence-based online information [30]. While sexual health questions may be uncomfortable for adolescents to bring up in clinical settings, practitioners may be able to initiate useful conversations by asking about particular topics that patients have been googling. This may lead to opportunities for imparting useful sexual terminology to contextualize future online searches.

Mental and Behavioral Health

Approximately 10–20% of adolescents seek online information on topics related to mental or behavioral health (Fig. 2.1). In this realm, the "stress and anxiety" category is most often endorsed as "very important" and is also the most commonly searched for topic. Other important concerns include alcohol and substance abuse, depression and other mental health issues, smoking, and eating disorders. Information about attention deficit hyperactivity disorder is searched for by 9% of adolescents [2]. Concerningly, 14% of adolescents report having ever encountered online information about obtaining or making illegal drugs, whether they were seeking it or not [2].

Social Influences: Substance Use

In addition to searching for specific behavioral health information online, adolescents also likely engage in *social learning* in this milieu. For example, online platforms present novel opportunities for social learning about substance use. Websites like *erowid.org* provide background information and experiences of individuals experimenting with novel drugs. *Experience reports*, or "trip reports," can be quite detailed with regard to dosing and polysubstance use while sometimes including narratives about having spiritual experiences or gaining deep philosophical insights [31]. Erowid and online messaging have played a role in adolescents' dissemination of "innovative" substance use information [32]. Recently, social media platforms such as Reddit have provided a forum for popular, anonymous discussions devoted to drug use, "research chemicals" (i.e., newly emerging psychoactive substances), and experience reports [33]. Online message boards also provide information about "bad trips" [34]. These online resources may be compelling enough to encourage adolescents to experiment with mind-altering substances. However, cautionary tales may also dissuade some from engaging in risky behaviors. Therefore, clinicians working with adolescents who use substances may wish to ask about knowledge of online drug use resources. In-depth knowledge of these resources might indicate a willingness to engage with novel substances.

Social Influences: Mood Disorders

With respect to mood disorders, online communities can provide both *informational support* and *emotional support* [35]. Emotional support may be particularly valuable to adolescents who are suffering from mental health concerns by providing a sense of belonging with others who experience similar issues [36]. Personal characteristics such as age, gender, and education play a role in active participation within online support venues [37]. For adolescents in this milieu, it may be important to engage with a peer group that provides relevant information and offers encouragement to overcome personal challenges. Receiving online support is associated with reciprocally offering support to others [38]. This social reciprocity may offer a sense of personal agency. As such, there is potential for adolescents to engage in meaningful, potentially helpful, online peer support environments.

Adolescents generally prefer to get emotional support from parents and peers and informational support from health professionals [39]. These types of social support systems are ideal when readily available, which is not always the case for adolescents dealing with mental health concerns. This presents both an opportunity and a challenge to practitioners who advocate for adjunctive online support for adolescents. For example, it is possible that some adolescents may gravitate toward online support environments while drifting further from appropriate family, peer, and clinical guidance. Research into evidence-based, online peer support options for adolescent mental health remains ongoing. While it is premature to make objective recommendations about how adolescents should or should not seek online mental health support, it is clear that this is a serious consideration for practitioners who work with adolescents.

Optimal and Extreme Health Behaviors

Adolescent online searches about diet and nutrition are more than three times as prevalent as searches related to eating disorders (Fig. 2.1). However, the type of information available when searching for topics related to healthy eating can model unhealthy behaviors. Making dietary decisions around pop-health beliefs or setting ideals around strict goals of "clean eating" may contribute to *orthorexia* [40]. Orthorexia (literally "cor-

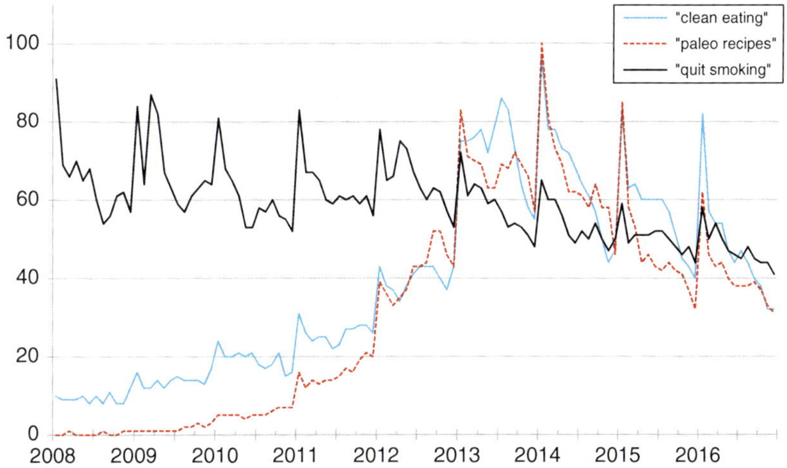

Fig. 2.2 Relative monthly prevalence of Google searches in the USA, 2008–2016. Source: http://trends.google.com/

rect appetite") is characterized by a preoccupation with the *quality* of food consumed [41], rather than concerns about quantity of calories or body image. Recent case studies have reported that malnourishment and associated negative health impacts are associated with severe orthorexic tendencies [42]. The availability and dissemination of pop-health content on social media is likely to be an exacerbating factor in disordered eating [43]. For example, image-sharing platforms such as Instagram can play a particularly influential role in the dissemination of unrealistic and unattainable health ideals [44]. As this is a relatively new and emerging health trend, there is still much to learn about how online information seeking may play a contributing role in adolescent eating disorders.

For a general sense of online search trends in this domain, Fig. 2.2 depicts Google Trends data about "clean eating" that are highly correlated with pop-health searches of "Paleo recipes" over time (Pearson $r = 0.97$). These searches peak around New Year's Day, much like other health resolutions such as "quit smoking." In contrast to the relatively constant pattern in searches related to quitting smoking, both "clean eating" and "Paleo recipes" rose from relative obscurity in 2008 to peak popularity in 2014. Monitoring the popularity of searches may provide new insights into emergent public health concerns surrounding pop-health trends and emerging patterns that may be related to orthorexia.

Other Health Topics

Adolescents also seek out online information about specific symptoms or health conditions affecting them (20%) or affecting friends or family members (23%) [2]. For these and other contributing reasons (e.g., school projects), 6% of adolescents seek online information about heart disease and 8% about diabetes. Online information about cancer is sought by 12% of adolescents, and this topic is endorsed as personally "very important" by 24%. In contrast, while the same proportion (12%) have sought online cold or flu information, this had the lowest comparable importance among all topics (17%) [2]. Initial searches for common, innocuous symptoms can sometimes escalate toward searches about symptoms or diseases that are more serious and less likely [45]. For individuals who are particularly concerned or anxious about their health, this "query escalation" may lead to increased anxiety rather than alleviating health concerns [45, 46].

Cyberchondria

Cyberchondria can be defined as health anxiety typified by Internet searches for medical information that (1) are repetitive or excessive, (2) increase negative affect or distress, (3) interrupt daily living or are compulsive, and (4) engender reassurance seeking [47]. While such searching may result in plausible explanations for health concerns, the results may not account for the established prevalence or likelihood of particular health conditions. This may lead adolescents to catastrophize about severe and chronic health conditions based on searches about common symptoms or transient experiences.

A suggested approach to mitigating the effect of cyberchondria in vulnerable adolescents is "Internet use education" to improve online health literacy [47]. Interventions that seek to improve online health literacy may also be useful in circumventing some of the challenges and biases associated with online health information seeking in general.

Online Health Literacy in Adolescent Health Information Seeking

The quality of health information that adolescents obtain is influenced by both extrinsic and intrinsic factors. Extrinsically, is there adequate and accurate information readily available? Intrinsically, what characteristics allow adolescents to locate reliable health information and formulate rational understandings from it? The level of *health literacy* that an adolescent possesses is a contributing factor to obtaining and synthesizing quality health information from online sources. The prevailing model of health literacy involves a tripartite framework of functional, interactive, and critical health literacy domains [48]. These domains build on one another as functional health literacy is requisite for developing interactive health literacy, which is a building block for critical health literacy.

Functional Health Literacy

While many adolescents seek health information online, particularly through search engines, they are not necessarily adept at doing so. Health-related information can be dense and can incorporate unfamiliar health terminology. Adolescents' limited grasp of health terminology may prevent them from searching for answers to health questions [13]. In some cases, search engines suggest corrections for minor misspellings. However, this still relies on the adolescent knowing succinct terminology for their health query. While googling "nosiatd" does display results for "nauseated," it still requires adequate conceptual knowledge to know what this word means. Deficits in functional health literacy may be particularly problematic in younger and socioeconomically disadvantaged populations [49].

As discussed earlier in the context of sexual health topics, adolescents with limited health vocabulary may encounter information that is irrelevant or unhelpful. Even when specific language is used, different health terminology can impact search results in nuanced ways. For example, searching for "vaccination" results in a significantly higher proportion of anti-vaccination websites compared to searching for "immunization" [50]. Therefore, low functional health literacy can be a major impediment to adolescents who are seeking health information online. In the mental health domain, few adolescents are likely to have an innate grasp of terminology like "anhedonia" or "depersonalization" and would thus describe such symptoms in lay language. When appropriate, providing adolescents with more precise health terminology that relates to their condition may help to steer them toward interacting with higher-quality online resources.

Interactive Health Literacy

While functional health literacy is related to knowledge about particular health-related terminology, interactive health literacy is focused on forming coherent thoughts and appropriate interactions around those topics. This could involve developing new heuristics for interacting with online platforms. For example, in a study of goal-directed online health searches, adolescents were found to use trial and error to formulate and refine search strings [10]. Adolescents who are particularly savvy may implement more advanced approaches such as using quotation marks to search for exact phrases or using Boolean operators (e.g., *this* AND *that*, *this* OR *that*, *that* AND NOT *this*) to further refine search parameters [51].

When applied to social media, the concept of interactive health literacy does not necessarily imply social interaction. For example, adolescents may "lurk" on social media sites where they can observe the communication of others and gain insights into particular health topics without actively posting content [52]. Lurking may be an effective way to assure a sense of normalcy and belonging without needing to self-disclose sensitive information. Observing social contexts can also influence adolescents' health decision-making. In one example, an adolescent male ultimately decided that it was not worth the risk of using a performance-enhancing supplement for body building after reading online discussions about side effects [13].

Interactive health literacy on social media may also take the form of active engagement (e.g., posting health questions), though it is less common among adolescents. Only 11% of adolescents report that they are likely to post a health query on a social networking site [2]. This represents one-third of those who report getting health information from social networking sites overall. Posting health queries is more likely to happen among adolescents from lower income brackets, racial and ethnic minorities, and those who recently engaged in risky behaviors [2]. This demographic pattern also holds true among adolescents following health-related links on social networking sites [2].

In addition to text-based interactions, video-sharing sites such as YouTube offer opportunities to view personal health stories or advice, featuring interactive comment sections. Furthermore, viewing messages from others of similar age or background may be more compelling. This may help to explain why YouTube is used to find health information by nearly a quarter of adolescents who seek health information online [2]. There are several popular young adult YouTube personalities ("YouTubers") who post personal videos about coping with mental illnesses. For example, Laura Lejeune and "LikeKristen" are young women who post videos about experiencing conditions such as anxiety, depression, seasonal affective disorder, and disordered eating. Googling "mental health youtubers" results in these and other examples that are highly popular and generate substantial online discussion about mental health. For some adolescents, engaging with this material may present a beneficial sense of emotional support and reduce perceived stigma. However, while health information from social media and YouTube may seem particularly relatable and compelling to adolescents, it is particularly important that such information is fact-checked against other reputable information sources.

Critical Health Literacy

Critical health literacy focuses on the ability to navigate and interpret the quality of available health information. This is similar to the concept of *information literacy*, which according to the American Library Association means a person has the ability "to recognize when information is needed and have the ability to locate, evaluate, and use effectively the needed information" [53]. Even when appropriate search results are found, adolescents may lack systematic approaches to reviewing those search results, such as considering the quality of the information source [10].

Critical health literacy relates to understanding the relevance and trustworthiness of information that is presented [13]. This is an important issue because many adolescents are likely to trust the first result appearing in online searches [2]. This reliance on primacy is problematic if the first results contain biased or misleading information. While large commercial websites employ expensive "search engine optimization" techniques to improve search rank, such advantages are not readily available for health advocacy organizations on tighter budgets [54]. Popular search engines are not currently adept at evaluating or organizing results by credibility of the source material, and search rankings can be manipulated in several ways [55].

While these extrinsic factors affect how information is presented, critical health literacy focuses on evaluation of information. For example, adolescents frequently access Wikipedia—an online encyclopedia where anyone can contribute or edit content—but they tend to trust health information from other types of websites more [2]. Perceptions of Internet sources' trustworthiness may also vary by gender. In one study of Chinese students, males tended to be more likely to incorporate information from Wikipedia based on appraisals of information accuracy, while females were more motivated by the perceived relevance of information [56].

Individuals with low health literacy tend to evaluate online health information based on factors such as position in search results, quality of pictures, and celebrity endorsements [57]. Compared with less educated online health consumers, more educated ones tend to trust information from medical universities and federal institutions [58]. Higher level of education has also been positively associated with checking credentials of health website authors [59].

Susceptibility to misinformation presents another challenge to effective health information seeking. For example, conspiracy theories related to vaccination are among the most widely circulated in the USA [60]. This is due in large part to the availability of unsubstantiated health claims and politicization around the topic (e.g., focusing narratives around civil liberties instead of health) [61, 62]. The majority of popular YouTube videos about vaccinations discourage their use and raise health concerns with little scientific substantiation [63]. Because YouTube videos are a staple of adolescent online health seeking, this warrants further investigation into how the concept of *media literacy* interrelates to broader understandings of critical health literacy. Recently proposed models of health literacy have incorporated aspects of media literacy and also considered online *eHealth literacy* as a unique construct [64, 65].

Case Report

Lucy is a 19-year-old college student. She presented to her primary care provider with complaints of persistent physical and psychological symptoms consistent with generalized anxiety. In the course of clinical evaluation, Lucy acknowledged anxiety as a serious personal concern and mentioned that she had been actively researching treatment options online. She explained that her online searches covered a variety of therapeutic approaches that led to more questions than answers. In particular, she felt confused about the potential risks and benefits of commonly accepted pharmaceutical treatments. This led her to be interested in "natural" remedies that might serve as alternative approaches in reducing her symptoms of anxiety.

Lucy's boyfriend, with whom she had previously discussed her mental health concerns, was adamant that natural remedies were safer than and just as effective as pharmaceutical "meds" that might be prescribed in the course of primary care. This led Lucy to turn to Google for confirmation. Given some of the common results of googling "dangers of anxiety meds," it is not surprising that Lucy had serious misgivings about pharmacological treatment options. For example, a prominent search result led to a *Psychology Today* editorial that states:

> …people who use anti-anxiety medication have a 36% increased mortality risk. That means persons using these drugs are almost 40% more likely to die than people who do not use them. Yikes. … Given the dire side effects, it does not make sense to pummel patients with these drugs when they are not needed. And even after an urgent situation has passed, many patients tend to remain on them indefinitely because doctors are not sure how to help patients wean off these, and/or prescribe non-pharmaceutical remedies.

The author's biography for this editorial links out to a private website that focuses on provision of naturopathic remedies and acupuncture services. This illustrates how commercial or self-promotional interests can leverage popular online health platforms to steer patients away from established primary care resources. Such circumstances may present challenges for providers who attempt to use evidence-based treatments. Patients who are skeptical of "unnatural" approaches may be predisposed to pop-health beliefs that discount the efficacy of evidence-based treatment modalities in favor of folk remedies. For example, individuals who contributed to the comment section for the editorial noted

Table 2.2 Example questions for adolescents to assess quality of online health information resources (higher values indicate better quality)

	No		Somewhat		Yes
High-quality indicators					
Does it clearly explain and link to some research studies?	1	2	3	4	5
Does it show how the author is an expert on this health issue?	1	2	3	4	5
Does it give many options for dealing with this health issue?	1	2	3	4	5
Does it suggest things to talk about with doctors or family?	1	2	3	4	5
Low-quality indicators					
Does it say that doctors or health experts have the wrong ideas?	5	4	3	2	1
Does it relate to selling a health product or service?	5	4	3	2	1

above touted Epsom salt baths as a standalone treatment for anxiety.

Clinicians may encourage patients like Lucy to use functional, interactive, and critical health literacy skills when interpreting online health information. Evaluation frameworks are increasingly available to help adolescents effectively engage with such resources. For example, the DISCERN instrument is a comprehensive tool for assessing the quality of online information [66]. While the DISCERN tool is lengthy and predates newer developments in social media, a clinician might review the DISCERN content and provide a similar tool that is tailored to a patient's particular situation and level of health literacy (e.g., Table 2.2). Using evaluation tools with accessible language may help patients gauge the quality of information, help improve health literacy, and subsequently foster evidence-based care.

Conclusions

Online resources offer a wealth of static and interactive information that adolescents can utilize to learn about health. Obtaining online health information can be done anonymously, offering adolescents a way to explore sensitive health topics. While adolescents might be considered technology-savvy "digital natives," their abilities to obtain reputable online health information may be hindered by biases in how information is portrayed and interpreted. Adolescents tend to gravitate toward health information that is popular or appears in top search results. Such information may run counter to clinical guidelines, omit important details, or be scientifically inaccurate.

Adolescents most frequently search for information about general well-being that might serve to improve health. However, when taken to extremes, this health-seeking behavior can also result in negative health impacts such as in extreme cases of "orthorexia" or "cyberchondria." Adolescents also commonly search for information around sexual, mental, and behavioral health. These topics present additional challenges such as heightened concerns about privacy, stigmatization, or modeling harmful behaviors. However, online health resources can also provide helpful emotional support and reputable informational support when approached thoughtfully.

Much research still needs to be done to better understand adolescents' online health information-seeking behaviors and associated health outcomes. In the meantime, helping adolescents to improve functional, interactive, and critical online health literacy skills is worthwhile. Clinicians might consider how such education might be creatively incorporated into interactions with patients.

References

1. Erikson EH. Identity: youth and crisis. New York: Norton; 1968.
2. Wartella E, Rideout V, Zupancic H, Beaudoin-Ryan L, Lauricella A. Teens, health, and technology: a national survey. Chicago, IL: Northwestern University Center on Media and Human Development; 2015.
3. Pew Research Center. Social media fact sheet. 2017. http://www.pewinternet.org/fact-sheet/social-media/.
4. Boyd D. White flight in networked publics: how race and class shaped American teen engagement with

MySpace and Facebook. In: Nakamura L, Chow-White PA, editors. Race after the internet. New York: Routledge; 2012. p. 203–22.
5. DeLegge A, Wangler H. Is this the end for Facebook? A mathematical analysis. Appl Math Comput. 2017;305:364–80.
6. Pew Research Center. Internet/broadband fact sheet. 2017. http://www.pewinternet.org/fact-sheet/internet-broadband/.
7. Bennett S, Maton K, Kervin L. The "digital natives" debate: a critical review of the evidence. Br J Educ Technol. 2008;39:775–86.
8. Wartella E, Rideout V, Zupanic H, Beaudoin-Ryan L, Lauricella A. Teens, health, and technology: a national survey. Media Commun. 2016;4:13–23.
9. Racey M, Machmueller D, Field D, Kulak V, Newton GS. Perceptions and use of sources of health knowledge by young adolescents. Int J Adolesc Med Health. 2016; [e-pub].
10. Hansen DL, Derry HA, Resnick PJ, Richardson CR. Adolescents searching for health information on the internet: an observational study. J Med Internet Res. 2003;5:e25.
11. Merriam-Webster Collegiate Dictionary. 11th ed. Springfield, MA: Merriam Webster; 2006.
12. Oxford English Dictionary. Oxford: Oxford University Press; 2006.
13. Gray NJ, Klein JD, Noyce PR, Sesselberg TS, Cantrill JA. The internet: a window on adolescent health literacy. J Adolesc Health. 2005;37:243.e1–7.
14. Senkowski V, Branscum P. How college students search the internet for weight control and weight management information: an observational study. Am J Health Educ. 2015;46:231–40.
15. Regan Á, Shan L, McConnon Á, Marcu A, Raats M, Wall P, et al. Strategies for dismissing dietary risks: insights from user-generated comments online health. Risk Soc. 2014;16:308–22.
16. St. Jean B, Subramaniam M, Taylor NG, Follman R, Kodama C, Casciotti D. The influence of positive hypothesis testing on youths' online health-related information seeking. New Libr World. 2015;116:136–54.
17. Ong AS-J, Frewer L, Chan M-Y. Cognitive dissonance in food and nutrition—a review. Crit Rev Food Sci Nutr. 2015; [e-pub].
18. Chang ML, Nowell A. How to make stone soup: is the "Paleo Diet" a missed opportunity for anthropologists? Evol Anthropol Issues News Rev. 2016;25:228–31.
19. Fenton TR, Fenton CJ. Paleo diet still lacks evidence. Am J Clin Nutr. 2016;104:844.
20. Manheimer EW. Reply to TR Fenton and CJ Fenton. Am J Clin Nutr. 2016;104:845.
21. Knight C. We can't go back a hundred million years. Food Cult Soc. 2015;18:441–61.
22. Caulfield TA. Is Gwyneth Paltrow wrong about everything? how the famous sell us elixirs of health, beauty & happiness. Boston, MA: Beacon Press; 2015.
23. Nordheim L, Pettersen KS, Flottorp S, Hjälmhult E. Critical appraisal of health claims: science teachers' perceptions and practices. Health Educ. 2016;116:449–66.
24. Selkie EM, Benson M, Moreno M. Adolescents' views regarding uses of social networking websites and text messaging for adolescent sexual health education. Am J Health Educ. 2011;42:205–12.
25. Knopf A, Groves D, Miller W, Fortenberry D, Priest C. Adolescents' anonymous sexual health queries to the ChaCha question and answer service. J Adolesc Health. 2016;58:S100.
26. Harvey KJ, Brown B, Crawford P, Macfarlane A, McPherson A. "Am I Normal?" teenagers, sexual health and the internet. Soc Sci Med. 2007;65:771–81.
27. LY F, Zook K, Spoehr-Labutta Z, Hu P, Joseph JG. Search engine ranking, quality, and content of web pages that are critical versus noncritical of human papillomavirus vaccine. J Adolesc Health. 2016;58:33–9.
28. Harris K, Byrd K, Engel M, Weeks K, Ahlers-Schmidt CR. Internet-based information on long-acting reversible contraception for adolescents. J Prim Care Community Health. 2016;7:76–80.
29. Buhi ER, Daley EM, Fuhrmann HJ, Smith SA. An observational study of how young people search for online sexual health information. J Am Coll Health. 2009;58:101–11.
30. Ragonese M, Bowman CP, Tolman DL. Sex education, youth, and advocacy: sexual literacy, critical media, and intergenerational sex education(s). In: Allen L, Rasmussen ML, editors. The Palgrave handbook of sexuality education. London: Palgrave Macmillan; 2017. p. 301–25.
31. Monteith A. "The words of McKenna": healing, political critique, and the evolution of Psychonaut religion since the 1960s counterculture. J Am Acad Relig. 2016; 84:1081–109.
32. Boyer EW, Lapen PT, Macalino G, Hibberd PL. Dissemination of psychoactive substance information by innovative drug users. CyberPsychol Behav. 2007;10:1–6.
33. Martinotti G, Lupi M, Carlucci L, Cinosi E, Santacroce R, Acciavatti T, et al. Novel psychoactive substances: use and knowledge among adolescents and young adults in urban and rural areas. Hum Psychopharmacol Clin Exp. 2015;30:295–301.
34. Valeriani G, Corazza O, Bersani FS, Melcore C, Metastasio A, Bersani G, et al. Olanzapine as the ideal "trip terminator"? Analysis of online reports relating to antipsychotics' use and misuse following occurrence of novel psychoactive substance-related psychotic symptoms. Hum Psychopharmacol Clin Exp. 2015;30:249–54.
35. Deetjen U, Powell JA. Informational and emotional elements in online support groups: a Bayesian approach to large-scale content analysis. J Am Med Inform Assoc. 2016;23:508–13.
36. Ali K, Farrer L, Gulliver A, Griffiths KM. Online peer-to-peer support for young people with mental health problems: a systematic review. JMIR Ment Health. 2015;2:e19.

37. Mattsson S, Olsson EMG, Alfonsson S, Johansson B, Carlsson M. Measuring use of health-related support on the internet: development of the health online support questionnaire (HOSQ). J Med Internet Res. 2015;17:e266.
38. Lin T-C, Hsu JS-C, Cheng H-L, Chiu C-M. Exploring the relationship between receiving and offering online social support: a dual social support model. Inf Manag. 2015;52:371–83.
39. Biggs BK, Lebow J, Smith CM, Harper KL, Patten CA, Sim LA, et al. Adolescents' preferences for social support for healthful eating and physical activity. J Dev Behav Pediatr. 2014;35:494–509.
40. Koven N, Abry A. The clinical basis of orthorexia nervosa: emerging perspectives. Neuropsychiatr Dis Treat. 2015;11:385–94.
41. Moroze RM, Dunn TM, Craig Holland J, Yager J, Weintraub P. Microthinking about micronutrients: a case of transition from obsessions about healthy eating to near-fatal "Orthorexia nervosa" and proposed diagnostic criteria. Psychosomatics. 2015;56:397–403.
42. Dunn TM, Bratman S. On Orthorexia nervosa: a review of the literature and proposed diagnostic criteria. Eat Behav. 2016;21:11–7.
43. Holland G, Tiggemann MA. Systematic review of the impact of the use of social networking sites on body image and disordered eating outcomes. Body Image. 2016;17:100–10.
44. Tiggemann M, Zaccardo M. 'Strong is the new skinny': a content analysis of #fitspiration images on Instagram. J Health Psychol. 2016; [e-pub].
45. Singh K, Brown RJ. From headache to tumour: an examination of health anxiety, health-related internet use and query escalation. J Health Psychol. 2016;21:2008–20.
46. McManus F, Leung C, Muse K, Williams JMG. Understanding "cyberchondria": an interpretive phenomenological analysis of the purpose, methods and impact of seeking health information online for those with health anxiety. Cogn Behav Ther. 2014;7:e21.
47. Alpaslan AH. Cyberchondria and adolescents. Int J Soc Psychiatry. 2016;62:679–80.
48. Nutbeam D. Health literacy as a public health goal: a challenge for contemporary health education and communication strategies into the 21st century. Health Promot Int. 2000;15:259–67.
49. Subramaniam M, Taylor NG, St. Jean B, Follman R, Kodama C, Casciotti D. As simple as that?: tween credibility assessment in a complex online world. J Doc. 2015;71:550–71.
50. Wolfe RM, Sharp LK. Vaccination or immunization? The impact of search terms on the internet. J Health Commun. 2005;10:537–51.
51. Guinee K, Eagleton MB, Hall TE. Adolescents' internet search strategies: drawing upon familiar cognitive paradigms when accessing electronic information sources. J Educ Comput Res. 2003;29:363–74.
52. Osatuyi B. Is lurking an anxiety-masking strategy on social media sites? The effects of lurking and computer anxiety on explaining information privacy concern on social media platforms. Comput Hum Behav. 2015;49:324–32.
53. American Library Association. Presidential Committee on information literacy: final report. Washington, DC; 1989.
54. Dunne S, Cummins NM, Hannigan A, Shannon B, Dunne C, Cullen W. A method for the medical or health care information websites to optimize search engine results page rankings on Google. J Med Internet Res. 2013;15:e183.
55. Lewandowski D. Is Google responsible for providing fair and unbiased results? In: Taddeo M, Floridi L, editors. The responsibilities of online service providers. London: Springer; 2017. p. 61–77.
56. Huang J, Shi S, Chen Y, Chow WS. How do students trust Wikipedia? An examination across genders. Inf Technol People. 2016;29:750–73.
57. Mackert M, Kahlor L, Tyler D, Gustafson J. Designing e-health interventions for low-health-literate culturally diverse parents: addressing the obesity epidemic. Telemed e-Health. 2009;15:672–7.
58. Dutta-Bergman M. Trusted online sources of health information: differences in demographics, health beliefs, and health-information orientation. J Med Internet Res. 2003;5:e21.
59. Gauld R, Williams S. Use of the internet for health information: a study of Australians and new Zealanders. Inform Health Soc Care. 2009;34:149–58.
60. Oliver JE, Wood T. Medical conspiracy theories and health behaviors in the United States. JAMA Intern Med. 2014;174:817.
61. Kata AA. Postmodern Pandora's box: anti-vaccination misinformation on the internet. Vaccine. 2010;28:1709–16.
62. Madden K, Nan X, Briones R, Waks L. Sorting through search results: a content analysis of HPV vaccine information online. Vaccine. 2012;30:3741–6.
63. Basch CH, Zybert P, Reeves R, Basch CE. What do popular YouTube videos say about vaccines? Child Care Health Dev. 2017; [e-pub].
64. Manganello JA. Health literacy and adolescents: a framework and agenda for future research. Health Educ Res. 2008;23:840–7.
65. Paige SR, Krieger JL, Stellefson M, Alber JM. eHealth literacy in chronic disease patients: an item response theory analysis of the eHealth literacy scale (eHEALS). Patient Educ Couns. 2017;100:320–6.
66. Charnock D, Shepperd S, Needham G, Gann R. DISCERN: an instrument for judging the quality of written consumer health information on treatment choices. J Epidemiol Community Health. 1999;53:105–11.

3 How Mental Health Conditions Affect Online Use and Access

Yolanda N. Evans

Case

Maddie is a 17 year old with a chief complaint of anxiety and weight loss. You spend time speaking with her confidentially, and she tells you that she switched schools last year due to significant bullying (including face to face and cyberbullying). Rumors were spread, and negative comments were made continuously on her social media platforms. Now attending an alternative school, she has become increasingly socially isolated and states, "I don't have friends." She begun having panic attacks a few months ago and lacks any appetite. Her weight has dropped by 10 pounds in the past month, and she is only sleeping about 4 h a night. Her time is spent on her smartphone, watching anime online and following others on social media. She often compares herself to the people she follows and comments to you, "I'm worthless, if a 12 year old can have 1000 followers on this video blog and I only have a few, I have no talent and don't see the point of going on."

Introduction

Adolescents have regular access to the Internet. It is estimated that over 90% of teens have smartphones and ~75% of US households have Internet access [1].While the Internet may be a source of harm (including cyberbullying, access to information on how to proceed with self-harm, and a source of social supports that encourage risky behavior), it also has the potential to be a great resource for health information and for receiving positive social support [2, 3]. With suicide being in the top three causes of US adolescent and young adult mortality [4] and an estimated 18% of US high school students seriously considering a suicide attempt [5], access and receipt of behavioral health services is extremely important. Despite these statistics, young adults and teens are less likely to receive health care than younger children [6]. The Internet may provide an opportunity for prevention, screening, and intervention in this population.

The case illustrates many of the challenges adolescents can face including being a victim and/or perpetrator of bullying, anxiety and other mood disorders, distorted body image, and maladaptive eating behaviors, as well as low self-esteem and social isolation. Teens may turn to the Internet for validation and social support and to look up information, while at the same time, social media and Internet resources can exacerbate behaviors or become a source of aggressive

Y.N. Evans, M.D., M.P.H.
Seattle Children's Hospital, University of Washington, Seattle, WA, USA
e-mail: Yolanda.Evans@seattlechildrens.org

M.A. Moreno, A. Radovic (eds.), *Technology and Adolescent Mental Health*,
https://doi.org/10.1007/978-3-319-69638-6_3

behavior. As providers who care for teens, many questions may come to mind. How should I screen for harmful Internet usage? Is it my responsibility to ask teens how they are accessing information online? Are teens with mood disorders using the Internet differently than those without mental health concerns? The following chapter will attempt to summarize the literature on this final question: are adolescents with mental health disorders using the Internet differently than those without?

Seeking Information

Adolescents have been described as "early adopters" of new technologies, including the Internet for access to health information. They seek information for a variety of reasons including social contexts, medical questions, body and nutrition concerns, personal safety, and reproductive health information [7]. Adolescents with mood disorders use the Internet as a way to find information on their health condition(s) as well. The information they encounter may help or it may hinder their emotional well-being. If exposed to inaccurate content, misinformation, or non-evidence-based recommendations for treatment, teens may be at risk for harm. For example, among adolescents with eating disorders, the Internet can be a source of harmful information if they search so-called "pro-ana" or "pro-mia" sites that share information on how to progress in more maladaptive eating behaviors [8, 9]. Even if teens are looking for information on how to improve their condition(s), the websites encountered may not give specific advice on how to avoid harm. A study conducted in 2015 searched 314 websites for terms related to suicide in order to evaluate whether the websites directed users to supportive information or promoted harmful behaviors [10]. The researchers found that sites accessed by the terms "self-harm/suicide" were mostly positive or preventative in tone, that is, the sites discouraged the behavior, and sites accessed by search terms "ways to kill yourself" were more likely to have a negative tone. Advice for how to find help was very limited, with only 56% of encountered sites having information on helpful resources.

Youth may be seeking information online, but they may not be finding information healthcare providers would encourage or expect. As practitioners, attempting to keep up with the ever-changing vocabulary teens use to search the Internet may feel daunting. Fortunately, search Internet engines can aid providers in keeping up with changes. As an example, Moreno et al. (2016) described useful strategies for determining which search terms may be popular for online information on self-harm [11]. As we work with youth around diagnosis, management, and treatment of mood disorders, asking about Internet usage should become a routine part of care. Both the youth and their parents/caregivers should be provided with information on reputable websites (such as hospital-sponsored information), and they should be encouraged to avoid slang when searching online resources in order to avoid disturbing or inappropriate content. If possible, discussion should be had on how to determine if a website is providing accurate, reliable, and trustworthy information. Examples include review of the website for author credentials and looking for cited resources in content.

Cyberbullying as a Cause or Source of Anxiety and Depression

There is a growing body of literature on the phenomenon of Internet aggression, electronic harassment, or cyberbullying. Studies report a prevalence of up to 26% of youth as perpetrators and over 42% as targets [12]. Unlike traditional bullying, cyberbullying can occur anonymously, has a widespread audience, and persists outside of school hours that may make it more harmful to adolescents than bullying that occurs face to face [13, 14]. It is known that cyberbullying is associated with negative effects on mood such as depression, anxiety, and thoughts of suicide [15–17], and those who are victims of cyberbullying are more likely to report depressive symptoms like feeling down, sad, or hopeless [18], but are those with mental health disorders, such as clinically diagnosed depression and anxiety, more likely to be victims or perpetrators of online harassment than peers without mood disorders?

The answer to this question is likely "yes." A longitudinal study of middle and high school students in the USA sought to evaluate this connection. In the study, those who had depression and anxiety (separately) in the beginning of the study were more likely to be victims of cyberbullying later in their academic years than those who did not report these mood disorders at all [19].These findings should prompt those who actively work with adolescents, whether in health care or education, to consider screening for Internet harassment among teens with mood disorders. An example of how to ask about bullying, including cyberbullying, is to ask the question: "Has there ever been anyone at home, school, or anywhere else who hurt you or made you feel afraid or threatened or who bullied you (this includes cyberbullying)?"

Are teens with mood disorders more likely to be cyberbullying perpetrators? Among adolescent males in Taiwan, those who were older teens had combined attention deficit hyperactivity disorder, and more severe Internet addictions were more likely to be perpetrators of traditional and cyberbullying [20]. Internet addiction in and of itself may be a risk factor for victimization. The following section will delve into the possible associations between mental health and problematic Internet usage.

Problematic Internet Usage and Depression/Anxiety

With Internet access being nearly universal for adolescents, questions of overuse arise. The *Diagnostic and Statistical Manual of Mental Disorders* (DSM-V) does not include a diagnosis of Internet addiction disorder; however if a teen feels a lack of control over or preoccupation with Internet use and the use is leading to mood changes, tolerance, social isolation, or declines in academic performance, Internet usage may be significantly impacting their life. It is estimated that problematic Internet usage is fairly uncommon (3.6%) [21], and significant associations between Internet addiction or problematic Internet usage and depression, aggression, and substance abuse have been found [22]. In a longitudinal study of Korean youth, those with high problematic Internet usage had associated relationship with social withdrawal and anxiety/depression [21]. Among US females in a university setting, problematic Internet usage was significantly associated with depression. Young women, who met the criteria for depression, using the validated Patient Health Questionnaire-9 (PHQ-9) [23], were significantly more likely to be at risk of problematic Internet usage. Those with severe depression were over eight times more likely than nondepressed peers to be at risk; moderately depressed youth were four times more likely to be at risk, and even those with mild depression were over twice as likely to be at risk for problematic Internet usage as those without depression [24]. Social anxiety may also be a predictor of problematic Internet usage. Youth with significant social anxiety, after controlling for generalized anxiety disorder and depression, have perceptions of greater control and decreased negative evaluation of communication when talking online [25]. Why might adolescents with mood disorders be at risk for problematic Internet usage? The Internet may offer adolescents suffering from anxiety a source of relief as well as the opportunity to have social networking groups without needing to leave the comfort of home and with the ease of communication on their own terms (e.g., replying to a message after they can think about a response) [26].

For youth with depression, social networking online and the amount of time spent on the Internet may impact mental health. While not all studies have found an association between social networking displays of mood and clinical depression [27], there does appear to be an association between depression, social networking websites, and the amount of time spent online. In a study that examined Internet use patterns of 189 older adolescents (mean age 18.9 years), those who had low or normal (30 min or 30 min to 3 h) Internet use did not have statistically significant differences in PHQ-9 score, but those with very high Internet use (>3 hours) had significantly higher PHQ-9 scores (higher score is correlated with increased severity of depression). The results support the idea that spending more time online is associated with depression [28].

In youth who may already have social withdrawal or limited communication with peers, the Internet may contribute to depression; however it also has the potential to serve as a vehicle for communicating with peers, forming a sense of community, and allow for access to mental health professionals outside of office hours.

Online Social Support for Adolescents with Mood Disorders

The evidence is growing that Internet-based interventions for adolescents with chronic medical concerns can lead to improved adherence to treatment and provide information on health conditions [29]. Social media has tremendous potential to engage youth in health education, the receipt of health services, and self-care [2]. Youth with mood disorders also have chronic ongoing challenges with health that have potential to be improved by the Internet. In one qualitative study, youth with psychotic and nonpsychotic disorders were asked about the role of the Internet in their pathway to care. While those with nonpsychotic mood disorders (such as depression) were more likely to search for information on how to stop their symptoms and those with psychotic disorders were more interested in what could have caused their disorder, both groups were open to the idea of providers using social media and the Internet as a way to provide them with information [30].

Communication with Health-Care Providers

As providers, the use of social media may allow a mode of addressing health that reaches beyond the confines of the office setting. Benefits include not being limited to strict business hours and the possibility of both static (but updated) information on resources and live chat or question and answer sessions. But there are drawbacks to its use. Social media may lead to challenges in maintaining professional boundaries for health-care providers [31] and can create a level of anxiety if providers are unable to immediately respond to the concerns of a teen in crisis; however, it does allow for instant and potentially constant access to mental health providers which may ease anxiety and allow for communication in a way that is on the "condition and terms of the teen" instead of at the convenience of providers [32].

Online Communication and Peer Connections

Teens not only use the Internet to search for information related to health, they also use it as a means of social connection. The benefits include, but are not limited to, self-perceived social support, increased self-esteem, increased opportunities for self-disclosure, and opportunity for identity experimentation [33]. There are a large variety of possibilities for social connection online including the vast array of social networking sites, blogs, and video blogs that adolescents have at hand. Therapeutic benefits of blogging about emotional and social struggles have been described and include increased self-esteem and a feeling of social connection [34].

The patterns of social networking and social media use may differ for teens with mood disorders. Young adult women with a childhood diagnosis of attention deficit hyperactivity disorder (ADHD) had an associated preference for online social communication versus in-person discussions; they also had a tendency toward increased interactions with strangers online and fewer "friends" on Facebook [35]. In a systematic review that examined the use of social networking and online tools by people with psychosis, it was found that people with psychosis spent more time in chat rooms or playing online video games and had less use of communication tools, such as email or Facebook. Despite the lower communication use, patients with psychosis were more likely to use the Internet for establishing and maintaining peer connection [36]. Though there are risks (exposure to cyberbullying, increased social isolation from lack of in-person encounters, increased interactions with unknown persons, exposure to self-harm, or negative commentary), the benefits may outweigh these inherent potentials for harm for a youth who is already suffering from the negative effects of a mental health disorder.

Sexuality and Relationships

As youth with mental health conditions go online to develop social connections, they may also be at risk for meeting with strangers, providing personal identifying information, and putting themselves at risk for unwanted sexual solicitation. In a study of over 1500 youth completing the Youth Internet Safety Survey (YISS), depressive symptoms were associated with using the Internet more frequently than nondepressed peers, being more likely to converse online with a stranger, meeting with a stranger they met online, and disclosing personal information (for males, posting a phone number or address; for females, posting a picture of themselves) [37]. This risky behavior places these adolescents at risk for unwanted sexual contact. Indeed, a separate study that used data from the YISS found that youth who reported major depressive-like symptoms was over 3 times as likely to report unwanted sexual solicitation than youth with no or mild symptoms. Among those who reported an Internet solicitation incident, those with depressive symptoms were twice as likely to report feeling emotionally distressed by the incident [38].

Summary

The case at the beginning of this chapter illustrated a teen confronted with multiple challenges: a history of anxiety, body image concerns, and poor school performance, experiencing social isolation, cyberbullying, and a need for both physical and emotional intervention. The Internet and social media provide opportunities for teens, such as Maddie from the case, to have access to health information, a connection with peers in a setting that is comfortable and convenient, as well as the potential for communication with mental health resources. Though there are risks, including exposure to websites that encourage maladaptive behavior, possible increased risk of sexual solicitation, and exacerbation of social isolation, those benefits should not be ignored. Adolescents with mood disorders do have patterns of Internet use that are unique. Their use of the Internet to form social connection may be more influential, and they may be at increased risk for problematic Internet usage (or Internet addiction). They may also be more likely to search for health-related topics online and use the Internet and social media (if available) to stay connected with mental health providers. The Internet has a number of advantages that health-care providers should consider using when caring for adolescents with mood disorders.

References

1. Pew Research Center. [Online] [Cited: 02.19.2017]. www.pewinternet.org/topics/social-networking/.
2. Wong C, Merchant R, Moreno M. Using social media to engage adolescents and young adults with their health. Healthcare (Amst). 2014;2:220–4.
3. Nickels A, Dimov V. Innovations in technology: social media and mobile technology in the care of adolescents with asthma. Curr Allergy Asthma Rep. 2012; 12:607–12.
4. Centers for Disease Control. [Online] [Cited: 02.22.2017]. https://www.cdc.gov/injury/images/lc-charts/leading_causes_of_death_age_group_2014_1050w760h.gif.
5. Centers for Disease Control. [Online] [Cited: 02.22.2017]. https://www.cdc.gov/healthyyouth/data/yrbs/pdf/trends/2015_us_suicide_trend_yrbs.pdf.
6. Lau J, et al. Young Adults' health care utilization and expenditures prior to the Affordable Care Act. J Adolesc Health. 2014;54:663–71.
7. Skinner H, et al. How adolescents use technology for health information: implications for health professionals from focus group studies. J Med Internet Res. 2003;5:e32.
8. Borzekowski D, et al. e-Ana and e-Mia: a content analysis of pro-eating disorder web sites. Am J Public Health. 2010;100:1526–34.
9. Arseniev-Koehler A, et al. Proana: pro-eating disorder socialization on Twitter. J Adolesc Health. 2016;58: 659–64.

10. Singaravelu V, et al. Information-seeking on the internet. Crisis. 2015;36:211–9.
11. Moreno M, et al. Secret society 123: understanding the language of self-harm on Instagram. J Adolesc Health. 2016;58:78–84.
12. Hamm M, et al. Prevalence and effect of cyberbullying on children and young people: a scoping review of social media studies. JAMA Pediatr. 2015;169:770–7.
13. Sticca F, Perren S. Is cyberbullying worse that traditional bullying? Examining the differential roles of medium, publicity, and anonymity for the perceived severity of bullying. J Youth Adolesc. 2013;42:739–50.
14. van Geel M, Vedder P, Tanilon J. Relationship between peer victimization, cyberbullying, and suicide in children and adolescents: a meta-analysis. JAMA Pediatr. 2014;168:435–42.
15. Kowalski R, Limber S. Psychological, physical, and academic correlates of cyberbullying and traditional bullying. J Adolesc Health. 2013;53:S13–20.
16. Hinduja S, Patchin J. Bullying, cyberbullying, and suicide. Arch Suicide Res. 2010;14:206–21.
17. Sourander A, et al. Psychosocial risk factors associated with cyberbullying among adolescents: a population-based study. Arch Gen Psychiatry. 2010;67:720–8.
18. Wang J, Nansel T, Iannoti R. Cyber and traditional bullying: differential association with depression. J Adolesc Health. 2011;48:415–7.
19. Rose C, Tynes B. Longitudinal associations between cybervictimization and mental health among U.S. adolescents. J Adolesc Health. 2015;57:305–12.
20. Yen C, et al. Cyberbullying among male adolescents with attention-deficit/hyperactivity disorder: prevalence, correlates, and association with poor mental health status. Res Dev Disabil. 2014;35:543–3553.
21. Cho S, et al. Does psychopathology in childhood predict internet addiction in male adolescents? Child Psychiatry Hum Dev. 2013;44:549–55.
22. Liu T, et al. Problematic internet use and health in adolescents: data from a high school survey in Connecticut. J Clin Psychiatry. 2011;72:836–45.
23. Richardson LP, et al. Evaluation of the Patient Health Questionnaire-9 Item for detecting major depression among adolescents. Pediatrics. 2010;126:1117–23.
24. Moreno M, Jelenchick L, Breland D. Exploring depression and problematic internet use among college females: a multisite study. Comput Human Behav. 2015;49:601–7.
25. Lee B, Stapinski L. Seeking safety on the internet: relationship between social anxiety and problematic internet use. J Anxiety Disord. 2012;26:197–205.
26. Wegemann E, Stodt B, Brand M. Addictive use of social networking sites can be explained by the interaction of internet use expectancies, internet literacy, and pyschopathological symptoms. J Behav Addict. 2015;4:155–62.
27. Jelenchick LA, Eickhoff JC, Moreno MA. "Facebook depression?" Social networking site use and depression in older adolescents. J Adolesc Health. 2013;52:28–30.
28. Moreno MA, et al. Depression and internet use among older adolescents: an experience sampling approach. Psychology. 2012;3:743–8.
29. Bass A, Farhangian M, Feldman S. Internet-based adherence interventions for treatment of chronic disorders in adolescents. Adolesc Health Med Ther. 2015;26:91–9.
30. Birnbaum M, et al. Role of social media and the internet in pathways to care for adolescents and young adults with psychotic disorders and non-psychotic mood disorders. Early Interv Psychiatry. 2015.
31. Kind T, Patel P, Lie D. Opting in to online professionalism: social media and pediatrics. Pediatrics. 2013;132:792–5.
32. van Rensburg S, et al. Patient-provider communication over social media: perspectives of adolescents with psychiatric illness. Health Expect. 2016;19:112–20.
33. Best P, Manktelow R, Taylor B. Online communication, social media and adolescent wellbeing: a systematic narrative review. Children Youth Services Rev. 2014;41:27–36.
34. Boniel-Nissim M, Barak A. The therapeutic value of adolescents' blogging about social-emotional difficulties. Psychol Serv. 2013;10:333–41.
35. Mikami A, et al. Online social communication patterns among emerging adult women with histories of childhood attention-deficit/hyperactivity disorder. J Abnorm Psychol. 2015;124:76–588.
36. Highton-Williamson E, Priebe S, Giacco D. Online social networking in people with psychosis: a systematic review. Int J Soc Psychiatry. 2015;61:2–101.
37. Ybarra ML, Alexander C, Mitchell KJ. Depressive symptomatology, youth internet use, and online interactions: a national survey. J Adolesc Health. 2005;36:9–18.
38. Ybarra ML, Leaf PJ, Diener-West M. Sex differences in youth-reported depressive symptomatology and unwanted internet sexual solicitation. J Med Internet Res. 2004;6:e5.

4 Technology Use Among Special Populations

Allison Schimmel-Bristow and Kym R. Ahrens

Introduction

This chapter presents extant research on how the use of technology influences, both positively and negatively, mental health of adolescents in special populations. As technology is a prominent part of today's society, particularly among adolescents, we need to consider the role technology plays in adolescents with higher risks of victimization and mental health concerns. This chapter reviews evidence on three categories of special populations: (1) sexual and gender minority youth (SGM), (2) adolescents exposed to early adversity, and (3) adolescents with health problems and disabilities. This literature review is not meant to be exhaustive but provides an overview of the research that exists in each of these populations. In addition to presenting literature on the "natural" risks and benefits of technology use in these populations, we also present research on how technology can be used as an intervention tool. Finally, the chapter concludes with a summary of common themes within these special groups, an illustrative case example, and recommendations for clinicians.

Sexual and Gender Minority (SGM) Adolescents

SGM youth are youth who identify as lesbian, gay, bisexual, transgender, gender nonconforming, queer, or questioning. Cisgender youth are youth for whom gender identity aligns with their sex assigned at birth. SGM youth are at higher risk of exposure to prejudice, verbal and/or physical attacks, and social rejection compared with their heterosexual or gender-conforming peers and consequently experience higher levels of isolation, homelessness, substance abuse, school failure, depression, and anxiety [1]. As examples, lesbian, gay, and bisexual youth are four times as likely to attempt suicide as heterosexual peers, and 40% of transgender adults in a national survey reported attempting suicide. Almost all (92%) of these adults reported that their attempt occurred at the age of 25 or younger [2, 3]. We review literature elucidating the ways in which SGM youth interact with technology, the potential positive and negative consequences of these

A. Schimmel-Bristow, M.S. (✉)
Department of Counseling, Education Psychology and Research, The University of Memphis, Memphis, TN, USA
e-mail: schmmlbr@memphis.edu; aschimmelbristow@loyola.edu

K.R. Ahrens, M.D., M.P.H.
Division of Adolescent Medicine, Department of Pediatrics, Center for Child Health Behavior and Development, Seattle Children's Hospital and Research Institute, Seattle, WA, USA

M.A. Moreno, A. Radovic (eds.), *Technology and Adolescent Mental Health*, https://doi.org/10.1007/978-3-319-69638-6_4

experiences, and the ways in which technology could be used as an intervention tool to promote positive mental health outcomes in this group.

Seeking Information Online

Nationwide, it is uncommon for youth to receive SGM-inclusive sexual education or other resources through school curriculums. Only five states/jurisdictions (California, Colorado, Iowa, Washington, and Washington, D.C.) have laws or regulatory guidance requiring SGM-inclusive sexual education [4]. Therefore, the Internet can sometimes be a key source of information on these topics. Several studies have described ways in which SGM youth use online resources sites to educate themselves and find information they need during the coming out and transitioning process. For example, Fox et al. [5] conducted a qualitative study in which adolescent and young adult SGM participants were interviewed regarding the ways in which participants used social media for learning purposes, as well as what characteristics of the sites shaped their experiences. Adolescents and young adults described using the Internet to seek specific information such as identity labels and meaning. Commonly used sites were easy to find using general terminology, displayed local resources, and allowed participants to remain anonymous offline. Participants also described using online sources to seek information more frequently during the coming out and/or gender transition process compared with after being out/transitioning. In another qualitative study conducted with transgender youth and caregivers of transgender youth conducted by Evans et al. [6], participants similarly reported using the Internet to find terminology to describe their identity as well as options for medical and mental healthcare, locating providers and finding social support [6, 7]. Some participants described using a hospital or clinic-based website as sources of information. However, compared with the Fox et al. [5] study, participants in this study reported that they mainly used sites such as Wikipedia, Tumblr, group forums, and YouTube; these sites may be less reliable because they are not necessarily reviewed by medical professional [6].

A number of studies have also explored the use of the Internet among SGM youth for sexual health education. Mitchell et al. [8] used the cross-sectional Teen Health and Technology (THT) study aimed to determine the extent that youth sought sexual health information and whether it varied by sexual orientation. This study incorporated 5542 youth ranging from 13 to 18 years old, 2162 of which identified as bisexual, gay, lesbian, queer, or questioning. SGM youth were more likely to access sexual health information, information about sexuality, and information about sexual attraction compared to their heterosexual peers. They were also two times more likely than heterosexual peers to seek sexual health information for "privacy-related reasons" in comparison with "curiosity." Finally, results also indicated that there was a significant relationship between reason for seeking information online (e.g., no one to talk to) and engagement in sexual behaviors. Thus, this study shows the importance of having accurate and relevant SGM-specific sexual health information online and highlights a potential link between seeking online information and engagement in risk behaviors.

Although the Internet has potential to be a valuable resource for SGM youth, online information may not be accurate and in some cases may be frankly harmful. In one study designed to understand available sources of lesbian sexual and relational health online, researchers found an overall lack of quality related to the message and comprehensiveness of information [9]. Unfortunately, the issue of quality is not one restricted to lay sites. One gender minority youth in a qualitative study by Gridley et al. [10] reported finding providers online that claimed they were SGM-friendly when, in fact, they had minimal knowledge/experience working with transgender youth. It is not difficult to imagine the potential negative impacts of this challenging experience.

Expressing Sexuality and Seeking Romantic Partners

SGM youth also use the Internet to express their sexuality and seek partners. Ybarra et al. [11] evaluated a sample of 5907 cisgender (i.e., not transgender or gender nonconforming) participants ages 13–18 in the THT dataset to examine how young people use the Internet to express themselves sexually. Results indicated that sexual minority youth (lesbian, gay, bisexual, or questioning) were more likely to have sexual conversations and share sexual pictures than nonsexual minority youth. Results also looked at gender differences for cisgender male and female participants among sexual minority youth and found that nonheterosexual cisgender males were three times more likely than heterosexual cisgender male peers to find online sexual partners; however this difference was not found among cisgender females.

DeHaan et al. [12] also conducted a qualitative study with SGM youth aged 16–24 to explore how the use of the Internet impacts offline behaviors and identities. Participants reported using the Internet to reflect on or understand their identities which influenced their offline expression. The Internet was also found to be an important setting for participants to forge social and romantic connections, especially for youth living in more isolated geographical areas or with unsupportive peers and family.

Online Identity Exploration and Social Support

Studies suggest that the Internet is also used by SGM youth as a place to explore their identity and develop non-romantic social connections [13]. SGM youth may be in particular and unique need of this type of online support. A study by Howard [14] evaluated three different online forums (a cancer survivors group, a Harry Potter forum, and a forum for SGM youth). Researchers found that purpose for the forum varied across each group. Main results found that members of the "support group" (i.e., the cancer survivors group) and the "stigmatized group" (i.e., the SGM forum) reported higher online group identity (i.e., sense of community within the online group) as compared to members of the "avocation group" (i.e., the Harry Potter group). Also, the SGM group members had less offline social support and lower well-being ratings than the other two groups.

Similarly, Ceglarek et al. [15] conducted a study in which 146 sexual minority youth and 477 heterosexual youth completed an online survey measuring social support, identity development, social networking site use, and mental health and well-being. Although both sexual minority and heterosexual youth use networking sites at equal rates, sexual minority youth used sites more purposefully for identity development and social communication. When using sites for sexual identity development, results indicated that sexual minority participants had increased positive mental health outcomes (i.e., decreased experiences of paranoia, anxiety, and hostility).

In-person identity expression for SGM youth may be particularly challenging when the youth does not have family support; thus SGM youth who are in unsupportive families may turn to online resources more often than their SGM peers with more familial support. Radovic et al. [16] conducted a qualitative study with adolescents aged 13–20 regarding parental monitoring. The study found SGM youth that were not open about their sexual or gender identity to their families frequently described the Internet as a safe space to explore who they are and get support from other supportive adults.

SGM youth also turn to the Internet to find and learn from supportive peers with similar experiences. For example, the Fox et al. study described above [5] also found that SGM youth use the Internet as a tool to learn from what other sexual minority individuals have experienced. Ybarra et al. [17] conducted another analysis using a cohort of 5907 youth from the THT study, aged 13–18 years, and completed an online survey of SGM youth. Results indicated the SGM youth were more likely than non-SGM youth to have friends they only know online and rate these online friends as more supportive than their in-person friendships. Taken together, these studies highlight the potential benefit of SGM youth using online resources for identity development and social support, especially when in-person social support is less available.

Online Mental Health Risks

Not all online interactions result in positive identity development and/or social connections. Unfortunately, social media sites can be used as tools to bully vulnerable youth. A number of studies illustrate the prevalence of cyberbullying over social media, text messages, and other applications among SGM youth. In a study conducted with SGM or SGM-allied adolescent participants, 39% of SGM and 32% of SGM-allied participants reported receiving angry, rude, or vulgar messages at least one to two times per week. Most commonly, these events occurred over social networking sites or instant messaging systems. The participants' emotional responses to being cyberbullied indicated that 56% of SGM and 33% of SGM-allied youth experienced feeling depressed, with 35% of SGM participants reporting suicidal thoughts as a result of being cyberbullied [18]. A study conducted by Varjas et al. with 18 lesbian-, gay-, or bisexual-identified participants 15–18 years old also reported several themes around cyberbullying in the sexual minority community [13]. During the semi-structured interviews, 14 of the 18 participants reported cyber victimization. This study also found that many of the participants reported engaging in cyberbullying or other negative behaviors over the Internet themselves. For example, five participants reported verbally harassing others due to losing patience, while another four reported sharing personal identifying information online with strangers. These results indicate SGM are commonly cyberbullying victims; however, at times SGM youth may also participate in cyberbullying themselves.

Technology as an Intervention Tool

Finally, technology could be used as an intervention tool to promote positive mental health and reduce high-risk behaviors for SGM youth. Individuals in the SGM community are at higher risk for sexually transmitted infections (STIs) and unwanted pregnancies [19]. Due to stigma, many individuals with STIs, including and especially those living with human immunodeficiency virus or acquired immune deficiency syndrome (HIV/AIDS), have difficulty seeking treatment and support. DiNapolim et al. [19] argues that by using technology to create a safe, anonymous space for SGM members with HIV/AIDS, individuals in this community would be able to receive mental health help and support in healthy lifestyle practices. This theory-based paper presents reasons to conduct technology-based support and group interventions for SGM individuals. The authors argue that through the use of computer-mediated self-help groups, individuals in the SGM community, especially those dealing with HIV/AIDS, would be able to have safe and open communication experiences fostering healthier well-being. In support of this premise, Ybarra et al. [20] conducted two online focus groups with lesbian, gay, or bisexual youth 14–18 years old to moderate discussions about HIV prevention. The participants were posed with a daily question/topic in which they were instructed to respond to at least twice a day. Results indicated that most participants benefited from participating in the focus group due to the self-reflection needed to respond to the forum; however sexually inexperienced youth reported perceiving the group as more beneficial. Similarly, Mustanski et al. [21] conducted an online comprehensive sexual health intervention study for SGM youth ages 16–20 years. Participants completed a pretest, and then five intervention modules followed by posttest assessments. Intervention effects were significant for all outcomes (e.g., HIV knowledge, STD knowledge, sexual arousal response, and technique) with the exception of two (i.e., male sexual knowledge inventory and sexual agreement self-efficacy); however these measures were still in the direction of positive intervention effects. Female participant scores showed a significant difference on the HIV knowledge scale. Results indicated that delivery of the intervention online was feasible, well received, and effective to increase knowledge.

Finally, mobile apps are starting to be used as a strategy to reduce risk behaviors in this population. For example, SGM youth and young adults have a higher prevalence rate of smoking compared to non-SGM peers. Baskerville et al. [22] conducted a qualitative study with SGM participants ages 16–29 years to explore perception of a culturally tailored mobile app for smoking cessation. The majority of participants felt a mobile app would be an appealing and accessible form or intervention. They also felt positively about the app being for SGM individuals specifically so they could have confidence in it being a safe space and discuss challenges specifically related to their experiences. Therefore, although technology use as a strategy to promote positive outcomes among SGM youth is a rapidly evolving field, given the fact that these youth seem to turn to technology more often for support, this may be a particularly important strategy for these youth.

Conclusions

Technology affords significant benefits and risks to the SGM youth community. Benefits include that the Internet can be a powerful tool to identify resources, cultivate social support, and develop a positive identity, especially for youth who have limited in-person resources on these fronts. However, the information that exists online is not always accurate and at times can be frankly harmful. An additional, significant risk of technology use in these youth is that social media exposes a group of youth who are already at risk of negative mental health outcomes to cyberbullying, which has the potential to further increase negative mental health sequelae. Another interesting finding of this literature is that SGM youth are not immune to perpetrating cyberbullying themselves. Overall, these studies suggest that SGM youth, like many other groups, may likely benefit from training on safe and respectful Internet use. This is likely to be especially important in this group, given their apparent increased use of the Internet to seek social support. Finally, the use of technology as an intervention tool to reduce risks and promote resilience is understudied among SGM youth; however theoretically technology has potential to be of great use as an intervention tool for this population. For example, it is possible that technology could be used to provide mental health treatment to those with limited access due to stigma or location. More research should focus on potential technology-based interventions to improve mental health outcomes for this vulnerable group.

Adolescents Exposed to Early Adversity

Adolescents that are exposed to significant early-life adversities such as abuse, neglect, poverty, parental and substance abuse are another group that is at a significantly increased risk of many negative mental health and related outcomes during adolescence and young adulthood. Specifically, they have been demonstrated in longitudinal studies to be at high risk of depression, suicidality, anxiety, substance use, and risky sexual behaviors [23–26]. Often, youth with high rates of exposure to early-life adversities have limited access to economic and social resources, which has the potential to compound the effects of exposures to adversity and existing mental health problems and result in a further risk of negative outcomes during the transition to adulthood [27]. The Internet offers easy access to information, education, and social support, which may be especially important for youth who underwent or are currently facing early-life adversities [27]. However, similar to SGM youth, this group has the potential to have increased negative impacts from media compared to their peers. Within this section, research that has been conducted exploring how technology may affect three specific populations of adolescents exposed to high rates of early adversity is discussed: (1) adolescents experiencing homelessness, (2) adolescents in foster care, and (3) juvenile justice-involved youth. Notably, the majority of research has been conducted in homeless youth, with very few studies conducted in the other two groups. Accordingly, we begin by summarizing studies in homeless youth and then briefly describe the limited studies that have been conducted in the other two populations.

Homeless Youth

Seeking Information Online

A qualitative study conducted by Jennings et al. [28] found that despite financial constraints, homeless youth had fairly consistent access to phones and the Internet. Several studies have explored the ways in which homeless youth use the Internet and their phones to access support-based information, including health and sexual health information, as well as looking for housing and job resources [27, 29, 30]. For example, Barman-Adhikari et al. [29] surveyed homeless adolescents to assess the frequency at which runaway and homeless youth seek sexual and other health information on the Internet. Approximately 61% of the sample sought general health information, 47% sought information regarding HIV or other STIs, 40% sought information about sex or sexuality, and 23% used the Internet to locate an HIV testing service. Rice et al. [30] also surveyed homeless youth, exploring their Internet use and reasons for using the Internet. This study also highlighted the use of technology for information and resources but had a more general focus rather than concentrating specifically on health-related information. Authors found that of the participants using the Internet, 28% used the Internet attempting to locate short-term shelters/housing for immediate needs, and 13% reported looking for housing for long-term needs. Additionally, participants that had easy access to the Internet were more likely to search for jobs. Similarly, these participants were also more likely to connect with potential employers and caseworkers. Thus, Internet availability may be a useful tool for homeless youth to access resources such as health-related information, housing, and employment.

Online Social Support

Prior research has suggested that homeless youth with increased rates of social support are less likely to engage in risky behaviors such as substance use and sexual risk behaviors and therefore less likely to experience negative health outcomes [31, 32]. Due to decreased avenues for accessing their social supports in person [27], technology may be an important means of social connection for this population, as it allows homeless youth an avenue to connect with family and friends during an otherwise isolating situation. In the Jennings et al. [28] study described above, youth also reported the benefits of connecting with peers and family via cell phones. Youth in the study highlighted the importance of having cell phones in order to connect with supportive adults, especially in the case of an emergency. Authors concluded that for many homeless youth, phones can be a critical way to stay connected and have the ability to reach out to support systems.

Online Mental Health Risks

A few studies have also explored potential mental health risks of technology use among homeless youth. A study by Barman-Adhikari et al. [33], in which 1046 homeless youth were surveyed, suggests that homeless youths' online interactions may be associated with an increase in their engagement in risky behaviors. Specifically, authors found that there were statistically significant associations between online connection with street friends and engagement in risky sexual behaviors such as having sex with someone they met online and engaging in sex with multiple concurrent partners. Similarly, homeless youth that talked about drinking, drugs, and partying online were also more likely to have sex with multiple, concurrent sex partners. The Jennings et al. [28] study also touched on this topic, with authors suggesting based on themes detected in their data that access to cell phones may place homeless youth at risk of vandalism and/or re-victimization by past perpetrators of trauma. This study described themes indicating that the financial responsibility associated with having a cell phone may negatively impact homeless youth, in that they may have obligations to talk to unsupportive family members that provided the phone or deal with the fear of theft.

Technology as an Intervention Tool

There is a small body of research that explores the use of technology as a means of prevention and treatment of mental health and behavioral issues in homeless youth. As homeless youth have disproportionately high rates of mental health, substance, and sexual risk behaviors compared to non-homeless youth, and they face potential logistical barriers to accessing healthcare, technology-based interventions may be a useful strategy to reach and support this vulnerable population [28, 34]. Much of the recent research on this topic has focused on the use of technology to make mental health and risk reduction interventions more accessible. In the Jennings et al. [28] study, homeless youth were asked about what content should be included in a phone app intervention called mHealth specifically pertaining to homeless youth. The youth's responses highlighted the importance of education and providing resources in regard to sexual health (i.e., risk reduction for HIV/STIs), reproductive health, and mental health. Another qualitative study conducted by Mutere et al. [35] engaged homeless youth in semi-structured interviews aimed to understand how popular culture, media, and art create barriers or aid homeless youth to obtain healthcare and gain a sense of self-efficacy. Some of the media barriers discussed included campaigns with culturally insensitive messages and ads using scare techniques. Although this study did not evaluate a specific intervention, youth responses highlighted the importance of having ongoing guidance by homeless youth in designing and implementing health promotion messages to make messages more accessible and effective.

One study by Bender et al. [36] tested the feasibility of providing electronic case management to homeless youth using prepaid cell phones. Case managers contacted youth over the phone every 2–3 weeks for a 3-month period. Engagement in sessions varied; however, the majority of youth (87.5%) engaged at least one time in case management. It should be noted that youth preferred texting to calling on the phone; however, the effectiveness of texting with case managers has not been studied. Another study conducted by Dang et al. [37] evaluated a project called *Healthshack*, a website that was developed in collaboration with homeless and runaway youth, that stores important information (medical records, social security card, school transcript, housing history, etc.) securely online so they can access it when working with health professionals, looking for jobs, or for a place to live. The study enrolled 149 youth participants, aged 9–24. Overall, youth participants felt positively about using *Healthshack* and were comfortable using technology to store and access their sensitive information.

Foster and Juvenile Justice-Involved Youth

Online Mental Health Risks and Benefits

There is limited research on media and mental health among foster youth and youth involved in the juvenile justice system. A study by Albertson et al. [38] aimed to understand how media affects foster youth. Data were collected qualitatively from 22 foster youth aged 15–21 via individual interviews and 86 foster and kinship caregivers engaged in focus groups. Participants from both studies shared the impact of media had on foster youths' views of social norms (i.e., relationships, sex, etc.). Themes were also described similar to studies conducted in homeless youth, indicating that foster youth tend to use social media to maintain connections with biological family members and peers, with some perceived positive effects (e.g., increased social support) and some perceived negative effects (e.g., unrealistic expectations of relationships with parents). Caregiver participants also reported feeling that due to their unique early-life experiences, foster youth were more susceptible to negative effects of media such as engaging in behaviors such as risky sexual behaviors commonly portrayed on media, viewing of pornography, and connecting with risky peers. In line with these findings, a literature review paper by Gustavsson et al. [39] discussed how the Internet could be used to support positive youth development for youth in foster care. Similar to the Albertson study, this study suggests that foster youth may have heightened risks related to their media use such as: (1) finding and using inaccurate online information, (2) remaining in contact with relatives who could be harmful to them, (3) posting and sending inappropriate material, or (4) providing identifying information to strangers. The authors argue by improving foster youths' digital literacy they may be able to better avoid these risks. The study also highlighted the importance of caretakers and case managers actively engaging in monitoring and discussing technology with foster youth.

There are a few states that have developed guidelines for caretakers and case managers to teach youth how to safely navigate and use the Internet as well as to limit and monitor their use. For example, one county in Georgia created a program that provided 23 foster youth with computers after completing a weekend digital literacy training aimed to better prepare the youth for adult independence [40]. No evaluation was conducted of this program; however authors concluded that this program may be useful in establishing media literacy among foster youth.

With respect to the connection between technology and juvenile justice-involved youth, there is strong evidence suggesting media portrayals contribute to violent and delinquent behaviors. Please see Escobar-Chaves [41] for a review of these findings as a description of these papers is out of scope for this chapter. However, in regard to impacts of technology on mental health among youth who are already involved in the juvenile justice system, we found a single study evaluating social media impacts among juvenile justice-involved youth. This study, conducted by Lim et al. [42] in Singapore, aimed to understand the role of online communication for juvenile male delinquents participated using semi-structured interviews. Participants mainly used the Internet for Facebook, which all participants accessed daily, as well as YouTube and other websites related to personal interests. Interviews highlighted some potential harms that social networking may have on this population including extended time and opportunity for unstructured and unsupervised peer socialization, peer reinforcement of delinquent behaviors, and pressures to display loyalty to a group, such as a gang, online.

Youth Exposed to Early Adversity: Conclusions

In summary, technology has unique mental health benefits and risks for youth exposed to early-life adversities. Benefits include access to information, education, and social support for youth that may otherwise be isolated. Further, it may be possible to improve mental health outcomes for these youth by providing more ubiquitous access to risk reduction education and case management as well as access to their providers and other resources. However, ease of access may put these youth more at risk to the dangers of technology, such as negative peer influences and re-victimization. Thus, technology-based mental health interventions would likely benefit from incorporation of strategies to mitigate these risks, such as media literacy training. This research is still in its infancy; more studies need to be done on media use impacts and potential benefits for these and other populations of youth exposed to early adversity.

Adolescents with Health Problems and Disabilities

Here, we present literature on technology and mental health among adolescents with health problems and disabilities. The empirical literature relating to media and mental health is primarily in three groups of adolescents with health problems and disabilities: adolescents with autism spectrum disorder (ASD), physical and intellectual disabilities, and attention deficit hyperactivity disorder (ADHD). These studies tended to focus on two specific areas: risks of cyberbullying and the use of technology as an intervention tool. Thus, the review of literature found relating to youth with these health problems and disabilities will focus on these specific issues.

Online Mental Health Risks

Adolescents with ASD are a group that faces unique challenges such as difficulties with face-to-face interactions, understanding social situations, and management of peer relationships [43]. As a consequence of these challenges, these youth often turn to technology as a less threatening way to interact with others [44]. Researchers have begun to explore how the age of technology has affected this population of youth. One emphasis of research has been this population's vulnerability to cyberbullying. For example, Robertson [45] conducted a qualitative study with autistic adolescents that examined how cyber and face-to-face bullying has affected participants' life perspectives, life experiences, and quality of life. The youth in the study reported varying experiences regarding cyberbullying experiences. A subset of participants experienced cyberbullying that specifically targeted their focused interest (i.e., an interest that an individual with ASD intensely engages in). For example, one participant who was passionate about playing Minecraft was targeted through the game. Participants poignantly described the impacts that bullying can have on their mental health or self-esteem. They also reported using ignoring as a strategy in dealing with the effects of bullying, although successfully ignoring the experience frequently did not negate negative impacts on the youth's emotional well-being.

In another study conducted by Kowalski et al. [46], individuals diagnosed with Asperger's syndrome and/or ADHD aged 10–20 and their parents participated in a survey. The study aimed to examine the prevalence of both traditional and cyberbullying and assess the social, psychological, and health effects. Results indicated that 21.4% of youth participants had experienced cyberbullying in the past 2 months. The most common venue was instant messaging and social networking sites. Although this study did not yield statistically significant effects regarding cyberbullying and experiences of anxiety and depression, the means were in the expected direction. Results also demonstrated that 5.8% of participants reported cyberbullying others at least once within the previous 2 months.

Several articles describe how youth with health problems and disabilities are affected by cyberbullying. These data suggest that similar to youth with ASD, cyberbullying is also higher among adolescents with ADHD and physical and intellectual disabilities. For example, in an online survey completed by college-aged students, cyberbullying occurred more often toward individuals with ADHD, mental health diagnoses, physical disabilities, or learning disabilities than toward students without these conditions. These increased rates of cyberbullying were, in turn, associated with low self-esteem and high rates of depression. Results indicated that likelihood of experiencing cyberbullying was associated with noticeability of disability (i.e., others ability to notice disability), amount of Internet use, and prior experiences with traditional (face-to-face) bullying [47]. Similarly, Didden et al. [48] surveyed adolescents between the ages of 12 and 19 with diagnoses of ADHD, pervasive developmental disorder, and other intellectual disabilities. Results showed 22% of participants experienced cyberbullying once a month and 9% experienced it once or more a week. It should also be noted that 16% of participants reported cyberbullying another peer. Consistent with prior studies, cyberbullying was found to be associated with low self-esteem and depressive feelings.

Finally, Heiman et al. [49] conducted a survey with 140 adolescents with ADHD and 332 adolescents without this diagnosis, with the goal of understanding differences in involvement in cyberbullying both as victim and perpetrator between these groups. Authors found significant differences in all types of cyber involvements, such that participants with ADHD were more likely to be both targets and perpetrators of cyberbullying. Participants with ADHD that experienced cyberbullying also reported higher levels of loneliness and lower levels of self-efficacy and social support than non-victims. Taken together, these studies demonstrate the vulnerability of individuals with a disability and how technology can increase the risk of mental health issues.

Technology as an Intervention Tool

Another body of research among youth with health problems and disabilities has focused on how technology can be used as an intervention tool. One area in which researchers have focused is improving communication. Burke et al. [50] conducted a qualitative study with participants ages 17–37 with high-functioning ASD to evaluate the use of currently available technology (i.e., email, test messaging, social networking sites, etc.). Technology was found to be beneficial for individuals with ASD in initiating social interactions with like-minded individuals. However, participants found difficulty in usability of certain technologies, maintaining connections with desired friends and romantic partners, knowing whom to trust and knowing how much to disclose. The authors also discussed ways computer-mediated communication could be improved to better support social outcomes for individuals with ASD. Authors suggest three potential ways computer-mediated communication training or tools could be improved: (1) teaching social skills including how to deal with predatory requests online; (2) creating a way for individuals with ASD to visually see statistics of their Internet use and patterns such as how long they have been on, what sites, and number of forum posts; and (3) developing a way to display trustworthiness of potential companions such as displaying a legitimate email address, ages of individuals they socialize with on the site, and average length of communication with other users. In the previously discussed qualitative study by Robertson [45], another aim of the study was to determine how the information gathered could have implications on the development of software to teach autistic youth to address and report all types of bullying. A few of the important themes included the importance of teaching youth how to walk away/ignore bullying, how to deal with the fear of reporting bullying, and how to report bullying. The author suggests that development of educational software could be a promising strategy to help teach autistic youth how to identify and deal with bullying as a way to teach and reinforce appropriate response skills.

Researchers are also attempting to use virtual worlds to help teach social and other skills with youth with ASD. For example, Kandalaft et al. [51] conducted a small study with late adolescents/young adults diagnosed with autism. The study aimed to explore the effectiveness of a virtual reality social skills intervention. Results indicate that participants' scores improved on measures assessing verbal and nonverbal recognition of social perception and ability to generate inferences about the thoughts and feelings of others. Didehbani et al. [52] conducted an extension of Kandalaft et al.'s [51] study with child and adolescent participants diagnosed with autism. The participants completed ten online scenarios, through an interactive interface, regarding real-world social situations such as bullying, bonding with friends, confronting conflict, consoling a friend, or handling social dilemmas. Results support the idea that emotion recognition, social attribution, and executive function of analogical reasoning can all be improved through practice in virtual worlds. In another study, Wang et al. [53] used a 3D collaborative learning environment to help youth with autism learn social competence. Participants included youth ages 11–14, diagnosed with Asperger's syndrome. Each participant had their own avatar (i.e., figure representing them in the online learning environment) and used the avatar to complete game-like learning activities. Participants were able to understand that the avatar was a representation of them and that other avatars represented other people and to understand collaborative engagement when working with other avatars on tasks across activities. Authors indicated that findings are promising; however, further research is needed to determine the translational benefit to real-life interactions.

Technology-based intervention methods have also been studied in youth with learning disabilities (LD) and youth with ADHD. Waight et al. [54] looked at a number of websites catered toward this population and found that sites varied in accessibility to individuals with difficulties in reading. Most commonly, these sites had a mixture of text and video. It was recommended that sites catered toward these individuals create similar layout designs across all sites so that individuals can navigate the pages more easily.

Finally, one study tested a technology-based intervention for youth with ADHD. Youth with

ADHD can have difficulties academically and socially due to impulsivity and lack of self-regulation. Vogelgesang et al. [55] completed a study regarding an iPad application (SCORE IT) to help promote self-regulation among adolescents with ADHD. Students and their teacher recorded academic engagement at different intervals. The intervention resulted in considerable improvements regarding academic engagement and teacher's perception of student. The author noted that the research is promising regarding the use of technology to record accomplishments and distractions so that we can not only better understand the experience of ADHD youth but help individuals with ADHD improve their productivity and success.

Conclusions

In summary, research regarding technology and youth with health problems and disabilities has focused on risk of cyberbullying and technology-based intervention strategies. Cyberbullying is a major concern for these vulnerable populations due to social skill difficulties for some of the subgroups of youth described above (e.g., youth with ASD, ADHD, and some youth with developmental disabilities), with potentially dire mental health consequences such as decreased self-esteem and increased risk of depression and anxiety. As a group, research suggests that youth with health problems and disabilities may benefit immensely from accessing technology-based interventions from both academic and mental health perspectives that are tailored to their specific needs.

General Conclusions

Overall, the body of literature for most of the special populations reviewed is best classified as being in the exploratory stage. More research needs to be completed for each population to understand the natural risks, benefits, and potential technology-based intervention strategies. However, there were several consistent themes. First, there is a clear trend in the literature for each specific group that suggests youth in these special populations use technology to (1) gather health and other types of information and (2) seek social support, particularly when it is difficult to find in their in-person lives. Second, there was also consistent evidence suggesting that most of the populations were at increased risk of being victims and, at times, perpetrators of cyberbullying. Further, being a victim was linked with negative mental health outcomes such as low self-esteem, depression, and anxiety in these groups.

Intervention strategies varied widely based on the needs of the individual groups, from case management to social support. Based on the natural risks and benefits that appear to be afforded by technology, it seems likely that youth in these groups would universally benefit from training to understand how to find accurate sources of online information, avoid predators, and respond to episodes of bullying. Future studies should continue to evaluate these and other intervention approaches as strategies to improve the mental health outcomes of these vulnerable youth populations. We conclude this chapter by presenting an illustrative case example summarizing some of the main themes described in this chapter and providing recommendations for clinicians working with the above populations.

Case Study

Ezra is a 19-year-old teen. He identifies as gay. He was placed in foster care at age 4 due to neglect and parental substance use. He was reunited with his biological family at age 11 and then put back in foster care again at 15. At age 18, he left his foster care placement and became homeless. He couch-surfed with friends for a while but eventually ended up on the streets. Prior to becoming homeless, he became very connected with social media as a teen because it was a way to keep in touch with his biological family members and friends. He mostly feels that social media has been a positive force in his life because it allowed him to stay connected with his biological mother and friends. However, he has also experienced cyberbullying several times by other former high school classmates because of his sexual orientation, which lead to a significant depressive episode at age 17 years. Just before his 19th birthday, Ezra connected with a case manager named Tim from a local agency serving homeless youth and young adults while staying in a temporary shelter. Tim helped Ezra get connected with a transitional housing program. Ezra feels that Tim has been very helpful, especially because Ezra feels comfortable texting Tim for help when he needs it. Tim has particularly helped him to fill out community college and job applications and enroll in extended foster care so that he can get economic and housing support from the state. He also found Ezra an SGM-friendly transitional housing program, which has allowed Ezra to develop a stronger in-person community, as well as a new therapist named Beth. Beth has been helping Ezra achieve several goals including processing through some of his early experiences, learning skills to deal with strong emotions, and developing goals for his future. As part of this work, she has also helped Ezra to develop a list of "safe" online forums and health resources for SGM youth and to recognize early warning signs for cyberbullying so that Ezra can avoid having more trauma due to difficult online experiences.

Recommendations for Clinicians

Clinicians should be aware that online platforms are a common source of information, identity exploration, and social support for many of the populations described in this section. Additionally, risks that are common to all teens, such as cyberbullying and online victimization, may be even more salient and/or impactful in these groups. However, research also suggests that for these groups, the Internet may be a critical lifeline of social support. Thus, advising these patients to avoid technology is not likely to be helpful. Developing strategies to coach youth on safe and effective use is likely to be the most effective way to reduce potential harms. Thus, mental health clinicians working with these populations should regularly screen for the types and frequency of the use of online platforms as well as potential negative consequences of this use. They should also provide regular psychoeducation around how to determine the accuracy of online information, given that many youth in these special populations use online resources to seek information more often that other groups of youth. Additionally, clinicians will benefit from continually educating themselves on positive, supportive sources of information and social support for their clients as well as on potential evidence-based mobile and/or online intervention resources as these platforms continue to be developed and evaluated. As an example, the use of text messaging may be an effective adjunct to in-person case management for these groups, particularly for homeless youth who may have difficulty access in person resources.

References

1. Health risks and needs of lesbian, gay, bisexual, transgender, and questioning adolescents position statement. J Pediatr Health Care. 2011;25(6):A9–10. [cited January 17, 2017]. http://www.sciencedirect.com/science/article/pii/S0891524511002276. https://doi.org/10.1016/j.pedhc.2011.07.002.
2. CDC. Sexual identity, sex of sexual contacts, and health-risk behaviors among students in grades 9–12: youth risk behavior surveillance. Atlanta (GA): U.S. Department of Health and Human Services; 2016 [cited January 17, 2017]. 133 p. https://www.cdc.gov/mmwr/preview/mmwrhtml/ss6007a1.htm.
3. James SE, Herman JL, Rankin S, Keisling M, Mottet L, Anafi M. The Report of the 2015 U.S. Transgender Survey. Washington, DC: National Center for Transgender Equality; 2016 [cited January 17, 2017]. 302 p. http://www.transequality.org/sites/default/files/docs/USTS-Full-Report-FINAL.PDF.
4. A call to action: LGBTQ youth need inclusive sex education. Human Rights Campaign. [cited January 17, 2017]. 10 p. http://hrc-assets.s3-website-us-

east-1.amazonaws.com//files/assets/resources/HRC-SexHealthBrief-2015.pdf.
5. Fox J, Ralston R. Queer identity online: informal learning and teaching experiences of LGBTQ individuals on social media. Comput Hum Behav. 2016 [cited January 14, 2017];65:635–42. http://www.sciencedirect.com/science/article/pii/S074756321630437X. https://doi.org/10.1016/j.chb.2016.06.009.
6. Evans Y, Gridley S, Crouch J, Wang A, Moreno M, Ahrens K, et al. Understanding online resources use by transgender youth and caregivers. In preparation. 2016.
7. Schimmel-Bristow A, Breland D, Crouch J, Evans E, McCarty C. Youth experiences of gender identity transition: a qualitative study. Psychol Sex Orientat Gend Divers. Forthcoming 2018.
8. Mitchell KJ, Ybarra ML, Korchmaros JD, Kosciw JG. Accessing sexual health information online: use, motivations and consequences for youth with different sexual orientations. Health Educ Res. 2013 [cited March 8, 2017];29:147–57. https://academic-oup-com.proxy1.library.jhu.edu/her/article/29/1/147/711147/Accessing-sexual-health-information-online-use.
9. Faulkner SL, Lannutti PJ. Representations of lesbian and bisexual women's sexual and relational health in online video and text-based sources. Comput Hum Behav. 2016 [cited January 14, 2017];63:916–21. http://www.sciencedirect.com/science/article/pii/S0747563216304678. https://doi.org/10.1016/j.chb.2016.06.039.
10. Gridley S, Crouch J, Evans Y, Eng W, Antoon E, Breland D, et al. Youth and caregiver perspectives on barriers to gender-affirming health care for transgender youth. J Adolesc Health. 2016 [cited January 14, 2017];59(3):254–61. http://www.sciencedirect.com/science/article/pii/S1054139X16000963. https://doi.org/10.1016/j.jadohealth.2016.03.017.
11. Ybarra ML, Mitchell KJ. A national study of lesbian, gay, bisexual (LGB), and non-LGB youth sexual behavior online and in-person. Arch Sex Behav. 2016 [cited March 8, 2017];45:1357–72. http://link-springer-com.proxy1.library.jhu.edu/article/10.1007/s10508-015-0491-7.
12. DeHaan S, Kuper LE, Magee JC, Bigelow L, Mustanski BS. The interplay between online and offline explorations of identity, relationships, and sex: a mixed-methods study with LGBT youth. J Sex Res. 2013 [cited March 8, 2017];50:421–34. http://eds.a.ebscohost.com/ehost/pdfviewer/pdfviewer?sid=b00aaaa4-6dd9-4337-b7f5-c85bad1db43e%40sessionmgr4008&vid=8&hid=4102.
13. Varjas K, Meyers J, Kiperman S, Howard A. Technology hurts? Lesbian, gay, and bisexual youth perspectives of technology and cyberbullying. J Sch Violence. 2013 [cited January 14, 2017];12(1):27–44. http://eds.b.ebscohost.com/ehost/pdfviewer/pdfviewer?sid=56de8eeb-5f73-4d6b-963a-c8bbc3530f3b%40sessionmgr101&vid=22&hid=113. https://doi.org/10.1080/15388220.2012.731665.
14. Howard MC. An epidemiological assessment of online groups and a test of typology: what are the (dis)similarities of the online group types? Comput Hum Behav. 2014 [cited January 14, 2017];31:123–33. http://www.sciencedirect.com/science/article/pii/S0747563213003713. https://doi.org/10.1016/j.chb.2013.10.021.
15. Ceglarek PJD, Ward LM. A tool for help or harm? How associations between social networking use, social support, and mental health differ for sexual minority and heterosexual youth. Comput Hum Behav. 2016 [cited January 14, 2017];65:201–09. http://www.sciencedirect.com/science/article/pii/S0747563216305416. https://doi.org/10.1016/j.chb.2016.07.051.
16. Radovic A, DeMand A, Gmelin T, Stein B, Miller E. Design of a Stakeholder Informed Social Media Website for Depressed Adolescents and their Parents. Society of Adolescent Health and Medicine Annual Meeting, Washington, D.C. Poster presentation. 2016.
17. Ybarra ML, Mitchell KL, Palmer NA, Reisner SL. Online social support as a buffer against online and offline peer and sexual victimization among U.S. LGBT and non-LGBT youth. Child Abuse Negl. 2015 [cited March 8, 2017];39:123–36. http://www.sciencedirect.com.proxy1.library.jhu.edu/science/article/pii/S014521341400283X.
18. Cooper RM, Blumenfeld WJ. Responses to Cyberbullying: a descriptive analysis of the frequency of and impact on LGBT and allied youth. J LGBT Youth. 2012 [cited January 24, 2017];9(2):153–77. http://www.tandfonline.com/doi/full/10.1080/19361653.2011.649616?scroll=top&needAccess=true. https://doi.org/10.1080/19361653.2011.649616.
19. DiNapolim JM, Gracia-Dia MJ, Garcia-Ona L, O'Flaherty D, Siller J. A theory-based computer mediated communication intervention to promote mental health and reduce high-risk behaviors in the LGBT population. Appl Nurs Res. 2014 [cited January 14, 2017]:27:91–3. http://www.sciencedirect.com/science/article/pii/S089718971300102X. https://doi.org/10.1016/j.apnr.2013.10.003.
20. Ybarra ML, DuBois Z, Parsons JT, Prescott TL, Mustanski B. Online focus groups as an HIV prevention program for gay, bisexual, and queer adolescent males. AIDS Educ Prev. 2014 [cited March 8, 2017];2696:554–64. http://eds.a.ebscohost.com/ehost/pdfviewer/pdfviewer?sid=b00aaaa4-6dd9-4337-b7f5-c85bad1db43e%40sessionmgr4008&vid=13&hid=4102.
21. Mustanksi B, Greene GJ, Ryan D, Whitton SW. Feasibility, acceptability, and initial efficacy of an online sexual health promotion program for LGBT youth: the queer sex ed Intervention. J Sex Res. 2015 [cited March 8, 2017];52(5):220–30. http://eds.a.ebscohost.com/ehost/pdfviewer/pdfviewer?sid=b00aaaa4-6dd9-4337-b7f5-c85bad1db43e%40sessionmgr4008&vid=17&hid=4102.
22. Baskerville NB, Dash D, Wong K, Smuh A, Abramowicz A. Perceptions toward a smoking cessation app targeting LGBTQ+ youth and young adults: a qualitative framework analysis of focus groups. JMIR Public Health Surveill. 2016 [cited March 8,

2017];2(2):e165. https://www.ncbi.nlm.nih.gov/pmc/articles/PMC5135733/.
23. Courtney ME, Terao S, Bost N. Midwest evaluation of the adult functioning of former foster youth: conditions of youth preparing to leave state care. Chicago (IL): Chapin Hall Center for Children; 2004. [cited January 15, 2017]. http://www.chapinhall.org/sites/default/files/CS_97.pdf.
24. Courtney ME, Dworsky A, Ruth G, Keller T, Havlicek J, Bost N. Midwest evaluation of the adult functioning of former foster youth: outcomes at age 19 [internet]. Chicago (IL): Chapin Hall Center for Children; 2005. [cited January 15, 2017]. http://www.chapinhall.org/sites/default/files/ChapinHallDocument_4.pdf.
25. Ammerman SD, Ensign J, Kirzner R, Meininger ET, Tornabene M, Warf CW, et al. Homeless young adults ages 18–24: Examining service delivery adaptations. Nashville, TN: National Health Care for the Homeless Council, Inc; 2004. [cited January 15, 2017]. p 50. http://www.nhchc.org/wp-content/uploads/2011/10/younghomelessadult1.pdf.
26. Federal Advisory Committee on Juvenile Justice. Federal Advisory Committee on Juvenile Justice Annual Report 2010. Washington, DC: Office of Juvenile Justice and Delinquency Prevention; 2010 [cited January 15, 2017]. http://www.facjj.org/annualreports/00-FACJJ%20Annual%20Report-FINAL%20508.pdf.
27. Rice E, Monro W, Barman-Adhikari A, Young SD. Internet use, social networking, and HIV/AIDS risk for homeless adolescents. J Adolesc Health. 2010 [cited January 15, 2017];47(6):610–13. http://www.sciencedirect.com/science/article/pii/S1054139X10002247. https://doi.org/10.1016/j.jadohealth.2010.04.016.
28. Jennings L, Lee N, Shore D, Strohminger N, Allison B, Cheskin L, et al. U.S. minority homeless youth's access to and use of mobile phones: implications for mHealth intervention design. J Health Commun. 2016 [cited January 15, 2017];21(7):725–33. http://www.tandfonline.com/doi/full/10.1080/10810730.2015.1103331?scroll=top&needAccess=true. https://doi.org/10.1080/10810730.2015.1103331.
29. Barman-Adhikari A, Rice E. Sexual health information seeking online among runaway and homeless youth. J Soc Social Work Res. 2011 [cited January 15, 2017];2(2):88–103. https://www.ncbi.nlm.nih.gov/pmc/articles/PMC3256925/. https://doi.org/10.5243/jsswr.2011.5.
30. Rice E, Barman-Adhikari A. Internet and social media use as a resource among homeless youth. J Comput Mediat Commun. 2014 [cited January 17, 2017];19(2):232–47. http://eds.b.ebscohost.com/ehost/pdfviewer/pdfviewer?sid=a7cb6796-4503-4a46-8849-6b3f0273deb0%40sessionmgr101&vid=16&hid=113. https://doi.org/10.1111/jcc4.12038.
31. Rice E, Stein JA, Milburn N. Countervailing social network influences on problem behaviors among homeless youth. J Adolesc. 2008 [cited January 17, 2017];31(5):625–39. http://www.sciencedirect.com/science/article/pii/S0140197107001017. https://doi.org/10.1016/j.adolescence.2007.10.008.
32. Wenzel SL, Tucker JS, Golinelli D, Green HD, Zhou A. Personal network correlates of alcohol, cigarette, and marijuana use among homeless youth. Drug Alcohol Depend. 2010 [cited January 15, 2017];112(1–2):140–49. http://www.tandfonline.com/doi/full/10.1080/10810730.2016.1177139?scroll=top&needAccess=true. https://doi.org/10.1016/j.drugalcdep.2010.06.004.
33. Barman-Adhikari A, Rice E, Bender K, Lengnick-Hall R, Yoshioka-Maxwell A, Rhoades H. Social networking technology use and engagement in HIV-related risk and protective behaviors among homeless youth. J Health Commun. 2016 [cited January 17, 2017];21(7):809–17. http://www.tandfonline.com/doi/full/10.1080/10810730.2015.1103331?scroll=top&needAccess=true. https://doi.org/10.1080/10810730.2016.1177139.
34. Marshall B D, Kerr T, Shoveller JA, Patterson TL, Buxton JA, Wood, E. Homelessness and unstable housing associated with an increased risk of HIV and STI transmission among street-involved youth. Health Place. 2009 [cited January 19, 2017];15(3):783–90. http://www.sciencedirect.com/science/article/pii/S1353829209000045. https://doi.org/10.1016/j.healthplace.2008.12.005.
35. Mutere M, Nyamathi A, Christiani A, Sweat J, Avila G, Hobaica L. Homeless youth seeking health and life-meaning through popular culture and the arts. Child Youth Serv. 2014 [cited January 19, 2017];35(3):273–87. http://www.tandfonline.com/doi/full/10.1080/0145935X.2014.950416?scroll=top&needAccess=true. https://doi.org/10.1080/0145935X.2014.950416.
36. Bender K, Schau N, Begun S, Haffejee B, Barman-Adhikari A, Hathaway J. Electronic case management with homeless youth. Evaluation Program Plann. 2015 [cited January 15, 2017];50:36–42. http://www.sciencedirect.com/science/article/pii/S0149718915000117. https://doi.org/10.1016/j.evalprogplan.2015.02.002.
37. Dang MT, Whitney KD, Virata MCD, Binger MM, Miller E. A web-based personal health information system for homeless youth and young adults. Public Health Nurs. 2012 [cited March 14, 2017];29(4):313–19. http://eds.a.ebscohost.com/ehost/pdfviewer/pdfviewer?sid=b00aaaa4-6dd9-4337-b7f5-c85bad1db43e%40sessionmgr4008&vid=25&hid=4102.
38. Albertson KM, Moreno MA, Garrison MA, Evans YN, Ahrens KR. Impacts of media on sexual behavior and relationships among youth in foster care. Child Family Soc Work. In press.
39. Gustavsson N, MacEachron A. Positive youth development and foster care youth: a digital perspective. J Hum Behav Soc Environ. 2015 [cited January 18, 2017];25(5):407–15. http://www.tandfonline.com/doi/full/10.1080/10911359.2014.966223. https://doi.org/10.1080/10911359.2014.966223.
40. Petrovic W. Free computers for county foster children helps bridge the digital divide. Net Literacy. 2011

[cited January 20, 2017]. http://www.netliteracy.org/?s=foster+children.
41. Escobar-Chaves SL, Anderson CA. Media and risky behaviors. Future Child. 2008 [cited March 14, 2017];18(1):147–80. http://eds.a.ebscohost.com/ehost/pdfviewer/pdfviewer?sid=b00aaaa4-6dd9-4337-b7f5-c85bad1db43e%40sessionmgr4008&vid=29&hid=4102.
42. Lim SS, Chan YH, Vadrevu S, Basnyat I. Managing peer relationships online—investigating the use of Facebook by juvenile delinquents and youths-at-risk. Comput Hum Behav. 2012 [cited January 15, 2017];29(1):8–15. http://www.sciencedirect.com/science/article/pii/S0747563212001732. https://doi.org/10.1016/j.chb.2012.04.025.
43. Dziuk MA, Larson JC, Apostu A, Mahone EM, Denckla MB, Mostofsky SH. Dyspraxia in autism: association with motor, social, and communicative deficits. Dev Med Child Neurol. 2007 [cited January 18, 2017];49(10):734–39. http://search.proquest.com/docview/195601991/fulltextPDF/23E59F02AA014CC5PQ/1?accountid=11752. https://doi.org/10.1111/j.1469-8749.2007.00734.x.
44. Davidson J. Autistic culture online: virtual communication and cultural expression on the spectrum. Soc Cult Geogr. 2008 [cited January 18, 2017];9(7):791–806. http://www.tandfonline.com/doi/full/10.1080/14649360802382586?scroll=top&needAccess=true. https://doi.org/10.1080/14649360802382586.
45. Robertson SM. Online and offline bullying of autistic youth: anti-bullying strategies, reporting, and technological solutions [dissertation on the internet]. Philadelphia, PA: The University of Pennsylvania; 2014. [cited January 19, 2017]. http://search.proquest.com/docview/1511999790.
46. Kowalski RM, Fedina C. Cyber bullying in ADHD and Asperger syndrome populations. Res Autism Spectr Disord. 2011 [cited January 19, 2017];5(3):1201–8. http://www.sciencedirect.com/science/article/pii/S1750946711000134. https://doi.org/10.1016/j.rasd.2011.01.007.
47. Kowalski RM, Morgan CA, Drake-Lavelle K, Allison B. Cyberbullying among college students with disabilities. Comput Hum Behav. 2016 [cited January 20, 2017];57:416–27. http://www.sciencedirect.com/science/article/pii/S0747563215303150. doi:https://doi.org/10.1016/j.chb.2015.12.044.
48. Didden R, Scholte RHJ, Korzilius H, de Moor JMH, Vermeulen A, O'Reilly M, et al. Cyberbullying among students with intellectual and developmental disability in special education settings. Dev Neurorehabil. 2009 [cited January 20, 2017];12(3):146–51. http://eds.b.ebscohost.com/ehost/pdfviewer/pdfviewer?sid=377f1ac7-ada6-4afb-8c46-e55c0b0a41bf%40sessionmgr104&vid=18&hid=113. https://doi.org/10.1080/17518420902971356.
49. Heiman T, Olenik-Shemesh D, Eden S. Cyberbullying involvement among students with ADHD: relation to loneliness, self-efficacy and social support. Eur J Spec Needs Educ. 2014 [cited January 20, 2017];30(1):15–29. http://www.tandfonline.com/doi/full/10.1080/08856257.2014.943562?scroll=top&needAccess=true. https://doi.org/10.1080/08856257.2014.943562.
50. Burke M, Kraut R, Williams D. Social use of computer-mediated communication by adults on the autism spectrum. In: Proceedings of the 2010 ACM conference on Computer supported cooperative work. ACM. 2010. pp. 425–434. http://thoughtcrumbs.com/publications/Burke_CSCW2010_CMC_and_Autism.pdf.
51. Kandalaft MR, Didenbani N, Krawczyk DC, Allen TT, Chapman SB. Virtual reality social cognition training for young adults with high-functioning autism. J Autism Dev Disord. 2013 [cited January 20, 2017];43(1):34–44. http://eds.b.ebscohost.com/ehost/pdfviewer/pdfviewer?sid=9722fc34-6078-4f95-90aa-0951afdc1499%40sessionmgr101&vid=6&hid=113. https://doi.org/10.1007/s10803-012-1544-6.
52. Didehbani N, Allen T, Kandalaft M, Krawczyk D, Chapman S. Virtual reality social cognition training for children with high functioning autism. Comput Hum Behav. 2016 [cited January 18, 2017];62:703–11. http://www.sciencedirect.com/science/article/pii/S0747563216303089. https://doi.org/10.1016/j.chb.2016.04.033.
53. Wang X, Laffey J, Xing W, Ma Y, Stichter J. Exploring embodied social presence of youth with Autism in 3D collaborative virtual learning environment: a case study. Comput Hum Behav. 2016 [cited January 18, 2017];55(Part A):310–21. http://www.sciencedirect.com/science/article/pii/S0747563215301370. https://doi.org/10.1016/j.chb.2015.09.006.
54. Waight M, Oldreive W. Accessible websites—what is out there? Br J Learn Disabil. 2016 [cited January 20, 2017];44(2):122–29. http://onlinelibrary.wiley.com/doi/10.1111/bld.12119/abstract;jsessionid=5FFE8A6F12151E150E1A757174D2886D.f03t02. https://doi.org/10.1111/bld.12119.
55. Vogelgesang K, Bruhn AL, Coghill-Behrends W, Kern M, Troughton L. A single subject study of a technology-based self-monitoring intervention. J Behav Educ. 2016 [cited January 18, 2017];25(4):478–97. http://link.springer.com/article/10.1007%2Fs10864-016-9253-4. https://doi.org/10.1007/s10864-016-9253-4.

Part II

Associations Between Mental Health Symptoms and Technology Use

5 Positive and Negative Associations Between Adolescent Mental Health and Technology

Linda Charmaraman, Tracy Gladstone, and Amanda Richer

Research on the psychological implications of using and being exposed to social technologies is an emerging area of inquiry, given that digital communication is increasingly and intricately tied to adolescent daily behavior. Ninety-two percent of adolescents aged 13–17 go online daily [1]. Facebook, which is by far the most popular and well-researched social networking site [2], surpassed Google.com in March 2010 as the most visited site in the USA [3]. As of 2015, Facebook remains the most used social media site in adolescents aged 13–17 (71%), followed by Instagram (52%), Snapchat (41%), and Twitter (33%) [1]. Since the early years of mobile communication, adolescents have helped drive the mass adoption of mobile technologies in society [4] and remain the most active users today, relying on texting and voice mails to develop and maintain friendships and romantic relationships [5]. Eighty-eight percent of adolescents now own or have access to a mobile phone [6]. The current Generation M were born in the twenty-first century and do not remember a time without access to mobile devices or to the Internet [7]. A nationally representative study of video game play demonstrates that 97% of adolescents aged 12–17 play computer, web-based, or portable video games [6]. Gentile [8] found that youth aged 8–18 play video games on an average of 13.2 h per week.

To date, both problematic and beneficial implications of social technologies have been identified; however, the literature is heavily dominated by negative outcomes related to adolescents using social technologies too soon, too often, or inappropriately. For instance, adolescence researchers in social and developmental psychology have primarily examined the negative consequences (over 20 studies) of adolescent video game use such as addiction [9], aggression [10], and decreased empathy [11], while research on positive outcomes in adolescence alone is limited with just a few empirical studies [12, 13].

The early adolescent years between age 10 and 15 are marked by pubertal development, cognitive maturation, school transitions, social identity redefinitions, and the emergence of sexuality. This developmental period is one of increased vulnerability because many problems experienced in young adulthood begin in the early adolescent years [14]. At no other stage in development are people more susceptible to the influence of peers than in early adolescence [15]. Early adolescence is a particularly vulnerable age period due to the heightened awareness of peer status, approval, and rejection, and it is associated with a drop in self-esteem, weaker academic performance, and increased anxiety and competition with others [16]. During early adolescence,

L. Charmaraman (✉) • T. Gladstone • A. Richer
Wellesley Centers for Women, Wellesley College, Wellesley, MA, USA
e-mail: lcharmar@wellesley.edu

M.A. Moreno, A. Radovic (eds.), *Technology and Adolescent Mental Health*,
https://doi.org/10.1007/978-3-319-69638-6_5

researchers have noted that there is a temporary increase in family conflict, particularly over issues of autonomy and control [17, 18]. Social media sites and mobile phones offer an opportunity for family members who are concerned or vigilant to become "friends" on the adolescent's profile page, where they can overtly (or covertly) monitor their adolescent's online behavior during the tumultuous early adolescent struggles with independence and peer approval.

A majority of adolescents use the Internet as a healthy venue for social interaction, online journaling, blogging, photography, and other pursuits [19]. Social technologies such as Facebook or mobile phones can facilitate an ability to define their peer community or "friendship network." Electronic interactions have been positively associated with emancipation from parental surveillance [20], adolescents' friendship quality, and feeling of closeness with friends [21–24]. Use of Facebook has been positively associated with building and maintaining social capital, particularly for at-risk young people, women of color [25], and those experiencing low self-esteem and life satisfaction [26].

On the other hand, due to young adolescents' limited capacity to self-regulate and susceptibility to peer pressure [27], potentially perilous online and social networking behaviors (e.g., lying about their age to gain access to certain sites) may increase as adolescents seek autonomy and separation from their familial networks [28–32]. Being susceptible to peer influences, adolescents are particularly vulnerable to the influence of what they see on social technologies [19, 26, 33, 34]. Risks include higher exposures to inappropriate sexual references or substance use [35–37], bullying [38], and psychosocial consequences such as anxiety, depression, and loneliness [39, 40], which may lead to higher likelihoods of substance abuse or unsafe sex [27]. In a national study of over 1500 students aged 10–15, 33% experienced online harassment in the past year, of which 9% were directly linked to a social media site [41]. Although not as frequent as in-person bullying, cyberbullying impacts on psychosocial health can be devastating. The negative impact of online victimization has been demonstrated to increase the number of detentions, suspensions, and truancy incidents as well as increases the likelihood of a student carrying a weapon to school in the past 30 days [41]. This is why it is critical to understand the online peer environments that adolescents experience as an avenue for parental consideration and clinical intervention.

In this chapter, we will provide an overview of both positive and negative psychological associations with adolescent use of social technologies, focusing mainly on interactive digital communication between peers, such as through social media and mobile use.

Hierarchy

Social Connectivity and Sense of Belonging

It is well established that a sense of social connection forms the basis for creating meaningful, enduring interpersonal bonds [42]. Humans have an innate psychological drive to belong to groups and participate in social interactions—the sense of belongingness is almost as compelling a need as food [43], particularly in the normative developmental trajectory between adolescence and adulthood. Research conducted over the past decade demonstrates that more frequent online communication is associated with higher quality friendships. For instance, Valkenburg and Peter [23] found significant associations among time spent online, time spent with friends in person, frequency of online chats with friends, friendship quality, and well-being. Reasons given for this link between online communication and social connectedness stems from the promotion of self-disclosure and feelings of belonging [24, 44]. Davis [44] conducted a qualitative study of 32 adolescents, which found that casual exchanges through texting, posting on social network sites, and instant messaging fostered a sense of belonging and a feeling of validation regardless of physical location or time of day. In terms of gender differences, Quinn and Oldmeadow [45] surveyed 443 early adolescents demonstrating that sense of belonging was associated with social networking for boys but not for girls. The researchers argued that boys might find online spaces as safe rehearsal venues for caring relationships and to feel more connected. However, in another study, girls were found to be less lonely than boys following use of social media [46], suggesting that girls may benefit from being connected to others through social media differently than for boys.

Colwell and Kato [12] conducted a study with 12- and 13-year-old Japanese students demonstrating that the preference of playing video games over spending time with friends was unrelated to friendship quality. They concluded that preferring video games might be an emotional substitute for in-person friendships when they are alone, as opposed to a preference for social isolation. More cross-cultural comparative studies can examine whether the "emotional substitution" hypothesis of interactive video gaming carries over into different cultural contexts. Contrary to popular sentiment, Durkin and Barber [13] demonstrated that 16-year-old adolescent video game players had higher levels of family closeness, activity involvement, attachment to school, and positive mental health, regardless of gender, when compared to non-video game players. This demonstrates that video gaming is not as antisocial as many people assume, because a lot of gaming is interactive with live players that form new communities to belong to and new ways of achieving a flow and personal contentment [47].

Personal Contentment and Self-Esteem

In our Media and Identity Study, which collected online survey data from 747 adolescents in 47 US states aged 12–18, we examined relationships between personal contentment and social technologies. Four items were used to create the personal contentment mean for each participant using their self-report answers about how well they get along with their parents, how many friends they have, and how often they feel bored and sad. Our results showed Facebook habits were significantly related to personal contentment. For example, as the number of Facebook friends increased, particularly friends they knew well on Facebook, so did personal contentment. Higher personal contentment was associated with more likelihood of texting and calling about having a bad day with peers, but we did not find any significant relationships between personal contentment and instant messaging, emailing, tweeting, or posting on Facebook. These findings demonstrate that even though social media is one forum to provide support in times of need, it does not preclude the use of other more traditional ways of connecting with people during difficult times.

Davis [48] collected survey data on over 2000 students aged 11 to 19, demonstrating that students who communicated online with their friends had higher friendship quality which was in turn associated with greater self-concept clarity, that is, a clear, well-defined sense of self across social situations. In one of the few experimental studies that induced social exclusion while using technology, adolescents and young adults were assigned to either a solitary game play versus playing games while instant messaging others. The ones who could instant message others during the task had higher self-esteem, perceptions of being valued, accepted, and respected [49] compared to those who could not communicate their thoughts with others.

The human need for affiliation and self-disclosure is highlighted in other forms of computer-mediated communication, such as blogging [50]. According to the 2015 Pew Research Center Teens, Social Media, and Technology overview [1], only 5% of boys use microblogging sites like Tumblr; however, 23% of girls aged 13–17 use Tumblr to curate and share their thoughts with a specified audience [1]. There is evidence suggesting that the motivation behind blogging for women is not just about self-expression but also about gaining influence in the blogosphere and forming connections with other people [50]. In a study examining MySpace bloggers and non-bloggers after 2 months' time, researchers demonstrated that compared to the control group, bloggers experienced higher levels of social integration (e.g., sense of belonging to like-minded communities) and counting on others for assistance (e.g., reliable alliance) [51]. In a more recent experimental study of the psychological effects of blogging, researchers found that bloggers who had an open, active audience who could submit feedback had the most positive effect on participants' self-esteem, mental health, and social behaviors, particularly when writing about their social-emotional difficulties [52].

Emotional Expression/Control

Those with existing vulnerabilities (such as shy introverts) may use online communication, such as instant messaging to build their social skills, increase interpersonal contacts, improve fluency of conversations, and decrease loneliness [53]. Texting provides adolescents with a greater sense of control with their interactions in emotional situations [54]. Bonetti, Campbell, and Gilmore [55] collected data on 626 Australian adolescents aged 10–16 and found that lonely students were significantly more likely than non-lonely students to use online chat spaces to discuss private topics such as emotions, problems, or secrets they may be experiencing. Lonely students were also more likely to admit meeting new people online since face-to-face encounters are too uncomfortable. Online communication reduces anxiety-inducing stimuli such as making eye contact or having to respond instantaneously [56] and thus allows vulnerable adolescents, such as those with social anxieties or learning disabilities [57] to experience less loneliness and improve their well-being [58].

Identity Development

Social identity gratification [59, 60] proposes that individuals tend to seek out information and experiences that affirm their preexisting social identities. Adolescents use social media for this purpose—to establish and maintain positive self-images, to express their sexuality, individuality, and "self-branding" [61]. Social media can be a forum for developing, maintaining, and highlighting social identities, particularly for unique or stigmatized groups. Online spaces may offer safer spaces for young people to explore sensitive topics and their identity and sexuality [62]. For instance, Ceglarek and Ward [63] demonstrated that sexual minority youth who engage in lesbian, gay, bisexual, transgender, and/or queer (LGBTQ) online communities experience reduced levels of paranoia associated with their "coming out" and identity development. Gajaria and colleagues [61] revealed that Facebook support groups for adolescents with attention deficit hyperactivity disorder (ADHD) tended to portray those with ADHD in a flattering light; thus group membership was used as a form of self-branding to ward off social stigma. Dolev-Cohen and Barak [64] argue that repressing emotions through nondisclosure can have a negative impact upon well-being; thus online disclosure opportunities can benefit stigmatized groups and encourage them to connect with mental health resources [65]. For instance, individuals with severe mental illness can find a support network through YouTube, thereby reducing isolation, improving hope, sharing strategies for coping with day-to-day challenges, and learning from shared experiences of medication use [66, 67].

Negative Associations

Negative Self-Concept

Although a prior study of 134 participants found that MySpace bloggers and non-bloggers did not differ in terms of anxiety or depression levels [51], our correlational study of 747 adolescents found lower levels of personal contentment for those creating characters online and writing blogs—both of which require personal investment in generating an audience for self-disclosures. In a sense, adolescents can be considered brave to be able to reveal such hidden truths about themselves to a public audience; however, there are a number of studies that correlate blogging with low self-esteem [68, 69]. Perhaps low self-esteem coincides with the compulsive need to self-disclose. Further research is needed to unpack whether the platform of blogging is primarily a forum for venting one's personal feeling and frustrations or if the act of blogging may negatively impact one's contentment or if the desire to blog in the first place is related to one's self-concept.

Alienation and Social Anxiety

Cyberostracism has been coined to describe the alienation that can occur in online social environments due to exclusion, rejection, or being ignored [70], a construct that is believed to be as hurtful as the equivalent in offline situations often threatening one's sense of belonging [71]. In a study comparing cyberostracism among 8–14-year-olds and adults playing an online interactive game of Cyberball where social inclusion or exclusion was manipulated, Abrams et al. [71] demonstrated that adolescents aged 13–14 were the most strongly affected by cyberostracism, suggesting that adolescents place more priority on inclusion by their peers compared to children and adults. Whereas online communication may help build networks and self-confidence for some, other individuals find that it exacerbates existing mental health concerns. When using technology for entertainment rather than communicative purposes, adolescents with poor friendship quality offline experienced heightened feelings of loneliness, isolation, and social anxiety [72]. Turkle [73] has warned of the dangers of adolescents who need to script a "flawless narrative" about their lives, echoing the sentiments of Bortree [74] who suggested that adolescents struggle to reconcile wanting to present their lives truthfully while wanting to impress others. Thus, there is a tension between being anxious about fitting in and belonging to an in-group versus being unnoticed and ignored altogether.

Body Dissatisfaction and Eating Disorders

It is estimated that approximately half of adolescent girls are unhappy with their bodies [75], and these feelings can begin as young as 6 years of age among individuals of various body shapes and cultural backgrounds [76, 77]. Despite the higher prevalence of women and girls to experience body dissatisfaction and disordered eating compared to male counterparts in the USA and Australia [78], in studies that examine the relation between social media sites and body image or disordered eating, there are no significant gender differences [79]. For instance, Facebook use was a predictor of body consciousness and greater body shame across gender [80], and both males and females are less satisfied with their bodies after being exposed to attractive Facebook profiles [81]. In a large study involving 1087 girls aged 13–15 years, Tiggemann and Slater [82] showed significant positive relationships among using social media sites, the number of friends in the online network, and body image concerns. Body dissatisfaction can lead to maladaptive consequences such as depression, anxiety, low self-esteem, and eating disorders [83–85].

Triggering of Emotions

The accumulation of digital data from adolescents' online communication in the form of posts, photos, and videos, termed as "digital dossier" by Palfrey and Gasser [7], may influence adolescents' evolving sense of self. This is particularly salient if review of these online archives could cause discomfort or reliving of charged experiences, whereas prior generations of adolescents had the benefit of fading memories that were not recorded online [84].

The term *Facebook depression* was coined by authors citing websites that argued for a relationship between depression and social media use [85–88, 105, 106]. Researchers have found statistically significant correlations between time spent on social media sites and scores on the Beck Depression Inventory; however, these findings do not support causation or directionality [89]. Other studies have found no association between social network use and depression, one of which used a rigorous design of real-time assessment of Internet use and a validated clinical screening instrument for depression [90].

Instant messaging was found to be associated with increased depression in one study [91]. Underwood's et al. [92] observational study of adolescent text messages revealed that adolescents who send texts with more negative content are more likely to suffer from self-reported internalizing and depressive symptoms. Similarly, texts with antisocial messages are strongly associated with self-reported, parent-reported, and teacher-reported antisocial behavior over time [93].

Although studies have shown that frequency of Facebook use bears no relation to depression, the *quality* of interactions on Facebook is key [94]. For instance, negative social interactions on Facebook are associated with greater levels of depressive symptoms, and positive interactions are associated with fewer depressive symptoms. In addition, if a young person is well-adjusted, he or she is more likely to experience enhanced feelings of connectedness on social media sites, whereas someone who is prone to depression will likely feel more disconnected [94]. More research is needed to determine the nature of the relationship between social technologies and triggering of intense emotions like depression [95].

Discussion and Implications

In this chapter, we provided an overview of positive and negative aspects of adolescents using social technologies that can bolster or hinder mental health depending on the intended use (solo entertainment vs. communication with others) as well as preexisting social and emotional conditions, such as quality of social networks offline and sense of self-worth. An important element of peers' online influence can be understood in the context of *social comparison processes*, the impetus to gain accurate self-evaluations [96, 97] which are major sources of influence on adolescent health attitudes, intentions, and behaviors [98]. Social technologies allow such social comparisons to take place. For instance, adolescents who are connected to each other online may learn through observation or vicarious experiences as they read about others' experiences, which can reduce (or intensify) feelings of isolation or provide role modeling to increase socially supportive interactions. Prior research has shown that youth who engage in more social comparison tend to use Facebook more frequently, have poorer self-perceptions, lower self-esteem, and more negative affect [99]. Rumination has been proposed as a key component to the negative effects of social comparison, resulting in more depressive symptoms [100]. In addition, passive or "surveillance" uses of social networking sites (i.e., viewing of others' posts without commenting or not making it known that they are observing others' online activities) predicts social anxiety, brooding, and envy [101, 102].

Despite the fact that 95% of adolescents are now online, 81% of them are using social media sites [1], and 80% of adolescents sleep with their mobile phones [103], little is known about the long-term effects of social technologies on psychosocial and behavioral health outcomes in adolescence, particularly early adolescence (aged 10–15). In a review of mobile use and reducing risk of harm [104], the following factors were identified as critical: personality factors (sensation-seeking, low self-esteem, moral disengagement, psychological difficulties), social factors (peer norms, lack of parental engagement), and digital factors (digital skills, online practices, affordances of online sites). These factors might be critical as a checklist for counselors, social workers, and practitioners to assess when to be concerned about online behaviors and how to identify the behavioral markers that can flag an emerging problematic situation. For instance, with the knowledge that higher levels of digital fluency, more frequent social media use, and greater exposure to more social network sites that feature anonymity is more likely to lead to online risk, practitioners can ask both parents and adolescents about digital skill levels, frequency of use, and the types of sites they use, to obtain a broad assessment of potential online risk. When clinicians see an adolescent showing signs of distress, they could inquire about possible online as well as offline contexts, particularly any indication that mental well-being is diminished due to use or misuse of social technologies by the patient/client or an online peer. Additionally, clinicians should also be aware of the adolescent's fear of losing phone or computer privileges, which can detract them from reporting harmful occurrences. The same devices can also be a source of private information or social support for the adolescent [104]. The age of digital devices that pervade our social interactions is here to stay; thus it would be of practical and clinical importance for clinicians and health practitioners to become more literate in social technologies that their adolescent populations use and to provide resources for parents, family members, educators, and adolescents to become media literate consumers who know when to pull the plug when mental health is at stake.

Case Study

Sixteen-year-old Dave presented for treatment with symptoms of depression and anhedonia, reportedly following a difficult season on his high school hockey team. According to Dave's mother, he recently became aware of a private group within his team Slack, which included disparaging comments about him and about his younger sister, who is developmentally delayed. Dave reported that he did not realize his teammates were teasing him about his tall skinny frame, nor did he know they were making inappropriate sexual comments about his sister. As a result, Dave reports quitting his hockey team and now finds himself bored and angry. His grades have dropped. He spends all of his time in his room, with the door shut, and is irritable toward family members.

In an initial meeting with Dave, the clinician begins by checking in about his family and social relationships, in order to evaluate the degree to which he is connected to his parents and peers. It quickly becomes clear that, while Dave felt close to his parents last year, he has drawn less engaged with them as he has become more and more reliant on digital communications with his peers. He now spends most of his time separate from family members, on his phone, or computer, where he is vulnerable to criticism and taunting by his peers. While Dave has no history of significant psychological difficulties, he reports that he has long been anxious about his school performance and feels pressure to be independent and successful. He admits that, when friends post about their grades, it makes him feel worried that he can't keep up academically and that he will never be able to go to a good enough college.

In working with Dave, the clinician utilizes behavioral activation strategies as well as a cognitive behavioral approach. Her first goal is to help him increase social activities with peers and family members, as a way to counter some of the negative effects of his difficult digital interactions with peers, decrease his reliance on digital communications, and address his isolation from family members. They plan two family dinners weekly and also schedule a fun activity for the family each weekend (e.g., a meal out, a baseball game). She similarly helps him to plan to meet friends one evening each weekend and also to see friends after school. The clinician also works on cognitive restructuring with Dave around media and technology, helping him to recognize that material that is posted is highly edited, and that it is likely that, when a peer posts a good grade, it is the highlight of an otherwise less stellar report card. The clinician likewise works with Dave to rethink the definition of success and the meaning of a "good" college. Finally, the clinician talks with Dave about the reality that adolescents are more likely to post negative comments than say them. She helps Dave to rank the types of negative comments he sees or hears from peers, from those that he can respond to with humor, such as those about his skinny frame, to those that are simply unacceptable, such as taunting comments about his sister. They plan ways that Dave can respond lightly to some comments and make clear that he will no longer be a friend to those who make unacceptable comments.

Acknowledgments Funding for the Media & Identity Project was provided by the 35th Anniversary Fund at Wellesley Centers for Women and Robert Wood Johnson Foundation New Connections. We wholeheartedly thank Megan Moreno and Ana Radovic for insightful feedback on this chapter. We are grateful for Ineke Ceder's editorial expertise and the students who made the data collection possible for the first wave of the Media & Identity Project: Temple Price, Huiying Bernice Chan, Budnampet Ramanudom, and Betsy Eriksen.

References

1. Lenhart A. Pew Research Center. Teen, social media and technology overview 2015. Pew Research Center Report, 2015. http://www.pewinternet.org/files/2015/04/PI_TeensandTech_Update2015_0409151.pdf.
2. Wilson RE, Gosling SD, Graham LT. A review of Facebook research in the social sciences. Perspect Psychol Sci. 2012;7(3):203–20. https://doi.org/10.1177/1745691612442904.
3. Dougherty H. Facebook reaches top U.S. ranking. Experian Hitwise. 2010. http://www.experian.com/blogs/marketing-forward/2010/03/05/facebook-reaches-top-ranking-in-us/.
4. Ling R. The mobile connection. San Francisco: Morgan Kaufman; 2004.
5. Ling R, Bertel T. Mobile communication culture among children and adolescents. In: The Routledge international handbook of children, adolescents, and media; 2015. p. 127–33.
6. Lenhart A, Kahne J, Middaugh E, Macgill AR, Evans C, Vitak J. Teens, video games, and civics. Washington, DC: Pew Internet and American Life Project; 2008. Report No. 202-415-4500.
7. Palfrey JG, Gasser U. Born digital: understanding the first generation of digital natives. New York: Basic Books; 2008.
8. Gentile DA. Pathological video-game use among youth ages 8 to 18: a national study. Psychol Sci. 2009;20:594–602. https://doi.org/10.1111/j.1467-9280.2009.02340.x.
9. Rehbein F, Kleimann M, Mößle T. Prevalence and risk factors of video game dependency in adolescence: results of a German nationwide survey. Cyberpsychol Behav Soc Netw. 2010;13:269–77. doi:10.1089=cyber.2009.0227.
10. Konijn EA, Bijvank MN, Bushman BJ. I wish I were a warrior: the role of wishful identification in the effects of violent video games on aggression in adolescent boys. Dev Psychol. 2007;43:1038–44. https://doi.org/10.1037/0012-1649.43.4.1038.
11. Krahe B, Moller I. Longitudinal effects of media violence on aggression and empathy among German adolescents. J Appl Dev Psychol. 2010;31:401–9.
12. Colwell J, Kato M. Investigation of the relationship between social isolation, self-esteem, aggression and computer game play in Japanese adolescents. Asian J Soc Psychol. 2003;6:149–58. https://doi.org/10.1111/1467-839X.t01-1-00017.
13. Durkin K, Barber B. Not so doomed: computer game play and positive adolescent development. Appl Dev Psychol. 2002;23:373–92. https://doi.org/10.1016/S0193-3973(02)00124-7.
14. Carnegie Council on Adolescent Development. Turning points: preparing American youth for the 21st century. New York: Carnegie Corporation; 1989.
15. Steinberg L, Silverberg SB. The vicissitudes of autonomy in early adolescence. Child Dev. 1986;57:841–51.
16. Brinthaupt TM, Lipka RP. Understanding early adolescent self and identity: applications and interventions. New York: SUNY Press; 2012.
17. Buchanan CM, Eccles JS, Becker JB. Are adolescents the victims of raging hormones? Evidence for the activational effects of hormones on moods and behavior at adolescence. Psychol Bull. 1992;111:62–107.
18. Steinberg L. Interdependence in the family: autonomy, conflict, and harmony in the parent-adolescent relationship. In: Feldman SS, Elliott GR, editors. At the threshold: the developing adolescent. Cambridge: Harvard University Press; 1990. p. 255–76.
19. Lenhart A, Purcell K, Smith A, Zickuhr K. Social media & mobile internet use among teens and young adults. Washington, DC: Pew Internet and American Life Project; 2010.
20. Clark LS. The parent app: understanding families in the digital age. Oxford: Oxford University Press; 2013.
21. Blais JJ, Craig WM, Pepler D, Connolly J. Adolescents online: the importance of internet activity choices to salient relationships. J Youth Adolesc. 2008;37:522–36.
22. Cummings JN, Lee JB, Kraut R. Communication technology and friendship during the transition from high school to college. In: Kraut R, Brynin M, Kiesler S, editors. Computers, phones, and the internet: domesticating information technology. New York: Oxford University Press; 2006. p. 265–78.
23. Valkenburg PM, Peter J. Preadolescents' and adolescents' online communication and their closeness to friends. Dev Psychol. 2007;43:267–77. https://doi.org/10.1037/0012-1649.43.2.267.
24. Valkenburg PM, Peter J. The effects of instant messaging on the quality of adolescents' existing friendships: a longitudinal study. J Commun. 2009;59:79–97. https://doi.org/10.1111/j.1460–2466.2008.01405.x.
25. Charmaraman L, Chan H, Price T, Richer A. Surviving and thriving: women of color cultivating virtual social capital. In: Tassie KE, Brown SM, editors. Women of color and social media multitasking: blogs, timelines, feeds, and community. New York: Lexington Books; 2015. p. 1–19.
26. Ellison NB, Steinfield C, Lampe C. The benefits of Facebook "friends": social capital and college students' use of online social network sites. J Comp Mediat Commun. 2007;12:1143–68. https://doi.org/10.1111/j.1083-6101.2007.00367.x.
27. O'Keefe S, Clarke-Pearson K. The impact of social media on children, adolescents, and families. Pediatrics. 2011;127(4):800–4. https://doi.org/10.1542/peds.2011-0054.
28. Bearman P, Brückner H. Power in numbers: peer effects on adolescent girls' sexual debut and pregnancy. Washington, DC: National Campaign to Prevent Teen Pregnancy; 1999.
29. Kinsman SB, Schwarz DF, Furstenberg F, Romer D. Peer influence and intention to initiate sexual intercourse in early adolescence. J Adolesc

Health. 1997;20(2):168. https://doi.org/10.1016/S1054-139X(97)87630-6.
30. Madden M, Lenhart A, Cortesi S, Gasser U, Duggan M, Smith A. Teens, social media, and privacy. Washington, DC: Pew Internet and American Life Project; 2013. http://www.pewinternet.org/2013/05/21/teens-social-media-and-privacy/
31. Miller B, Norton M, Curtis T, Hill J, Schvaneveldt P, Young M. The timing of sexual intercourse among adolescents: family, peer, and other antecedents. Youth Soc. 1997;29:54–83. https://doi.org/10.1177/0044118X97029001003.
32. Stanton B, Li X, Pack R, Cottrell L, Harris C, Burns JM. Longitudinal influence of perceptions of peer and parental factors on African American adolescent risk involvement. J Urban Health. 2002;79:536–48. https://doi.org/10.1093/jurban/79.4.536.
33. Lenhart A, Madden M. Social networking sites and teens: an overview. Pew Internet and American Life Project; 2007. http://htlab.psy.unipd.it/uploads/Pdf/lectures/technology_for_young/Social%20Networking%20Websites%20and%20Teens%20text.pdf.
34. Lenhart A, Madden M. Teen content creators and consumers. Washington, DC: Pew Internet and American Life Project; 2005. http://www.pewinternet.org/2005/11/02/teen-content-creators-and-consumers/
35. Livingstone S, Helsper E. Parental mediation and children's internet use. J Broadcast Electron Media. 2008;52(4):581–99. https://doi.org/10.1080/08838150802437396.
36. Moreno MA, Brockman L, Rogers CB, Christakis DA. An evaluation of the distribution of sexual references among "top 8" Myspace friends. J Adolesc Health. 2010;47:418–20.
37. Patchin JW, Hinduja S. Trends in online social networking: adolescent use of Myspace over time. New Media Soc. 2010;12:197–216. https://doi.org/10.1177/1461444809341857.
38. Ybarra M, Mitchell K, Espelage D. Comparisons of bully and unwanted sexual experiences online and offline among a national sample of youth. 2012. http://cdn.intechopen.com/pdfs/30834/InTech-Comparisons_of_bully_and_unwanted_sexual_experiences_online_and_offline_among_a_national_sample_of_youth.pdf. Accessed 10 Sept 2015.
39. Moreno MA, Jelenchick LA, Egan KG, Cox E, Young H, Gannon KE, Becker T. Feeling bad on Facebook: depression disclosures by college students on a social networking site. Depress Anxiety. 2011;28:447–55. https://doi.org/10.1002/da.20805.
40. Ybarra ML, Alexander C, Mitchell KJ. Depressive symptomatology, youth internet use, and online interactions: a national survey. J Adolesc Health. 2005;36:9–18.
41. Ybarra ML, Mitchell KJ. How risky are social networking sites? A comparison of places online where youth sexual solicitation and harassment occurs. Pediatrics. 2008;121(2):e350–7.
42. Maslow AH. A theory of human motivation. Psychol Rev. 1943;50:370–96. https://doi.org/10.1037/h0054346.
43. Baumeister RF, Leary MR. The need to belong: desire for interpersonal attachments as a fundamental human motivation. Psychol Bull. 1995;117(3):497–529. https://doi.org/10.1037/0033-2909.117.3.497.
44. Davis K. Friendship 2.0: adolescents' experiences of belonging and self-disclosure online. J Adolesc. 2012;35:1527–36.
45. Quinn S, Oldmeadow JA. Is the igeneration a 'we' generation? Social networking use among 9- to 13-year-olds and belonging. Br J Dev Psychol. 2013;31:136–42. https://doi.org/10.1111/bjdp.12007.
46. Apaolaza V, Hartmann P, Medina E, Barrutia J, Echebarria C. The relationship between socializing on the Spanish online networking site Tuenti and teenagers' subjective wellbeing: the roles of self-esteem and loneliness. Comput Hum Behav. 2013;29:4.
47. Weibel D, Wissmath B, Habegger S, Steiner Y, Groner R. Playing online games against computer- vs. human-controlled opponents: effects on presence, flow, and enjoyment. Comput Hum Behav. 2008;24:2274–91. https://doi.org/10.1016/j.chb.2007.11.002.
48. Davis K. Young people's digital lives: the impact of interpersonal relationships and digital media use on adolescents' sense of identity. Comput Hum Behav. 2013;29:2281–93. https://doi.org/10.1016/j.chb.2013.05.022.
49. Gross EF. Logging on, bouncing back: an experimental investigation of online communication following social exclusion. Dev Psychol. 2009;45:1787–93. https://doi.org/10.1037/a0016541.
50. Chen GM. Why do women write personal blogs? Satisfying needs for self-disclosure and affiliation tell part of the story. Comput Hum Behav. 2012;28:171–80.
51. Baker JR, Moore SM. Blogging as a social tool: a psychosocial examination of the effects of blogging. Cyberpsychcol Behav. 2008;11(6):747–9.
52. Boniel-Nissim M, Barak A. The therapeutic value of adolescents' blogging about social-emotional difficulties. Psychol Serv. 2013;10(3):333–41.
53. Bardi AC, Brady MF. Why shy people use instant messaging: loneliness and other motives. Comput Hum Behav. 2010;26:1722–6. https://doi.org/10.1016/j.chb.2010.06.021.
54. Madell DE, Muncer SJ. Control over social interactions: an important reason for young people's use of the internet and mobile phones for communication? Cyberpsychol Behav. 2007;10(1):137–40.
55. Bonetti L, Campbell MA, Gilmore L. The relationship of loneliness and social anxiety with children's and adolescents' online communication. Cyberpsychol Behav Soc Netw. 2010;13(3):279–85. https://doi.org/10.1089/cyber.2009.0215.
56. Valkenburg PM, Peter J. Social consequences of the internet for adolescents: a decade of research.

Curr Dir Psychol Sci. 2009;18:1–5. https://doi.org/10.1111/j.1467-8721.2009.01595.x.
57. Sharabi A, Margalit M. Virtual friendships and social distress among adolescents with and without learning disabilities: the subtyping approach. Eur J Special Needs Educ. 2011;26:379–94. https://doi.org/10.1080/08856257.2011.595173.
58. Allen KA, Ryan T, Gray DL, McInerney DM, Waters L. Social media use and social connectedness in adolescents: the positives and the potential pitfalls. Aust Educ Dev Psychol. 2014;31(1):18–31.
59. Barker V. A generational comparison of social networking site use: the influence of age and social identity. Int J Aging Hum Dev. 2012;74(2):163–87. https://doi.org/10.2190/AG.74.2.d.
60. Harwood J. Age identification, social identity gratifications, and television viewing. J Broadcast Electron Media. 1999;43:123–36. https://doi.org/10.1080/08838159909364479.
61. Gajaria A, Yeung E, Goodale T, Charach A. Beliefs about attention-deficit/hyperactivity disorder and response to stereotypes: youth postings in Facebook groups. J Adolesc Health. 2011;49:15–20. https://doi.org/10.1016/j.jadohealth.2010.09.004.
62. Harper GW, Bruce D, Serrano P, Jamil O. The role of the internet in the sexual identity development of gay and bisexual male adolescents. In: Hammack PL, Cohler BJ, editors. The story of sexual identity: narrative perspectives on the gay and lesbian life course. New York: Oxford University Press; 2009. p. 297–326.
63. Ceglarek PJD, Ward MA. Tool for help or harm? How associations between social networking use, social support, and mental health differ for sexual minority and heterosexual youth. Comput Hum Behav. 2016;65:201–9.
64. Dolev-Cohen M, Barak A. Adolescents' use of instant messaging as a means of emotional relief. Comput Hum Behav. 2013;29(1):58–63.
65. Best P, Manktelow R, Taylor B. Online communication, social media and adolescent wellbeing: a systematic narrative review. Child Youth Serv Rev. 2014;41:27–36.
66. Moorhead SA, Hazlett DE, Harrison L, Carroll JK, Irwin A, et al. A new dimension of health care: systematic review of the uses, benefits, and limitations of social media for health communication. J Med Internet Res. 2013;15:e85.
67. Naslund JA, Grande SW, Aschbrenner KA, Elwyn G. Naturally occurring peer support through the experiences of individuals with severe mental illness using YouTube. PLoS One. 2014;9(10):e110171. https://doi.org/10.1371/journal.pone.0110171.
68. Fioravanti G, Dèttore D, Casale S. Adolescent internet addiction: testing the association between self-esteem, the perception of internet attributes, and preference for online social interactions. Cyberpsychol Behav Soc Netw. 2012;15(6):318–23. https://doi.org/10.1089/cyber.2011.0358.
69. Huang HY, Leung L. Gratification-opportunities, self-esteem, and loneliness in determining usage preference of BBS and blog among teenagers in China. Atlantic J Commun. 2012;20(3):141–57.
70. D'Amato G, Cecchi L, Liccardi G, Pellegrino F, D'Amato M, Sofia M. Social networks: a new source of psychological stress or a way to enhance self-esteem? Negative and positive implications in bronchial asthma. J Invest Allerg Clin. 2012;22(6):402–5. http://www.ncbi.nlm.nih.gov/pubmed/23101183.
71. Abrams D, Weick M, Thomas D, Colbe H, Franklin KM. On-line ostracism affects children differently from adolescents and adults. Br J Dev Psychol. 2011;29:110–23. https://doi.org/10.1348/026151010494089.
72. Selfout MHW, Branje SJT, Delsing M, ter Bogt TFM, Meeus WHJ. Different types of internet use, depression, and social anxiety: the role of perceived friendship quality. J Adolesc. 2009;32:819–33. https://doi.org/10.1016/j.adolescence.2008.10.011.
73. Turkle S. Alone together: why we expect more from technology and less from each other. New York: Basic Books; 2011.
74. Bortree DS. Presentation of self on the web: an ethnographic study of teenage girls' weblogs. Educ Commun Inform. 2005;5:25–39. https://doi.org/10.1080/14636310500061102.
75. Bearman SK, Presnell K, Martinez E. The skinny on body dissatisfaction: a longitudinal study of adolescent girls and boys. J Adolesc. 2006;35:217–29. https://doi.org/10.1007/s10964-005-9010-9.
76. Dohnt HK, Tiggemann M. Body image concerns in young girls: the role of peers and media prior to adolescence. J Youth Adolesc. 2006;35:135–45. https://doi.org/10.1007/s10964-005-9020-7.
77. Grabe S, Hyde JS. Ethnicity and body dissatisfaction among women in the United States: a meta-analysis. Psychol Bull. 2006;132:622–40. https://doi.org/10.1037/0033-2909.132.4.622.
78. Ata RN, Ludden AB, Lally MM. The effects of gender and family, friends, and media influences on eating behaviors and body image during adolescence. J Youth Adolesc 2007;36:1024–1037. doi: 10.1007.
79. Holland G, Tiggemann M. A systematic review of the impact of the use of social networking sites on body image and disordered eating outcomes. Body Image. 2016;17:100–10.
80. Manago AM, Ward L, Lemm KM, Reed L, Seabrook R. Facebook involvement, objectified body consciousness, body shame, and sexual assertiveness in college women and men. Sex Roles. 2015;72:1–14. https://doi.org/10.1007/s11199-014-0441-1.
81. Haferkamp N, Kramer NC. Social comparison 2.0: examining the effects of online profiles on social-networking sites. Cyberpsychol Behav Soc Netw. 2011;14:309–14. https://doi.org/10.1089/cyber.2010.0120.
82. Tiggemann M, Slater A. NetGirls: the internet, Facebook, and body image concern in adolescent girls. Int J Eat Disord. 2013;46:630–3.

83. Dittmar H. How do "body perfect" ideals in the media have a negative impact on body image and behaviours? Factors and processes related to self and identity. J Soc Clin Psychol. 2009;28:1–8. https://doi.org/10.1521/jscp.2009.28.1.1.
84. Grabe S, Ward L, Hyde JS. The role of the media in body image concerns among women: a meta-analysis of experimental and correlational studies. Psychol Bull. 2008;134:460–76. https://doi.org/10.1037/0033-2909.134.3.460.
85. Groesz L, Levine M, Murnen S. The effect of experimental presentation of thin media images on body satisfaction: a meta-analytic review. Int J Eat Disord. 2002;21:1–16. https://doi.org/10.1002/eat.10005.
86. Irvine C. Excessive chatting on Facebook can lead to depression in teenage girls. Daily Telegraph. 2010. www.telegraph.co.uk/technology/facebook/4405741/Excessive-chatting-on-Facebook-can-lead-to-depression-inteenage-girls.html.
87. Herr J. Internet entangles college students in a web of loneliness and depression. Truman State University Index. www.trumanindex.com/2.10111/internet-entangles-collegestudents-in-a-web-of-loneliness-an-ddepression-1.1462681. Accessed 27 Feb 2007.
88. Sturm S. Social networking psych studies:research shows teen Facebook users prone to depression. TrendHunter. www.trendhunter.com/trends/depressionfrom-facebook.
89. Pantic I, Damjanovic A, Todorovic J, et al. Association between online social networking and depression in high school students: behavioral physiology viewpoint. Psychiatr Danub. 2012;24:90–3.
90. Jelenchick LA, Eickhoff JC, Moreno MA. Facebook depression? Social networking site use and depression in older adolescents. J Adolesc Health. 2013;52:128–30.
91. van den Eijnden RJJM, Meerkerk GJ, Vermulst AA, Spijkerman R, Engels RCME. Online communication, compulsive internet use, and psychosocial well-being among adolescents: a longitudinal study. Dev Psychol. 2008;44(3):655–65.
92. Underwood MK, Ehrenreich SE, More D, Solis JS, Brinkley DY. The BlackBerry project: the hidden world of adolescents' text messaging and relations with internalizing symptoms. J Res Adolesc. 2015;25:101–17.
93. Ehrenreich SE, Underwood MK, Ackerman RA. Adolescents' text message communication and growth in antisocial behavior across the first year of high school. J Abnorm Child Psychol. 2014;42:251–64. https://doi.org/10.1007/s10802-013-9783-3.
94. Davila J, Hershenberg R, Feinstein BA, Gorman K, Bhatia V, Starr L. Frequency and quality of social networking experiences: associations with depressive symptoms, rumination, and co-rumination. Psychol Pop Media Cult. 2012;2(3):72–8. https://doi.org/10.1037/a0027512.
95. Richards D, Caldwell PH, Go H. Impact of social media on the health of children and young people. J Paediatr Child Health. 2015;51:1152–7.
96. Festinger L. A theory of social comparison processes. Hum Relat. 1954;7(2):117–40.
97. Suls J, Martin R, Wheeler L. Social comparison: why, with whom, and with what effect? Curr Dir Psychol Sci. 2002;11(5):159–63. https://doi.org/10.1111/1467-8721.00191.
98. Keefe K. Perceptions of normative social pressure and attitudes toward alcohol use: changes during adolescence. J Stud Alcohol. 1994;55(1):46–54.
99. Vogel EA, Rose JP, Okdie BM, Eckles K, Franz B. Who compares and despairs? The effect of social comparison orientation on social media use and its outcomes. Personal Individ Differ. 2015;86:249–56. https://doi.org/10.1016/j.paid.2015.06.026.
100. Feinstein BA, Hershenberg R, Bhatia V, Latack JA, Meuwly N, Davila J. Negative social comparison on Facebook and depressive symptoms: rumination as a mechanism. Psychol Pop Media Cult. 2013;2(3):161–70. https://doi.org/10.1037/a0033111.
101. Shaw AM, Timpano KR, Tran TB, Joormann J. Correlates of Facebook usage patterns: the relationship between passive Facebook use, social anxiety symptoms, and brooding. Comput Hum Behav. 2015;48:575–80. https://doi.org/10.1016/j.chb.2015.02.003.
102. Verduyn P, Lee DS, Park J, Shablack H, Orvell A, Bayer J, et al. Passive Facebook usage undermines affective well-being: experimental and longitudinal evidence. J Exp Psychol. 2015;144(2):480–8. https://doi.org/10.1037/xge0000057.
103. Lenhart A, Ling R, Campbell S, Purcell K. Teens and mobile phones. Washington, DC: Pew Research Center; 2010.
104. Livingstone S, Smith PK. Annual research review: harms experienced by child users of online and mobile technologies: the nature, prevalence, and management of sexual and aggressive risks in the digital age. J Child Psychol Psychiatry. 2014;55(6):635–54.
105. George MJ, Odgers CL. Seven fears and the science of how mobile technologies may be influencing adolescents in the digital age. Perspect Psychol Sci. 2015;10(6):832–51. https://doi.org/10.1177/1745691615596788.
106. Melville K. Facebook use associated with depression. Science A Go Go. 2010;3. www.scienceagogo.com/news/20100102231001data_trunc_sys.shtml.

6 Social Media Use and Display of Depressive Symptoms Online by Adolescents and Young Adults

Ana Radovic, Olga Santesteban-Echarri, Mario Álvarez-Jiménez, John Gleeson, Simon M. Rice, and Megan A. Moreno

Introduction

Although social media use among adolescents is ubiquitous, there is a scarcity of high-quality studies regarding usage patterns among adolescents with depression. Of the available studies, findings regarding the possible benefits and harms of social media on depression are inconsistent. Although there has been discussion in the lay public regarding a "Facebook depression" phenomenon, the evidence has been mixed as several studies have not found a direct association between social media use and adolescent depression [1–3]. Studies that have found an association have been cross-sectional in design, limiting interpretation of causality of social media use on depression [4]. Evidence is emerging that specific types of activity within Facebook or other social media and individual-specific psychological and/or personality characteristics, rather than social media use per se, determine positive or negative outcomes in relation to mood. We know adolescents use a variety of social media sites, with 71% using more than one site [5]; how, when, and how often they use each site is complex and ever-changing—but social media is a trend that is not going away. Examination of social media use in depressed adolescents through more nuanced studies which examine the type of use and use qualitative designs and actual observational data of social media displays to understand this relationship as well as use longitudinal design and measure baseline psychological/personality characteristics may improve our understanding. In the following chapter, we will use some of these types of findings to describe how adolescents who have depression use social media and specifically how they display their depressive symptoms online.

A. Radovic (✉)
University of Pittsburgh School of Medicine, Children's Hospital of Pittsburgh of UPMC, Pittsburgh, PA, USA
e-mail: ana.radovic@chp.edu

O. Santesteban-Echarri
Orygen, The National Centre of Excellence in Youth Mental Health, Melbourne, VIC, Australia

Centre for Youth Mental Health, The University of Melbourne, Melbourne, VIC, Australia

Department of Psychology, Universitat Rovira i Virgili, Tarragona, Spain
e-mail: olga.santesteban@orygen.org.au, olga.santesteban@gmail.com

M. Álvarez-Jiménez • S.M. Rice
Orygen, The National Centre of Excellence in Youth Mental Health, Melbourne, VIC, Australia

Centre for Youth Mental Health, The University of Melbourne, Melbourne, VIC, Australia
e-mail: Mario.Alvarez@orygen.org.au; simon.rice@orygen.org.au

J. Gleeson
School of Psychology, Australian Catholic University, Melbourne, VIC, Australia
e-mail: John.Gleeson@acu.edu.au

M.A. Moreno
Department of Pediatrics, University of Wisconsin-Madison, Madison, WI, USA
e-mail: mamoreno@pediatrics.wisc.edu

M.A. Moreno, A. Radovic (eds.), *Technology and Adolescent Mental Health*, https://doi.org/10.1007/978-3-319-69638-6_6

Case

A nurse practitioner (NP) is working in a primary care office where adolescent patients are regularly seen for yearly visits and acute care. She works closely with an integrated behavioral health team consisting of social workers and a psychologist. Her next patient is a 15-year-old girl named Ivy, and the reason for the visit is "mother has concerns." The NP walks in the room and sees that Ivy's mother is distraught. She says that she brought her in today because she is concerned that Ivy might have depression. Ivy's mother asks to talk to the NP alone first, so the NP introduces Ivy to the social worker, Carol, and lets her get a psychosocial history and conduct routine screening questionnaires while the NP speaks to Ivy's mother alone. Ivy's mother reports she noticed Ivy was being somewhat defiant—recently she found out she had skipped school to hang out with some new older friends who had recently graduated and she thinks they may be smoking marijuana together because she smelled it when washing Ivy's clothes. She is worried that Ivy's new friends are exposing her to risky behaviors, but for the most part Ivy is still doing well in school—and so she attributed these changes to normal adolescence. She recently attended an after-school presentation for parents called, "A close look at social media and what it is doing to your teen" and became concerned about some recent reports on the harms of social media. She decided to secretly look at Ivy's phone and check out her accounts. She was shocked when she saw that Ivy was following accounts on Instagram which used the hashtag #MySecretFamily. These accounts would show images of a hand with cut marks smoking a cigarette or a quote that said, "Mommy, Daddy, Don't you know? You lost Your daughter Years ago…." When she confronted Ivy, they got into a heated argument because Ivy was upset her mother had invaded her privacy. Ivy's mother took away her phone and is extremely upset. She says, "this social media stuff is making my daughter depressed! I hate it! Life was so much simpler when I was a kid." They were not able to get past their argument and so came in to the primary care clinic to get help with what to do now.

Overview of Negative and Positive Outcomes of Social Media Use on Depression

Negative Outcomes of Social Media Use on Depression

Due to concerns regarding the association of social media use and psychological distress, it is important to understand how adolescents with symptoms of depression use social media [4]. Although some studies show that adolescents with depression appear to use social media more than their non-depressed counterparts [4, 6, 7] (i.e., increased symptom severity correlates with frequency of Facebook posting [8]), this has not been corroborated in other studies [9]. Demographic factors, such as age, may moderate associations. The probability of an association between the amount of social media use and negative outcome is higher for young people (age = 18–23) relative to adult users [10], and younger relative to older adolescents [11].

A recent systematic review into social networking site (SNS) use examined 70 studies, with 24 studies exploring the relationship between SNS use and depression (across all age ranges) [12]. The majority of studies included in the review were youth specific (late teens or early 20s, as defined by the authors). Only eight were adolescent-specific studies [13–20]. Among these, four studies reported on time spent on social media. A study within a community sample (age = 12–17) [18] and a study with high school students (mean age = 18) [13] did not find a relationship between a number of SNS friends, time spent in SNS, SNS-related activities, and depression symptoms. Contrary to these results, two studies within a community sample (mean age = 18 [19] and 16.7 [20]) found a significant relation between time spent in SNS (the second specifically reporting on addictive Facebook use) and depressive symptoms. The reverse relationship has also been reported, where problematic Facebook use is also more prevalent among adolescents and young people (age = 12–25) with depressive traits [17]. These differences may be related to study design, measurement tools, and country of origin. Among youth-specific studies, and in terms of the language and activity from social media, youth with depressive symptoms were found to have less positive interactions and more negative interactions such as co-rumination [21–23]. A recent study focusing on the type of interactions on Facebook also highlighted that first year college students experiencing higher psychological distress had less satisfaction with the result of the interaction and the responses received from peers than their non-distressed counterparts [24].

Certain mediating factors have been found to be important in the association between depressive symptoms and social media use. Passive use of social media (i.e., reading posts without interacting actively) as compared to active use (i.e., image management such as maintaining a profile and commenting on friends' statuses) does not, in general, increase the probability of showing symptoms of depression [12], but a positive relationship between passive use and depressive symptoms is found in specific situations, for example, when experiencing feelings of "Facebook envy" or feeling discontented when viewing or reading about others' curated lives on social media. A study undertaken with a community sample of 1840 Flemish high school students (mean age = 15.4) is one of the only longitudinal studies to date in adolescents to shed light upon the relationship between negative Facebook experiences and depressive symptoms at two time points 6 months apart [4, 16]. This study found that although depressive symptoms at time 1 predicted negative Facebook experiences at time 2, the opposite was not true: negative Facebook experiences at time 1 did not predict depressive symptoms at time 2 at the 6-month time point. This would suggest that depressive symptoms may lead to negative experiences on Facebook but not vice versa. However, when friend support was taken into account, both relationships were found—but only for those with low friend support outside of social media use (i.e., in real life). In other words, those with depression were more vulnerable to experiencing negative experiences on Facebook, and for those who were more lonely, negative Facebook experiences were found to be related to subsequent increases in depressive symptoms. In those with low friend support, negative Facebook experiences at time 1 *predicted* depressive symptoms at time 2; but if social support was perceived when using social media, it protected adolescents (mean age = 14.76) from peer victimization (which was highly increased among adolescents with depressive symptoms) [15]. A cross-sectional study in Canadian high school students (mean age 15) also found the relationship between psychological distress and amount of social media use may be mediated by cybervictimization [25]. This literature suggests three different types of experiences based on baseline adolescent characteristics and experiences using social media: (1) adolescents with depressive symptoms at baseline may be more likely to experience negative social media experiences such as peer victimization; (2) adolescents who may or may not have depressive symptoms but who have low friend support outside of social media, and use social media sites to seek online friend support but instead experience peer victimization, may experience an increase in depressive symptoms as a result; and (3) adolescents who have depressive symptoms but have high friend support outside of social media may experience a buffering against the effects of online peer victimization or cybervictimization. A cross-sectional study in almost 500 Scottish adolescents (age = 11–15) found a positive association between social media use and poorer sleep quality, anxiety, and depression; this association was more pronounced for adolescents who had higher levels of emotional investment in social media (e.g., agree with items such as "I get upset when I can't log on to social media") [26]. Specifically, the type of emotional investment may be due to one's self-worth being contingent on external validation—or seeking approval from others; in young adults who sought this external validation, they were more likely to use Instagram, an image-sharing platform, more intensely and use it for social comparison [27]. Certain activities on Instagram have been associated with higher levels of loneliness including broadcasting or sharing information with a public audience as opposed to interaction (i.e., commenting) or browsing (i.e., looking at profiles) which was related to less loneliness [28]. These findings differed for those young people who hold a social comparison orientation—or a tendency to compare themselves with others and therefore experience low self-esteem—they do not experience the benefit of lower levels of loneliness when they interact with others online. While one study showed that using image-based platforms (e.g., Instagram) as opposed to text-based platforms (e.g., Twitter) is associated with a decrease in loneliness potentially due to more intimacy with relation to picture sharing [29], these associations may not apply to depressed adolescents, who may tend to have a social comparison orientation due to feelings of low self-worth.

Therefore, helping adolescents gain insight on and reflect on their purposes for using social media (e.g., is it to compare with others?), their activity on social media (e.g., is it broadcasting to anyone—a potential sign of loneliness—or a specific interaction with a peer), and their emotions after using social media may be beneficial. Also, ensuring that adolescents with depression are also establishing real-life meaningful social connections—and accessing online communities, which are oriented toward providing social support and moderated, and also being more authentic (representing themselves more accurately) online [30]—may be protective from negative social media experiences.

In general, compared to their counterparts without depression, adolescents with depression may be more likely to experience cyberbullying [31, 32] and online peer victimization [15] and display risky online behaviors (i.e., engaging in communication with strangers [7], self-disclosure activities like sharing personally identifiable information on the Internet, or sending and posting pictures of oneself [29]). These risks appear particularly pronounced for adolescents given they tend to have larger numbers of people within their online networks [7]. Davis' (2001) cognitive-behavioral model of problematic Internet use proposes that problematic use may result from a depressogenic cognitive style [33] as individuals exhibit their preexisting psychopathology on the Internet. This model stresses the role of cognitions as both preceding and being the main source of abnormal behavior, which develop and maintain problematic Internet use. From a diathesis-stress conceptualization (i.e., predisposed vulnerability—life event), psychopathology would be a necessary distal cause, while maladaptive cognitions are the proximal cause of problematic Internet use symptoms [33].

Cognitive Biases Exhibited on Social Media by Young People with Depression

In line with Davis' model of problematic Internet use, some studies have identified biases in how young people with depression may interpret their social media interactions. For instance, although studies show that depression is associated with less offline social support and less diverse social networks [34], others report a positive association of depression and social support from Facebook when users reveal negative information [35]. Park and colleagues described that both young people with depression symptoms (mean age = 19.8) and older youth (mean age = 26.75) with a major depressive disorder had the perception they were not receiving sufficient social support, regardless of the actual social support received. Also, young people with depression may interpret communications as more negative, irrespective of the communication content [35]. Another possible bias faced by depressed young people using social media is related to social comparison and the way they rate their profile. Young people with depression tend to feel more inferior, less attractive, and more envious when asked to compare their profile relative to others without depression [36] and as having lower social rank compared to students without depression [37]. Consequently, communication interpretation, perceived support, and perceived attractiveness may be biased among youth with depression. These specific cognitive biases and how to restructure them may be explored by practitioners when discussing social media use.

Benefits and Positive Outcomes of Social Media Use on Depression

Despite the risk behaviors previously mentioned (i.e., self-disclosure activities), social support could be a protective factor against peer victimization [15], especially if groups are peer-selected (compared to larger groups where user has less control) [38]. Social media use has been associated with life satisfaction and lower levels of loneliness, promotion of supportive relationships, increased self-esteem, facilitation of communication, and feelings of group membership among young people with depression [39, 40]. Public sites can be used as a place to share and develop their identity. For example, changing or updating their profiles and sharing pictures [41], and especially when receiving positive feedback from peers [42], resulted in improved self-esteem. Beneficial outcomes highlight the potential importance of social media use in ameliorating social withdrawal commonly experienced by adolescents with depression, especially those at elevated risk of social isolation [39].

Being able to correctly classify adolescents at risk may be particularly useful for suicide prevention, especially taking into account that more than 80% of adolescents have public social media accounts such as Facebook [43]. A recent systemic review examined the findings of 30 studies (across all age groups) targeting the use of social media for suicide prevention that reported largely positive findings [44]. Among those, there were only four adolescent-specific studies [45–48]. Results showed that adolescents use public social media to share suicidal ideation, behaviors, and intentions [47] and also join social media sites in order to help-seek. It seems that over time, help-seekers offer their help to other distressed adolescents creating a reciprocal suicide prevention community [48]. Moreover, among adolescents assessed in an emergency room for chief complaint of suicidality, the great majority sent a previous electronic communication of suicidality via an electronic tool (social media, text, or email), and among those, 67% did so to a peer [45]. Among youth-specific studies [44], results showed that social media enable difficult-to-engage youth to be reached, and posts reflecting suicidal ideation were easy to notice, highlighting that intervention and prevention are possible through this medium. Further, social media platforms were well accepted by young people as they felt they could share, anonymously, difficult experiences with others. Sites reviewed were usually moderated, although users reported a preference for obtaining peer support rather than having professional help. While informative, the studies included in this review were descriptive or cross-sectional, highlighting the need for well-designed controlled studies. Despite the positive results in the potential prevention of suicidality, additional research is required in order to overcome challenges such as risk assessment, privacy, confidentiality, and the probability of contagion.

Displays of Symptoms on Social Media

Display of Depressive Symptoms on Social Media by Adolescents

The diagnosis of depression is made more by a clinical interview requiring an adolescent to share their thoughts and emotions, and less so by observation of physical attributes—for example, psychomotor retardation. This requires an adolescent to be willing to share personal information about themselves. Obtaining this information from an adolescent may be difficult as they may be hesitant at being forthcoming due to self or social stigma or embarrassment. Also, placing their symptoms in a developmental context and ruling out other comorbidities can lead to diagnostic uncertainty. Research and professional experience with those individuals who work closely with adolescents as well as public displays on readily accessible social media sites have revealed trends in how adolescents display their depressive symptoms online. Studying these displays may help to understand more about how adolescents experience depression in the digital age, as well as the nuanced ways adolescents with depression use social media. It also may help parents understand more about their child's symptoms as well as assist therapists with material that they may use (with the adolescent's consent) to support the adolescent with cognitive restructuring. For example, an adolescent's thought, based on their social media wall, may be that all of their friends have more exciting social lives than they do. The therapist can help them restructure this thought by helping them conclude that due to impression management, much of social media displays may not reflect actual life experiences. The sections below will take a more focused look at how adolescents display their depressive symptoms as well as self-harm behavior online, using research, which has applied qualitative and quantitative methods.

Displays of Self-Harm

About 10% of adolescents report that they have self-harmed before [49]. This involves intentional poisoning or injury to oneself and does not take into account the reason for harm and whether or not it was of suicidal intent [49]. A systematic review by Dyson et al. examined studies on social media use to discuss and view deliberate self-harm acts [50]. Most of the 26 studies reviewed focused on 19–21-year-olds. While these studies found multiple benefits including providing encouragement and empathy, developing a strong sense of community and belonging, with some evidence of reduction in self-harm behaviors when using these sites [51, 52], they also found harms such as normalizing and accepting the self-harm behavior, live depictions of self-harm acts, and open discussion of triggers, concealment, and suicidal plans [50]. Depictions of self-harm are well represented on popular video-based social media sites such as YouTube [53] and may provide advice on how to self-harm "safely" [54]. An analysis of Twitter messages on the term "self-harm" revealed themes of celebrities such as Demi Lovato sharing their story of overcoming self-harm, frustration at those who make fun of self-harm, support to and from others, as well as self-harm's relationship to eating disorders and self-harm videos and personal stories [55]. Although self-harm is not always related to suicidality, relatedly, the popularity of using public websites to reveal suicidal thoughts and behaviors is concerning due to possibilities of suicidal contagion [56, 57]. While some social media sites have incorporated alerts in response to concerning searches, adolescents have responded by creating ambiguous hashtags, which can be difficult to stay up to date with [58]. A paper by one of the co-authors, Moreno et al., included an algorithm that could be used by parents or providers to understand hashtag terms related to self-harm [58]. For example, the term #blithe (defined on urbandictionary.com to be used for "appearing to have a detached, yet cheerful, disposition") was found to be a keyword for self-harm, and a process is described in how to determine that by cross-referencing searches online. This study also found a popular image on social media called "My Secret Family" which details nicknames/hashtags commonly used to represent underlying mental health conditions including self-harm. This is recreated as Fig. 6.1.

It is important for providers to query adolescents about their use of these sites and discuss the consequences of interacting with triggering content

Repost if you battle with any of these and put the name in your profile

Disorder	Girls	Boys
Anorexia	Ana	Rex
Bulimia	Mia	Bill
Paranoia	Perry	Pat
Anxiety	Annie	Max
ADD/ADHD	Addie	Andy
OCD	Olive	Owen
Borderline	Bella	Ben
Bipolar	Bri	Bob
Schizophrenia	Sophie	Skip
Insomnia	Izzy	Isaiah
EDNOS	Ellie	Ed
Self Harm	Cat	Sam
Depression	Deb	Dan
Suicidal	Sue	Dallas

Fig. 6.1 #MySecretFamily

such as self-harm videos and how this can get in the way of their improvement. For example, as in the case, the nurse practitioner may ask Ivy regarding what social media sites she regularly uses, what her main purposes are for using these sites, whether she finds helpful content related to her mood, and whether she finds unhelpful content related to her mood. It may help to discuss specific times she has interacted with unhelpful content and use a mood journal to keep track of how she feels after using social media and what aspects make her feel better and what aspects make her feel worse. Is she triggered to self-harm when she views an image of self-harm? Can she cut down on these feelings by spending less time on social media, only doing things she knows have made her feel more positive in the past (e.g., following an inspirational person or directly communicating online with a close, supportive friend)?

Qualitative Outcomes of Social Media Use by Adolescents with Depression

Qualitative analysis is also necessary to meaningfully understand dynamics of social media use, engagement, subjective user experiences, and perceived benefits by specific populations. Qualitative research on the use of social media by adolescents diagnosed with depression has found that adolescents with depression use social media similarly (i.e., for social connection, seeking information, as an entertainment, a way to share their creative work) and also face similar negative outcomes (i.e., cyberbullying and feeling distressed due to social comparisons) relative to other adolescents [59]. Importantly, depression severity in some may trigger elevated social media use as a coping mechanism, where the adolescents seek to improve their mood, but how they use it may affect whether in fact their mood improves or not. Social media use patterns and purposes may also differ by type of site. In cases where use of social media sites was anonymous, adolescents with depression felt comfortable to share personal information regarding their mood and tended to create a network of people with a similar background facing similar difficulties [59]. A site which is mainly anonymous and used often by the depression community is Tumblr, which can be used for sharing text, images, video, and longer posts or blogs. A study by Cavazos-Rehg reviewed 17 popular depression-related Tumblr accounts held by mainly 14–20-year-olds and found major themes of self-loathing, loneliness and feeling unloved, self-harm, and suicide [60]. Out of 200 random posts, 18% showed graphic images and video clips with some posts glorifying dangerous behaviors. Although having potential to be harmful, these sites held a large online audience and also displayed some comforting messages of support and prevention.

In a study by one of the co-authors, Radovic et al., a group of 23 adolescents (mean age 16, range 13–20) currently in treatment for depression were interviewed about their current and past social media use [59]. These adolescents were also asked whether they change their social media use in response to a depressed mood. Some adolescents reported using social media less while others reported using it more. For those who used social media more, this would be in the hope to access social support to share their emotions and access online content (i.e., humorous media, inspirational quotes) to boost their mood. This is consistent with studies reporting that depression is related to lower levels of internal self-regulation, with social media use being used as a regulatory coping mechanism [61]. Radovic and colleagues found adolescents with depression described one of three types of posts that may be problematic: (1) *stressed posting* (sharing negative posts), as a way of venting their feelings and indirectly seeking social support; these types of posts could lead to a negative consequence if no one were to respond; (2) *oversharing* (posting excessively or sharing personal information such as mundane or private details) increasing the probability of misinterpretation and misuse of the posts by third parties such as leading to negative peer feedback; and (3) *viewing triggering posts* (posts generating a negative emotional response due to the reactivation of a traumatic experience related to the content of the post) (Table 6.1) [59].

As shown in Table 6.1, adolescents identified that they may self-disclose in order to enhance intimacy and satisfaction with others [62] and to find social support [63]. However, if self-disclosure is used excessively, or in the wrong contexts

Table 6.1 Adolescent descriptions of and opinions on specific negative experiences when using social media ($N = 23$)

Major category theme and example quote	Adolescent opinion on theme
Oversharing "Like however you're feeling like in that day or in that moment. Like if you're listening to like a good song and you like this one specific part of the song, you can put, like you tweet like those lyrics. Or if you're having like a really good day, just say, like, 'I had a really good day!' So yeah."—ID 1 "I literally will walk around, take a picture, and post it. Literally, I don't care what it is. I know my last picture that I posted on Instagram, I think, pretty sure it was one of my band t-shirts. Like literally, like, I'll take a picture of my band t-shirt, and I'll put it on Instagram. I'll be like, 'look at the new shirt I got.'"—ID 3 "I have two very close friends, female, both 18, and they'll take like these dumb like sink pictures, trying to make their butt look big and post those online. And I'm like, 'you know, like, I don't even have an Instagram. I don't have anything, and I can type in your name and see that because your page is public,' and they just don't care. They won't make it private."—ID 5	**Turns into gossip:** "Because once you let it out of your mouth, it'll travel and travel into stories and stories and no one will know the whole truth."—ID 15 **To get attention, increase self-esteem:** "I think maybe just for the attention. Even if it's negative attention, it's still attention. Like my one friend who I was talking about who was being bullied through online outlets and in school, when they put her on that website, she didn't even try very hard to get it taken down—some of the comments were like, 'nice ass,' whatever. Those boosted her ego, and she's kind of a narcissistic person, so I think that's why she left it up."—ID 5 **Annoyance:** *Interviewer:* "What do you think about that, you were just rolling your eyes?" "I feel like why does the whole world need to know your business? Like, why do I care if you went…if you went and got a bucket of fried chicken."—ID 8 "People use it as, like, publicity, like, and try to become, like, Facebook famous. And then complain about, if there's, like pictures of themselves like half-naked, and like, complain that people only like them for their body and want them for sex. So it just gets kind of annoying after a while."—ID 6
Stressed Posting "If I would to post, 'this is the worst day ever.' And then they would tweet at me and say, 'are you okay? Text me if you need anything.'"—ID 1 "There's this one kid and he always used to post like, 'I hate my life and I should just end things now.' And, like things like, 'I'm going to hell,' or, just really negative, scary things."—ID 26	**Emotional relief, seek social support:** "Yeah. I feel like it does. I don't know if it helps me like just get the weight off my shoulders because I've been thinking about it all day, and then just posting that. I don't know. Made you feel relieved. Because I know that my friends do see it. So then, like they all have one. So by them seeing that, then maybe they'll all talk to me."—ID 1 **Analyze thoughts:** "You might, in your head it might be way out of proportion to what actually happened. And it'll make you realize that it's not actually that bad. And I can, like you can analyze what you're feeling or whatever it is if you read it over when you're all out. "– ID 4
Triggering Material "I follow this account on Instagram, and it's a band account, and one day the girl took a picture of her arm, and it was all sliced, and there was blood down it, down her arm. And it just hurt me so bad. I was like, 'how could you post something like that?'"—ID 12	**Causes distress:** "They have the whole hashtags, #selfharm, #depression, and I mean like I've came across pictures, and I'll literally go to that person and I'll hit, 'Unfollow and block,' because I don't want to see pictures like that. Because it honestly makes me extremely upset that I have to see pictures like that."—ID 3

or without receiving the expected reward from the audience, adolescents may feel worse [59]. In contrast, other adolescents appear to be aware of their vulnerability when experiencing low mood and avoided social media due to the possibility of encountering triggering information (i.e., suicidal ideation or self-harm) or in order to avoid feeling socially excluded. Some studies conceptualize the negative association between depression and social media use as reflecting the social withdrawal feature of depression [64]. Nevertheless, in Radovic and colleagues' study, adolescents reported the use of social media changed as they matured and underwent treatment, and the experience of negative outcomes when using social media (i.e., cyberbullying, harassment) contributed to a change in their social media use (i.e., blocking or deleting unsporting users or the entire social media account) (Table 6.2) [59].

Table 6.2 Adolescents used social media in a more positive way after time, experience, and treatment for depression

Major category theme	Discontinued behavior	New behavior	Example quote
Risky online behavior	Posting about risky behavior (e.g., smoking, drinking, drugs, promiscuity, online arguing, gossip)	Knowing there will be consequences to negative online behavior	"So there was definitely negative consequences. And I was just trying to imagine, like if my dad read all my Facebook messages, I don't know what I'd do. Like I have them going back to when I was like 13. Like there were definitely some stuff on there that he would not be happy about *Interviewer: What kind of stuff would that be?* Just dumb decisions that I used to make. Stuff with guys or stuff with friends that I shouldn't have been doing and have outgrown by now. I guess maybe some drug and alcohol use and self-medicating. Things he definitely would not appreciate reading from guys."—ID 5
Interactions with strangers and acquaintances	Talking to strangers Accepting everyone who asks for a request to be a friend	Using only to connect with and get feedback from close friends and family Deleting unsupportive friends and bullies	"I just recently unfollowed them because I'm following people that don't even talk to me anymore, and seeing their photos just kind of makes me upset, so I'm like why am I following this person, and seeing their photos, and it just makes me upset? Since I basically just unfollowed these people I haven't really had any negatives since."—ID 28 "A few years ago, I would just add anyone. And then I was like, I've gone through that phase after that where I'm like, I don't know you so I'm not going to add you. So, I mean, I say every day, well I need to go through all my friends and delete people I don't know. But, there's just so many now. It might just be better to delete your Facebook andrestarteverything. Yeah."—ID 26

(continued)

Table 6.2 (continued)

Major category theme	Discontinued behavior	New behavior	Example quote
Privacy	"Oversharing"—Posting personal information	Increasing privacy settings and threshold for sharing personal information	"Well, I started, like whenever I start looking at other people and if they'll post personal stuff, I think, 'why would they do that?' I mean, I can see that. Anyone can see that. And then I'm like, 'well, I did that. Why would I do that?' And I think I matured a little bit. From last year to now. And I started thinking a little more clear. So I realized having social media, it can be fun, but you have to be very responsible with it or it can end very badly" "I was going through Tumblr, and I saw, I would post really stupid things. I was like, 'okay, I got to get rid of this. This is nobody else's business.'"—ID 12 "There's no point in putting all my business out there because either people just judge, or they'll just have something negative to say about it. So I don't want to do that anymore. I realize I need to be more careful with what info I send out to people."—ID 15
Using social media when in a low mood	"Stressed posting"—Posting about being in a low mood Using social media when upset	Taking breaks from using social media when it makes one feel worse or a conflict is starting	"When I'm sad, the last thing I need to know is how much fun other people are having or how great other people are having it. Or other people's situations. That doesn't really help my own mood. And it's mostly a waste of time. I mean I'm still—I'm still getting past that. Like sometimes I still go on twitter when I'm upset because I just want to see what's going on, but mostly I just get jealous of other people's lives."—ID 14 "If I do see something on it that will make me upset, I'll just exit out and avoid it for like an hour or two of the day, and then I'll go back on and be whatever about it. That's just how I do it."—ID 28

Table 6.2 (continued)

Major category theme	Discontinued behavior	New behavior	Example quote
Social media for self-esteem	Posting with the purpose to increase self-esteem Placing importance on number of friends or followers	Using with the goal of connecting with others versus getting approval	"Back then, Facebook just came out, and it was cool to have 700 friends. And I think the idea was just see how many people you can get to comment on things, see how many people you can get to like on something. I just feel like it's a really warped view once you start thinking about things in that kind of perspective. And now I don't really care what strangers' opinions are on my pictures. I really just care what my friends and family have to say."—ID 5 "It's just another way to connect with friends and family now. Versus this way to like kind of control your self-esteem and make yourself feel better."—ID 5
Responding to negative online interactions	Reacting to negative comments, starting fights	Using coping skills to control getting upset at a mean comment Speaking up for self if something bothers them—Being assertive	"I used to use it differently like basically I used to even, I would you know start fights and you know try to like post provocative photos. And like, I guess it affected me more. And I realized all I have to do now in my life is all I have to do is delete those people, block them, and they're out of my life, instead of seeing them, annoying me and ticking me off by their statuses every day on Facebook, I can just delete them, like it's that simple. And I guess it just affected me more like mentally, and emotionally. But I guess since I'm older now and I know better, I know how to handle it more, I can just say no, and ignore them, you know what I mean? I guess that's how I used to use it differently."—ID 28

The reflections that these adolescents had regarding changes in their social media use may offer some techniques that practitioners can use when discussing more positive social media use with depressed adolescents and which can be incorporated into future testable interventions (Table 6.3).

Table 6.3 Potential TIPS to provide adolescents with depression on social media use

Risky online behavior	Reflect on how others posting about risky behavior (e.g., drinking, gossip) may result in consequences for them *Tip*: **Before you post, think about what grandma would think if she saw it**
Interactions with strangers/acquaintances	Consider consequences to having online interactions with those you are not close to (e.g., unwanted stress from viewing an annoying or upsetting post) *Tip*: **Be picky with your online friends or who you follow. Weed out your "friend list" from everyone who is not actually a friend or modify settings to view less of their posts**
Privacy	When you share, do you think about who will see what you post? What types of consequences can occur if your privacy settings are too low? *Tip*: **Know and set your privacy settings, know who will see what you post**
Using social media when in a bad mood	Think about whether social media use helps your mood? If it does—does it depend on how you use it? For example, sending a private message helps but posting a status update doesn't? *Tip*: **Use social media to connect with people you know are there for you. Don't use it to get approval or compare yourself with others, especially when you are feeling lonely or in a low mood**
Negative people and comments	Online fights are not worth your time. When have you seen something good come out of one *Tip*: **Ignore or delete negative people, and stand up for yourself without being negative too. Screenshot cyberbullying and get help from a trusted adult**
Most importantly: **If it makes you feel worse, take a break. If it makes you feel better, remember what it was you did and why you felt better. Try your best to tailor your social media use to work best for you**	

Quantitative Outcomes of Social Media Use by Adolescents with Depression

In one previous study of college students, 25% of Facebook profiles disclosed one or more depressive symptoms that were consistent with *Diagnostic and Statistical Manual of Mental Disorders IV* (DSM-IV) criteria on status updates [63]. Participants who displayed depression symptoms were more likely to have updated their Facebook profile more recently, to be more senior in college, and to have received a response to a previous depression display on Facebook. This suggests that those who receive reinforcement to a depression disclosure from their online friends may be more likely to discuss their depressive symptoms publicly on Facebook. Another study found that those who displayed depression symptoms on Facebook were more likely to score in the depression range on the Patient Health Questionnaire (PHQ-9), particularly in the mild depression category [65].

Why might adolescents display feelings of depression in such a public online venue? Previous work illustrates that online interactions elicit higher levels of self-disclosure and uninhibited personal expression compared to offline interactions [66–68]. Adolescents report that they often disclose more about themselves on social networking sites than they do in person [69]. Further, the social risk hypothesis suggests that humans try to minimize social risks in order to maintain ties to a group. It has been posited that people with depression will change their behaviors to make "safer" social decisions in order to avoid social failures [70], and they may feel that using social media to share their depressive symptoms may be safer, although this might not actually be the case. Thus, social media may present a venue to those with depression that feels safer for expressing emotion during periods of isolation.

What Can Parents or Providers Do When They See Depression Disclosed on Social Media?

When a parent or provider notices a display on a social media site that suggests depression, it can be challenging to figure out how or whether to approach that young person. A previous study investigated who and how adolescents (mean age = 18.5) would want this communication to happen [71]. Almost all (93%) participants indicated that they would want a familiar adult, such as a parent or trusted role model, to approach them in response to a depression reference. The communication approach that was preferred was in person or by phone. And it was clear that participants wanted people to approach them by asking questions, even as simple as "I saw your post on Facebook, are you ok?" compared to making clinical judgments based on a social media post. Considering the sensitive nature of depression, it may be unsurprising that face-to-face communication from a trusted individual—friend or teacher—was preferred. These results underscore the point that online social environments are not viewed by young adults as a replacement for traditional, in-person interactions [72]. The study findings also suggest that communication about social media posts can be approached similar to many other clinical topics, by asking open-ended and nonjudgmental questions and following the patient's lead.

Case Continued

The nurse practitioner (NP) brings Ivy's mother back into the room. She discusses in private with the social worker, who has found that Ivy has screened positive for depression. While Ivy has had some thoughts of self-harm, she has not yet acted on these thoughts. Ivy disclosed some recent passive suicidal thoughts. The NP speaks to Ivy alone who states that she has been feeling depressed for some time now, and feels because she does well in school, no one really understands how she feels. Recently she started following depression accounts on Instagram and Tumblr, which she says make her feel better because "these people understand." She does recognize that her urge to self-harm became stronger when she recently viewed a self-harm video. The NP then meets with Ivy and her mother and proposes a treatment plan for depression and self-harm. The NP explains to Ivy's mother that depression is a complex illness and there are multiple factors involved in why some adolescents experience it. The NP discusses that there are some ways that social media can be helpful, and other ways it can be harmful, but part of the goal of therapy will be to address social media use and discover the impact of certain types of social media use on her symptoms and well-being. Ivy's mother still states she will take away Ivy's phone. The NP explains that an alternative strategy could be to help Ivy self-regulate her use, given the pervasiveness of social media and the possibility that adaptive use might assist in her recovery. After several therapy sessions, at which some time is dedicated to Ivy's social media use, Ivy's mother decides she will give the phone back on condition that Ivy is open about talking with her therapist or mother if her social media use starts to impact her mood or functioning.

Summary

In summary, the interplay between social media use and depressive symptoms is a complex one. Multiple factors including an individual's underlying personality traits, tendencies for social comparison, sense of loneliness, and the types of interactions they have with social media such as intensity of use, valance of interactions with others versus broadcasting updates to a wide audience, may affect potential emotional consequences experienced from its use. As we continue to learn more about social media use in depressed adolescents and young adults, we can learn something from them and the way they display their symptoms online. These displays can be used as a point of discussion with which to engage adolescents and young people to share their inner world, and how their social media use may be managed so that they experience less harm and greater benefit.

References

1. Jelenchick LA, Eickhoff JC, Moreno MA. Facebook depression? Social networking site use and depression in older adolescents. J Adolesc Health. 2013; 52:128–30.
2. Primack BA, et al. Using ecological momentary assessment to determine media use by individuals with and without major depressive disorder. Arch Pediatr Adolesc Med. 2011;165(4):360–5.
3. Selfhout MHW, et al. Different types of internet use, depression, and social anxiety: the role of perceived friendship quality. J Adolesc. 2009;32(4):819–33.
4. Sampasa-Kanyinga H, Lewis RF. Frequent use of social networking sites is associated with poor psychological functioning among children and adolescents. Cyberpsychol Behav Soc Netw. 2015;18(7):380–5.
5. Lenhart A. Teen, social media and technology overview 2015. Washington, DC: Pew Research Center; 2015.
6. Shaw AM, et al. Correlates of Facebook usage patterns: the relationship between passive Facebook use, social anxiety symptoms, and brooding. Comput Hum Behav. 2015;48:575–80.
7. Ybarra ML, Alexander C, Mitchell KJ. Depressive symptomatology, youth internet use, and online interactions: a national survey. J Adolesc Health. 2005;36:9–18.
8. Steers M-LN, Wickham RE, Acitelli LK. Seeing everyone else's highlight reels: how Facebook usage is linked to depressive symptoms. J Soc Clin Psychol. 2014;33:701–31.
9. van den Eijnden RJJM, et al. Online communication, compulsive internet use, and psychosocial well-being among adolescents: a longitudinal study. Dev Psychol. 2008;44:655–65.
10. Lin LY, et al. Association between social media use and depression among U.S. young adults. Depress Anxiety. 2016;33(4):323–31.
11. Tsitsika AK, et al. Online social networking in adolescence: patterns of use in six European countries and links with psychosocial functioning. J Adolesc Health. 2014;55(1):141–7.
12. Seabrook EM, Kern ML, Rickard NS. Social networking sites, depression, and anxiety: a systematic review. JMIR Mental Health. 2016;3:e50.
13. Banjanin N, et al. Relationship between internet use and depression: focus on physiological mood oscillations, social networking and online addictive behavior. Comput Hum Behav. 2015;43:308–12.
14. Dumitrache SD, Mitrofan L, Petrov Z. Self-image and depressive tendencies among adolescent Facebook users. Revista de Psihologie. 2012;58:285–95.
15. Frison E, Subrahmanyam K, Eggermont S. The short-term longitudinal and reciprocal relations between peer victimization on Facebook and Adolescents' well-being. J Youth Adolesc. 2016;45(9):1755–71.
16. Frison E, Eggermont S. The impact of daily stress on adolescents' depressed mood: the role of social support seeking through Facebook. Comput Hum Behav. 2015;44:315–25.
17. Moreau A, et al. Psychopathological profiles of adolescent and young adult problematic Facebook users. Comput Hum Behav. 2015;44:64–9.
18. Morin-Major JK, et al. Facebook behaviors associated with diurnal cortisol in adolescents: is befriending stressful? Psychoneuroendocrinology. 2016;63:238–46.
19. Pantic I, et al. Association between online social networking and depression in high school students: behavioral physiology viewpoint. Psychiatr Danub. 2012;24:90–3.
20. Hanprathet N, et al. Facebook addiction and its relationship with mental health among Thai high scool students. J Med Assoc Thail. 2015;98:81–90.
21. Davila J, et al. Frequency and quality of social networking among young adults: associations with depressive symptoms, rumination, and corumination. Psychol Popular Media Culture. 2012;1:72–86.
22. Feinstein BA, et al. Another venue for problematic interpersonal behavior: the effects of depressive and anxious symptoms on social networking experiences. J Soc Clin Psychol. 2012;31:356–82.
23. Moberg FB, Anestis MD. A preliminary examination of the relationship between social networking interactions, internet use, and thwarted belongingness. Crisis. 2015;36:187–93.
24. Bazarova NN, et al. Psychological distress and emotional expression on Facebook. Cyberpsychol Behav Soc Netw. 2017;20(3):157–63.
25. Sampasa-Kanyinga H, Hamilton HA. Social networking sites and mental health problems in adolescents: the mediating role of cyberbullying victimization. Eur Psychiatry. 2015;30(8):1021–7.
26. Woods HC, Scott H. #Sleepyteens: social media use in adolescence is associated with poor sleep quality, anxiety, depression and low self-esteem. J Adolesc. 2016;51:41–9.
27. Stapleton P, Luiz G, Chatwin H. Generation validation: the role of social comparison in use of Instagram among emerging adults. Cyberpsychol Behav Soc Netw. 2017;20(3):142–9.
28. Yang C. Instagram use, loneliness, and social comparison orientation: interact and browse on social media, but don't compare. Cyberpsychol Behav Soc Netw. 2016;19(12):703–8.
29. Alvarez-Jimenez M, et al. Online social media: new data, new horizons in psychosis treatment. Schizophr Res. 2015;166:345–6.
30. Grieve R, Watkinson J. The psychological benefits of being authentic on Facebook. Cyberpsychol Behav Soc Netw. 2016;19(7):420–5.
31. Rose CA, Tynes BM. Longitudinal associations between cybervictimization and mental health among U.S. adolescents. J Adolesc Health. 2015;57:305–12.
32. Gámez-Guadix M, et al. Longitudinal and reciprocal relations of cyberbullying with depression, substance use, and problematic internet use among adolescents. J Adolesc Health. 2013;53(4):446–52.

33. Davis RA. Cognitive-behavioral model of pathological internet use. Comput Hum Behav. 2001;17:187–95.
34. Homan CM, et al. Social structure and depression in TrevorSpace. In: 17th ACM Conference on Computer Supported Cooperative Work and Social Computing. 2014. Baltimore, MD, p 615–624.
35. Park J, et al. When perceptions defy reality: the relationships between depression and actual and perceived Facebook social support. J Affect Disord. 2016;200:37–44.
36. Appel H, Crusius J, Gerlach AL. Social comparison, envy, and depression on Facebook: a study looking at the effects of high comparison standards on depressed individuals. J Soc Clin Psychol. 2015;34:277–89.
37. Gilbert P. The relationship of shame, social anxiety and depression: the role of the evaluation of social rank. Clin Psychol Psychother. 2000;7(3):174–89.
38. Takahashi Y, et al. Potential benefits and harms of a peer support social network service on the internet for people with depressive tendencies: qualitative content analysis and social network analysis. J Med Internet Res. 2009;11(3):e29.
39. Collin P, et al. Literature review: the benefits of social networking services. Melbourne, VIC: CRC for Young People, Technology and Well being; 2011.
40. O'Keeffe GS, Clarke-Pearson K. The impact of social media on children, adolescents, and families. Pediatrics. 2011;127:800–4.
41. Gonzales AL, Hancock JT. Mirror, mirror on my Facebook wall: effects of exposure to facebook on self-esteem. Cyberpsychol Behav Soc Netw. 2011;14:79–83.
42. Moreno MA, Kolb J. Social networking sites and adolescent health. Pediatr Clin N Am. 2012;59:601–12.
43. Lenhart A. Teens, social media and technology overview 2015: smartphones facilitate shifts in communication landscape for teens. Washington, DC: Pew Research Center; 2015. p. 1–47.
44. Robinson J, et al. Social media and suicide prevention: a systematic review. Early Interv Psychiatry. 2016;10:103–21.
45. Belfort EL, Mezzacappa E, Ginnis K. Similarities and differences among adolescents who communicate suicidality to others via electronic versus other means: a pilot study. Adolesc Psychiatry. 2012;2:258–62.
46. Silenzio VMB, et al. Connecting the invisible dots: reaching lesbian, gay, and bisexual adolescents and young adults at risk for suicide through online social networks. Soc Sci Med. 2009;69:469–74.
47. Cash SJ, et al. Adolescent suicide statements on MySpace. Cyberpsychol Behav Soc Netw. 2013;16:1–9.
48. Greidanus E, Everall RD. Helper therapy in an online suicide prevention community. Br J Guid Counc. 2010;38:191–204.
49. Hawton K, Saunders KE, O'Connor R. Self-harm and suicide in adolescents. Lancet. 2012;379:2373–82.
50. Dyson MP, et al. A systematic review of social media use to discuss and view deliberate self-harm acts. PLoS One. 2015;11(5):e0155813.
51. Barak A, Dolev-Cohen M. Does activity level in online support groups for distressed adolescents determine emotional relief. Couns Psychol Q. 2006;6(3):186–90.
52. Murray CD, Fox J. Do internet self-harm discussion groups alleviate or exacerbate self-harming behaviour? Aust e-J Adv Mental Health. 2006;5(3):1–9.
53. Duggan J, et al. An examination of the scope and nature of non-suicidal self-injury online activities: implications for school mental health professionals. Sch Ment Heal. 2012;4(1):56–67.
54. Smithson J, et al. Membership and boundary maintenance on an online self-harm forum. Qual Health Res. 2011;21(11):1567–75.
55. Hilton CE. Unveiling self-harm behaviour: what can social media site Twitter tell us about self-harm? A qualitative exploration. J Clin Nurs. 2016;26:1690–704.
56. Pirkis J, Norderntoft M. Media influences on suicide and attempted suicide. In: O'Connor R, Platt S, Gordon J, editors. International handbook of suicide prevention. New York: Wiley-Blackwell; 2011.
57. Cash SJ, et al. Adolescent suicide statements on MySpace. Cyberpsychol Behav Soc Netw. 2013;16(3):166–74.
58. Moreno MA, et al. Secret society 123: understanding the language of self-harm on Instagram. J Adolesc Health. 2016;58(1):78–84.
59. Radovic A, et al. Depressed adolescents' positive and negative use of social media. J Adolesc. 2017;55:5–15.
60. Cavazos-Rehg P, et al. An analysis of depression, self-harm, and suicidal ideation content on Tumblr. Crisis. 2017;38(1):44–52.
61. Wegmann E, Stodt B, Brand M. Addictive use of social networking sites can be explained by the interaction of internet use expectancies, internet literacy, and psychopathological symptoms. J Behav Addict. 2015;4:155–62.
62. Sprecher S, Hendrick SS. Self-disclosure in intimate relationships self–disclosure in intimate relationships: associations with individual and relationship characteristics over time. J Soc Clin Psychol. 2004;23:857–77.
63. Moreno MA, et al. Feeling bad on Facebook: depression disclosures by college students on a social networking site. Depress Anxiety. 2011;28:447–55.
64. Andreassen CS, et al. The relationship between addictive use of social media and video games and symptoms of psychiatric disorders: a large-scale cross-sectional study. Psychol Addict Behav. 2016;30:252–62.
65. Moreno MA, et al. A pilot evaluation of associations between displayed depression references on Facebook and self-reported depression using a clinical scale. J Behav Health Serv Res. 2012;39:295–304.
66. Walther JB, Parks MR. Cues filtered out, cues filtered in: computer mediated communication and relationships. In: Miller GR, editor. The handbook of interpersonal communication. Thousand Oaks: Sage; 2002. p. 529–63.

67. Wallace P, et al. A randomized controlled trial of an interactive web-based intervention for reducing alcohol consumption. J Telemed Telecare. 2006;12(Suppl 1):52–4.
68. Fleming PJ. Software and sympathy: therapeutic interaction with the computer. In: Fish SL, editor. Talking to strangers: mediated therapeutic communication. Norwood: Ablex; 1990. p. 170–83.
69. Christofides E, Muise A, Desmarais S. Information disclosure and control on Facebook: are they two sides of the same coin or two different processes? Cyberpsychol Behav. 2009;12(3):341–5.
70. Dawson DA, et al. Another look at heavy episodic drinking and alcohol use disorders among college and noncollege youth. J Stud Alcohol. 2004;65:477–88.
71. Whitehill JM, Brockman LN, Moreno MA. "Just talk to me": communicating with college students about depression disclosures on facebook. J Adolesc Health. 2013;52(1):122–7.
72. Kujath CL. Facebook and MySpace: complement or Substitute for Face-to-Face Interaction? CyberPsychol Behav Soc Netw. 2011;14(1/2):75–8.

7 Cyberbullying and Mental Health

Rajitha Kota and Ellen Selkie

What Is Cyberbullying?

Before smartphones took over the world, teenagers used to pass notes in class, notes that could have been confessions about their crushes, spilling secrets, creating gossip, or maybe just making after-school plans. Today, these things are done via text message or social media, but the content is still the same. Hearts can still be broken, secrets can still be spilled, gossip can spread faster and farther than wildfire, and relationships can be forged and broken. It's easy to imagine how these interactions could become harsh and cruel in "real life," and unsurprisingly, the same kind of thing happens online.

When someone thinks of "bullying," the images that come to mind might be of a big kid pushing a little kid down on the playground, a bully shaking a kid down for lunch money, or maybe even a fight breaking out at school. "Traditional" bullying often involves harassment, teasing, or forcing another person to do something and happens when the parties involved meet face-to-face in the schoolyard. It includes components of physical bullying (e.g., hitting, kicking), which is an aspect that makes it distinct from cyberbullying. Traditional bullying also includes relational (e.g., spreading rumors to damage a person's reputation) and verbal (e.g., name-calling) bullying. So then what is cyberbullying? Broadly, cyberbullying can be defined as "an aggressive, intentional act or behavior that is carried out by a group or individual, using electronic forms of contact, repeatedly against a target who cannot easily defend him or herself." [1] Electronic forms of contact include social media, like Facebook, Twitter, Snapchat, or Instagram, e-mail, text messaging, and even online gaming. Online harassment can include behaviors such as insults, impersonation, exclusion, spreading rumors, hacking, stealing personal information, unwanted sexual advances, and creating damaging websites to defame others [2, 3].

Traditional Bullying Compared with Cyberbullying

Cyberbullying can be just as harmful as traditional bullying. Traditional bullying often has a physical component to the harassment, but online bullying offers perpetrators the benefit of anonymity. Often, perpetrators will then act without much regard for consequences, and this reduces

R. Kota, M.D., M.P.H. (✉)
University of Wisconsin School of Medicine and Public Health, Madison, WI, USA
e-mail: rkota@wisc.edu; rajithakota@gmail.com

E. Selkie, M.D., M.P.H.
Division of Adolescent Medicine, Department of Pediatrics, University of Michigan, Ann Arbor, MI, USA

M.A. Moreno, A. Radovic (eds.), *Technology and Adolescent Mental Health*,
https://doi.org/10.1007/978-3-319-69638-6_7

guilt and accountability for their actions [4]. Traditional bullying also often occurs at a specific time and place, often at school. Targets of cyberbullying, however, potentially must deal with harassing behaviors anytime and anyplace. Even if offline, targets often worry about what is being posted without their knowledge, especially because information can be spread so quickly and widely. However, the Internet and social media are integral to many adolescents' social identity and daily lives—this makes it nearly impossible for most teens to "just log off."

Although there are distinct differences between traditional bullying and cyberbullying, the fact remains that many individuals may be targets of both. Bullying that begins in the schoolyard can extend to messages online and vice versa. The National Academies of Sciences, Engineering, and Medicine concluded that cyberbullying should be considered within the context of traditional bullying rather than viewing the two as separate entities [5]. This is an important concept to understand, because screening efforts and interventions are often geared at only one type of bullying when in reality, a more global approach has the highest yield for prevention.

Technology and Social Media Use

Technology use among adolescents is nearly ubiquitous. 92% of teenagers aged 13–17 go online at least once a day, with a smaller subset of 24% who say they are online "constantly." Almost three-quarters of teens have smartphones, and 71% use more than one social networking site [6]. In terms of social networking sites, Facebook remains the most popular, with 71% of teens using the site daily, although Instagram and Snapchat continue to rise in popularity with 52 and 41% of teens on these platforms, respectively [6]. For more detailed demographic information, please see Chap. 2 of this book.

As a result of this tremendous use, cyberbullying has been an increasingly prominent topic of conversation in the popular media. Some high-profile examples of teens being driven to self-harm or suicide after experiencing severe cyberbullying have also caught the media's attention in recent years, and multiple movies, books, and television shows featuring cyberbullying as a main theme have been created in the last decade. For example, the popular book series and TV show *Gossip Girl* features an anonymous poster who exposes the secrets of a group of friends via social media, and a made for TV movie, *Cyberbully*, depicted a teenage girl driven to depression and a suicide attempt due to extreme cyberbullying [7, 8].

Prevalence

Cyberbullying can occur across all age groups, starting when adolescents first start using the Internet and extending into college and even adulthood. Assessing the prevalence of cyberbullying is challenging as an operational definition of the term is lacking, as well as a standardized way to measure it. For instance, one study that defined cyberbullying as "mean things" or "anything that someone does that upsets or offends someone else" found that 72% of 12–17-year-olds reported being targets. In contrast, another study that surveyed 10–17-year-olds about cyberbullying by framing it as "making rude or nasty comments to someone on the Internet or using the Internet to harass or embarrass someone with whom [they were] mad" found the prevalence rate to be 7%. A review of cyberbullying literature investigating prevalence found similar results, stating that while there is a robust quantity of literature on the topic, there are inconsistencies in the quality of the studies and reported prevalence rates [9].

Roles in Bullying

The *bullying circle* is a concept developed by Dan Olweus, a leader in bullying prevention and intervention research (Fig. 7.1) [10]. While it was initially developed in the context of traditional bullying, many of the same principles can be applied to cyberbullying when examining the roles that different involved parties play. At the

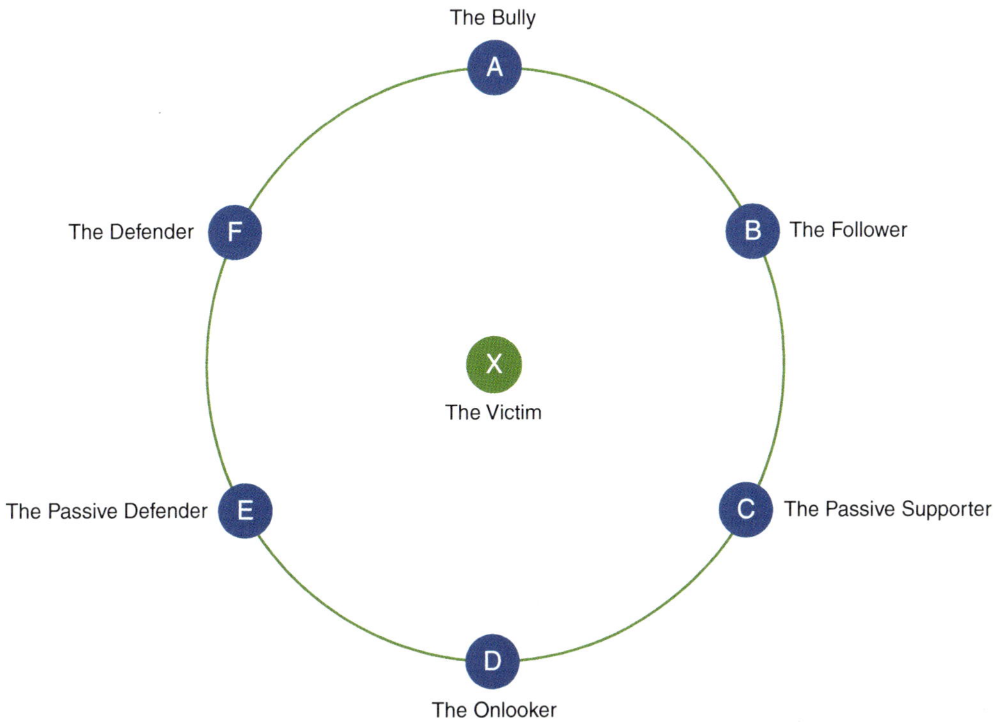

Fig. 7.1 The circle of bullying. Adapted courtesy of Olweus Bullying Prevention Program and Hazelden Publishing

center of the circle is the target or target of bullying (X). Surrounding the target are other potential roles that may be involved. The first (A) is the perpetrator, who directly engages with the target. In the context of cyberbullying, the perpetrator is the individual who texts, posts, or otherwise harasses the target on social media or some other electronic forms of contact. The second (B) are the followers of the perpetrator. In cyberbullying these individuals may become involved by distributing the perpetrator's messages or making further comments on the initial post. The third (C) are passive supporters of the perpetrator. An example of how they might get involved is by liking the perpetrator's post or otherwise engaging with it in some way that is on the side of the perpetrator. The fourth (D) are disengaged onlookers. These individuals might "scroll past" the instance of bullying without having one opinion or another in regard to the situation. The fifth (E) are passive defenders of the target. They may dislike the perpetrator and think they should defend the target but do not directly engage with the situation. In the context of cyberbullying, perhaps they would unfollow the perpetrator on social media. The sixth (F) are active defenders of the target, also known as positive bystanders. They directly engage with the perpetrator and defend the target, or they might engage with the target and offer support. On the Internet, this could involve making comments directly under the perpetrator's post or sending a positive message to the target. This framework places individuals in somewhat concrete roles but that is not to say that individuals cannot play multiple roles in the circle simultaneously, especially in cases when bullying occurs both online and offline. Adolescents may take on different roles in a situation when confronted with a situation in "real life" versus online or potentially even vacillate between defending the target and supporting the perpetrator depending on the context.

While the role of bystanders in traditional bullying has been extensively studied, less is known about bystanders of cyberbullying. Existing studies do suggest that many adolescents have witnessed cyberbullying and that many view these incidents passively without taking action [11]. One study among 12–15-year-olds found that adolescents may simultaneously play multiple roles in the "bullying circle." [12] Adolescents reported that they might support the perpetrator by liking a post but then comfort the target offline. They stated that possible ways to defend against a perpetrator would be to speak to them offline, asking the perpetrator for motives, providing comfort to the target, using humor to retaliate, or occasionally using physical retaliation. They also commented that defending the target forces them to risk themselves being bullied, but they were more likely to engage in the conflict if their friends were targets.

Cyberbullying Risk Factors

As with traditional bullying, participation in cyberbullying can be associated with certain risk factors. Perpetrators of cyberbullying have been shown to have lower empathy, increased conduct and hyperactivity problems, higher rates of substance use, and more antisocial tendencies compared to non-perpetrators [13]. Lack of social supports, as well as a negative view of school and learning, may also predispose an adolescent to become a cyberbullying perpetrator [14]. Interestingly, perpetrators are also more likely to have been targets; if a target has other characteristics such as low empathy or a high level of reactive aggression, they may turn their anger or fear onto others and thus become a perpetrator [15].

Adolescents who are targets of cyberbullying are more likely to be from families with other than their two biological parents; have psychosomatic problems such as headaches, sleeping difficulties, and abdominal pain; have high levels of perceived difficulties and peer problems; and may also feel unsafe at school and untrusting of teachers. They also have higher rates of mental health problems such as depression [16]. Remarkably, many of these risk factors also overlap with adolescents who act as bullies—namely, feeling unsafe at school, feeling uncared for by teachers, and having psychosomatic symptoms. A number of studies of Finnish adolescents have also found that those who engaged in bullying as both targets *and* bullies were the group most at risk for a wide range of psychiatric problems, crime, and even suicide [17–19].

Personality traits of bullying perpetrators and targets have also been well characterized. Three main personality traits, consisting of callous-unemotional traits, narcissism, and impulsivity, have been found to be associated with antisocial adolescents or adolescents with conduct problems including bullying [20]. Callous-unemotional traits are traits such as lack of remorse or guilt, lack of concern for others' feelings, and shallow emotions and have been found to be associated with adolescents who partake in traditional bullying [21]. A study done with Greek adolescents found that these traits are risk factors for cyberbullying, as well [22]. This is consistent with the idea that perpetrators often engage in behaviors because they lack concern for others' feelings or do not recognize it when they cause distress to others.

Mental Health Consequences of Cyberbullying

Cyberbullying can have significant psychological effects on both targets and bullies. Adolescent targets of cyberbullying have been found to have higher levels of depression and lower self-esteem [23]. The severity of depression in targets also seems to be associated with the severity of cyberbullying experienced [24]. Studies have also shown that cyberbullying is a predictor of suicide attempts in both targets and perpetrators, and being a member of either group is associated with increased suicidal ideation [25]. Higher rates of social anxiety have also been noted among individuals who have been targets of cyberbullying [26]. Further, emotional distress, anger, sadness, detachment, externalized hostility, and delinquency have been shown to be more common in targets of cyberbullying than in the general population [26]. Among perpetrators, factors such as headache, high levels of perceived difficulties, not feeling safe in school, behavior problems, hyperactivity, substance use, and reduced pro-social behavior have been shown to be more common [26].

Why can cyberbullying have such a powerful impact on mental health? Several explanations have been proposed. First, cyberbullying affords the perpetrator 24/7 access to the target, making it difficult for the target to find an escape. In the case of traditional bullying, the target may be able to find a safe place at home or at school [28]. In addition, in a digital setting, even if a target were to "log off," anxiety may still result since they may worry about continued harassment, i.e., through the perpetrator posting public, derogatory content about the target in the target's absence. Bullies may also attack their targets anonymously. This lack of face-to-face confrontation may cause some adolescents to engage in harmful behaviors that they would otherwise avoid—by not seeing their target's face and reactions in real time, it makes it easier to harass their target [28]. Supervision on electronic media is also generally lacking. Teachers or parents may intervene when bullying occurs in real life, but on social media, monitoring can be very difficult. In addition, younger adolescents may be more adept at using technology, which can result in a unique power differential between teachers or parents and the adolescent [29]. Finally, posting content on the Internet has the potential to very quickly reach a huge number of people. With traditional bullying, it is likely that the incident stays within a small group of people or, at the most, an entire school. With cyberbullying, any post can "go viral," and thus harmful content can rapidly spread [30, 31]. Depending on the nature of the cyberbullying attack—for example, when tactics result in widespread humiliation with a large viewing audience—targets may experience increased fear and decreased levels of trust for peers as well as other symptoms of post-traumatic stress disorder (PTSD) [32]. Targets may also fear for their physical safety as a result of cyberbullying, especially if the perpetrator is unknown or anonymous [16].

Academic Outcomes Related to Cyberbullying

Academic outcomes can be affected by cyberbullying, making it a priority for intervention in schools. Targets of both traditional bullying and cyberbullying are more likely to avoid attending school, have higher rates of truancy and absenteeism, say they dislike school, and even receive lower grades and standardized test scores [33, 34]. While cyberbullying has the potential to be anonymous, it may also occur between classmates; students may take their fights from the schoolyard online. This may cause the target's poorer concentration at school due to preoccupation and frustration, sadness, or anger with the perpetrator and the situation. Many targets also report that they do not feel safe at school [27, 35].

A Word About Sexting

Sexting is the act of sending, receiving, or forwarding sexually explicit messages or pictures over the Internet or a cell phone [36]. In most cases, these messages are meant to only be viewed by the intended recipient, usually a boyfriend or girlfriend that is also engaged with the sender in an offline relationship [37]. However, if these relationships turn sour, it is not difficult to imagine situations in which these images or messages may be distributed or used in ways to shame the sender. As a result, 21% of teens who have appeared in or created sexually explicit images report feeling extremely upset, embarrassed, or afraid, and up to 25% of youth who received the messages reported feeling this way [38].

Adolescents also use technology to flirt and express interest in a potential partner, with various levels of sexual suggestiveness [39]. About 14% of teens without dating experience have engaged in some sort of online sexual flirting behavior, while 63% of teens with offline dating experience have done this. This suggests that online sexual behavior is more likely to occur in those adolescents who are also engaging in sexual behavior in person. However, not all of these behaviors are appreciated or appropriate. In fact, 25% of all teens report having blocked or unfriended someone on social media who was sending them sexual messages or flirting in way that caused them discomfort. Teenage girls are twice as likely to experience this form of harassment as teenage boys [39].

Protective Factors

In order to be able to prevent cyberbullying, counsel adolescents who are both perpetrators and targets, and to gain a better understanding of the environments which might make cyberbullying more or less likely, it is important to characterize protective factors that prevent adolescents from developing these behaviors. Evidence suggests that a positive school climate and social support from friends are negatively related to both traditional and cyberbullying and may help prevent adolescents from being both perpetrators and targets [14, 40]. Adolescents who reported greater family support also reported fewer incidents involving cyberbullying both as perpetrators and targets [22]. Therefore, adolescents who do not have these protective factors in their lives may be more likely to engage in bullying or to be targeted and as such could potentially be screened for these behaviors when engaging with healthcare providers.

Cyberbullying Interventions

A number of interventions to combat cyberbullying have been proposed and trialed, with varying levels of success. Efforts include educational programs, antibullying websites, and distribution of information and resources to parents, teachers, and clinicians. However, researchers do not utilize a common definition of cyberbullying when conducting research, and the evidence base for developing an intervention specifically targeting cyberbullying is largely inadequate [2, 41]. However, research on traditional bullying may inform how to best develop interventions that also apply to cyberbullying [42]. Given that traditional bullying generally occurs at school, many effective bullying interventions favor a "whole school" approach that also addresses systemic factors on a wider scale. This is based on the idea that bullying is a systemic issue that is influenced by multiple factors such as the school environment as well as support of teachers, parents, and peers. Interventions include materials on improving awareness of bullying, discussing bullying in school as part of an evidence-based curriculum, and improving monitoring and supervision. Many states have laws mandating antibullying laws in schools, while individual school districts have the ability to implement specific programming to prevent bullying, support targets, and address consequences for perpetrators. Cyberbullying, however, may be more difficult to target in a school setting. Since many incidents occur outside of school property, it may not be within a school's jurisdiction to enforce rules against cyberbullying, even if incidents often occur between classmates from the same school [43]. However, research indicates that school climate and perception of teachers' ability to intervene in bullying can decrease rates of cyberbullying, so schools are still an important avenue to consider when designing interventions [44].

Most of the limited evaluations of school-based interventions on cyberbullying have been done in Europe. The ConRed program is one such school-based program that specifically addresses cyberbullying. It is a 3-month program with in-class activities and promotes collaboration between schools and communities. In Spain, it was shown to have a reduction in rates of both cyberbullying and victimization [45]. The 9-month KiVa program is another school-based antibullying curriculum that teaches students about conflict resolution, gives peers support tools, and encourages students to intervene if they see a classmate bullied. A study of the outcomes of this intervention showed that 4th–6th graders in the control group were on average 29% (5–57% at the 95% CI) more likely to be bullied than 4th–6th graders who went through the KiVa intervention [46]. The success of both of these interventions indicates that school climate is an important factor in influencing the rates of cyberbullying. Despite these successes, a review of existing cyberbullying prevention and intervention programs found mixed results in regard to the success of the programs, with only a little over half of the programs yielding positive results [41]. Given these results, it is clear that more research on cyberbullying interventions is needed.

Parents can also make an important contribution in cyberbullying prevention. Since cyberbullying can occur while an adolescent is at home, it is important to have parental involvement. Parents should discuss online etiquette with their children, starting as soon as the child begins using technology, and utilize negative incidents as teaching points. It should be emphasized that one should not say things online or via text message that they would not ordinarily say in person. One of the difficulties in involving parents is a difference in the knowledge base when using technology. Most adolescents are very proficient at using social media, have an understanding of "Internet culture," and may even have rewarding online relationships both with friends they have offline and friends they make online. However, some parents are not as well versed in these issues as their children, and thus it may be difficult to teach their children about subjects they themselves do not know much about. These issues can be mitigated by emphasizing that online interactions should mirror real-life ones and by questioning whether the content that they are posting or viewing would be appropriate in a face-to-face interaction. Parents should also feel free to ask their children to show them their social media accounts and teach them about the ways they communicate with peers in order to advance the parent's knowledge. Having open conversations about cyberbullying in a non-crisis situation is helpful, because another consideration when involving parents is the idea that some adolescents may not wish to report cyberbullying to their parents for fear of having technology taken away from them [47]. If an adolescent is forbidden from using social media or their cell phone, it can represent a cutoff from their social life and subsequently cause more harm than good. Creating an open atmosphere instead of a zero-tolerance policy is important for parents to keep in mind, as well as listening to their child's side of the story. Involving the child's school or law enforcement authorities should depend on the seriousness of the bullying, and in these instances, it can be helpful to capture screenshots of the incidents.

Strategies for Clinicians

In an era of ever-increasing technology use, it is critical for providers to be aware of the ways in which their patients are engaging with these forms of communication. The Internet is an extremely valuable tool, and there are many positive ways that adolescents use it, from homework to learning about current events and engaging in social justice, to creating supportive friendships, and to reinforcing their offline relationships. It may be tempting to write off adolescents' increasing use of social media and the Internet as a waste of time, but it is more important to remember that the way we communicate is simply changing. As a result, clinicians have the ability to ask their patients about the ways they are using these technologies and offer them advice about healthy and appropriate communication.

Anticipatory guidance about appropriate online conduct can begin as soon as the child begins interacting with online technology, and counseling parents about the risks *and* benefits of social media and Internet use can be done by the clinician. The Children's Online Privacy Protection Act prohibits websites from collecting information from children younger than 13 years without parental permission in the United States. As a result, the official terms of service for the majority of social media websites state that 13 is the minimum age to sign up for a site. However, it is not difficult for many children or even their parents to falsify a child's age in order to create a profile [36]. A recent survey in the United Kingdom showed that almost 50% of 10–12-year-olds have Facebook accounts, and 41% have an Instagram account—this information suggests that screening for social media use and cyberbullying could begin as early as age 10 [48].

Providers can implement screening for bullying and cyberbullying in the office as part of the social history. A discussion about general computer and Internet use could precede specifically asking about cyberbullying, and it is a good opportunity to educate children and their parents about healthy Internet use in general. A conversation about bullying and cyberbullying might include a provider saying, for example, "It's common for young people your age to see bullying or be involved in it. Some examples of bullying are when a person or group says mean things or spreads rumors about another person, hits or kicks them, threatens them, or excludes them from things (like not talking to them on purpose). A lot of times bullying happens frequently to the same person and can make people feel really bad. Have you ever seen that happen? Have you ever been part of bullying someone else, or have you been bullied?" When discussing cyberbullying, a provider could say, "Sometimes bullying also happens online and through social media. Do you have any experiences with this?" Should a patient endorse involvement in cyberbullying and/or traditional bullying either as a victim or perpetrator, providers should assess how the bullying has impacted the child's mood, physical well-being, as well as school attendance and performance. Assessing for mental health concerns including depression, anxiety, and suicidality in children involved in bullying is essential, as is referral to appropriate treatment such as psychotherapy.

The provider should be a trusted resource for both patients and parents, and part of being in such a role is to remain nonjudgmental and open to what their patients and parents tell them. It may be surprising to hear that a child or teen is disclosing information that seems very personal online, especially to people they may or may not know in real life, but these kinds of disclosures are becoming more commonplace. It is important to understand how these relationships affect youth and whether they are being safe in terms of the information they share, i.e., making sure not to reveal their address and other personal identifying information. Efforts should be made to advise patients about healthy and safe social media use instead of advising patients to stop using these websites. Information for providers, parents, and children and teenagers can be found on trusted resource websites such as commonsensemedia.com and stopbullying.gov and through the American Academy of Pediatrics (aap.org for providers and healthychildren.org for parents). These websites can help providers find handouts as well as bullying statistics, interventions, and information about leading these discussions with their patients.

It is important to keep in mind that for many children and young adults, "real life" does truly extend online; the opposite also holds true. For example, in some situations, it may even be appropriate for the clinician to reach out to their patient's school administrators to express concern about their patient's welfare and safety. Clinicians can also be important advocates in their communities by supporting the inclusion of cyberbullying in antibullying policies.

Case Example

Ally is a 14-year-old girl who recently started her first semester of high school. She comes in accompanied by her mother for an annual physical. Ally's mother does not have any health concerns regarding her daughter, but she does remark that her grades seem to be worse than when she was in middle school; Ally simply shrugs noncommittally. When her mom steps out of the room, Ally remains somewhat aloof but cooperates and answers questions when typical social history questions are asked. When she is asked how school is going and how her grades are, she becomes very quiet and finally says, "not great." She tearfully reveals that she is very distracted, depressed, and anxious because she is being verbally bullied by a group of older girls at school and mentions that the attacks continue when she gets home, on her Facebook page. She does not have any friends at school that she can confide in or get support from, and she has been feeling very lonely and isolated since school started. She has not told her parents or any adults because she fears she will draw undue attention to herself at school. Ally explains that she does have some close online friends that offer her support and a safe space to share her feelings on the Internet and is worried that any adult authority figures will simply tell her to delete her social media accounts.

What Can the Provider Do?

First, it is important to ensure Ally's physical safety. Is she being harmed physically at school? She endorses depression—does she have any suicidal ideation or has she tried to harm herself in any way? After her physical safety is ensured, the provider should address Ally's mental health concerns—namely, her depression and anxiety, which are leading to poor academic outcomes. If time is limited, it may be beneficial to have Ally come in for a follow-up appointment to discuss these matters further. Referral to a therapist or psychiatrist may be appropriate to help the patient explore further how she is feeling, build coping skills, and determine the best course of action. Communication with Ally's school may be needed if she and her parents feel that nothing is being done to address the problem. Most states have laws requiring schools to have antibullying policies. If a provider reaches out to the school to discuss health concerns related to a student's involvement in bullying, it calls attention to the seriousness of the problem and may help schools take next steps to ensure students' safety.

The provider should also delve more into how Ally is using social media. She states that she does have friends online, but is she being safe about the information she discloses to them? Has she ever met them offline? The provider should encourage Ally to tell either a parent or another trusted adult about the situation—if she is afraid of being punished, often providers can act as a mediator and guide parents to consider options such as frequent check-ins about social media content, rather than completely taking away Ally's devices. Providers can remind families that if bullying is occurring online, taking a screenshot of the bullying before deleting may be important if this information is requested later. While acute disclosure of bullying or cyberbullying may cause great concern for patients and families, healthcare providers have an important role in assessing for sequelae of bullying and cyberbullying as well as facilitating access to resources that can help youth who are involved.

References

1. Smith PK, Mahdavi J, Carvalho M, Fisher S, Russell S, Tippett N. Cyberbullying: its nature and impact in secondary school pupils. J Child Psychol Psychiatry. 2008;49(4):376–85.
2. Kota R, Schoohs S, Benson M, Moreno MA. Characterizing cyberbullying among college students: hacking, dirty laundry, and mocking. Societies. 2014;4(4):549–60.
3. Selkie EM, Kota R, Chan YF, Moreno M. Cyberbullying, depression, and problem alcohol use in female college students: a multisite study. Cyberpsychol Behav Soc Netw. 2015;18(2):79–86.
4. Li Q. New bottle but old wine: a research of cyberbullying in schools. Comput Hum Behav. 2007;23(4): 1777–91.
5. National Academies of Sciences, Engineering, and Medicine. Preventing Bullying Through Science, Policy, and Practice. National Academies Press; 2016 Oct 14.
6. Lenhart A. Teens, social media & technology overview 2015. Pew Research Center; 2015 Apr 9;9.
7. Booth T (Writer) and Binamé C (Director). Cyberbully [Motion Picture]. United States: Discovery—Gaiam. 2011.
8. Savage, Stephanie and Josh Schwartz, creators. *Gossip Girl*. Dist. Warner Bros Television, 2007.
9. Selkie EM, Fales JL, Moreno MA. Cyberbullying prevalence among US middle and high school–aged adolescents: a systematic review and quality assessment. J Adolesc Health. 2016;58(2):125–33.
10. Olweus D. Peer harassment: a critical analysis and some important issues. In: Peer harassment in school: The plight of the vulnerable and victimized. New York: Guilford Press; 2001. p. 3–20.
11. Vandebosch H, Van Cleemput K. Defining cyberbullying: a qualitative research into the perceptions of youngsters. Cyberpsychol Behav. 2008;11(4): 499–503.
12. DeSmet A, Veldeman C, Poels K, Bastiaensens S, Van Cleemput K, Vandebosch H, De Bourdeaudhuij I. Determinants of self-reported bystander behavior in cyberbullying incidents amongst adolescents. Cyberpsychol Behav Soc Netw. 2014;17(4):207–15.
13. Schultze-Krumbholz A, Scheithauer H. Social-behavioral correlates of cyberbullying in a German student sample. Zeitschrift für psychologie/J Psychol. 2009;217(4):224–6.

14. Williams KR, Guerra NG. Prevalence and predictors of internet bullying. J Adolesc Health. 2007;41(6):S14–21.
15. Beran T, Li Q. The relationship between cyberbullying and school bullying. J Student Wellbeing. 2008;1(2):16–33.
16. Sourander A, Klomek AB, Ikonen M, Lindroos J, Luntamo T, Koskelainen M, Ristkari T, Helenius H. Psychosocial risk factors associated with cyberbullying among adolescents: a population-based study. Arch Gen Psychiatry. 2010;67(7):720–8.
17. Sourander A, Jensen P, Rönning JA, Niemelä S, Helenius H, Sillanmäki L, Kumpulainen K, Piha J, Tamminen T, Moilanen I, Almqvist F. What is the early adulthood outcome of boys who bully or are bullied in childhood? The Finnish "from a boy to a man" study. Pediatrics. 2007;120(2):397–404.
18. Sourander A, Jensen P, Rönning JA, Elonheimo H, Niemelä S, Helenius H, Kumpulainen K, Piha J, Tamminen T, Moilanen I, Almqvist F. Childhood bullies and victims and their risk of criminality in late adolescence: the Finnish from a boy to a man study. Arch Pediatr Adolesc Med. 2007;161(6):546–52.
19. Klomek AB, Sourander A, Kumpulainen K, Piha J, Tamminen T, Moilanen I, Almqvist F, Gould MS. Childhood bullying as a risk for later depression and suicidal ideation among Finnish males. J Affect Disord. 2008;109(1):47–55.
20. Frick PJ, Dickens C. Current perspectives on conduct disorder. Curr Psychiatry Rep. 2006;8(1):59–72.
21. Fanti KA, Frick PJ, Georgiou S. Linking callous-unemotional traits to instrumental and non-instrumental forms of aggression. J Psychopathol Behav Assess. 2009;31(4):285.
22. Fanti KA, Demetriou AG, Hawa VV. A longitudinal study of cyberbullying: examining riskand protective factors. Eur J Dev Psychol. 2012;9(2):168–81.
23. Ybarra ML, Mitchell KJ, Wolak J, Finkelhor D. Examining characteristics and associated distress related to internet harassment: findings from the second youth internet safety survey. Pediatrics. 2006;118(4):e1169–77.
24. Ellison NB, Steinfield C, Lampe C. The benefits of Facebook "friends:" social capital and college students' use of online social network sites. J Comput-Mediat Commun. 2007;12(4):1143–68.
25. Hinduja S, Patchin JW. Bullying, cyberbullying, and suicide. Arch Suicide Res. 2010;14(3):206–21.
26. Suzuki K, Asaga R, Sourander A, Hoven CW, Mandell D. Cyberbullying and adolescent mental health. Int J Adolesc Med Health. 2012;24(1):27–35.
27. Kosciw JG, Diaz EM. Involved, Invisible, Ignored: The Experiences of Lesbian, Gay, Bisexual and Transgender Parents and Their Children in Our Nation's K-12 Schools. Gay, Lesbian and Straight Education Network (GLSEN). 121 West 27th Street Suite 804, New York, NY 10001; 2008.
28. DeHue F, Bolman C, Völlink T. Cyberbullying: Youngsters' experiences and parental perception. Cyberpsychol Behav. 2008;11(2):217–23.
29. Patchin JW, Hinduja S. Bullies move beyond the schoolyard a preliminary look at cyberbullying. Youth Violence Juvenile Justice. 2006;4(2):148–69.
30. Slonje R, Smith PK. Cyberbullying: another main type of bullying? Scand J Psychol. 2008;49(2):147–54.
31. Shariff S. Cyber-bullying: issues and solutions for the school, the classroom and the home. New York: Routledge; 2008.
32. Bauman S. Conventional bullying versus Cyberbullying. Cyberbullying. 2015:17–27.
33. Rigby K. Bullying in schools: and what to do about it. Aust Council for Ed Research; 2007.
34. Smith PK, Talamelli L, Cowie H, Naylor P, Chauhan P. Profiles of non-victims, escaped victims, continuing victims and new victims of school bullying. Br J Educ Psychol. 2004;74(4):565–81.
35. Juvonen J, Gross EF. Extending the school grounds?--bullying experiences in cyberspace. J Sch Health. 2008;78(9):496–505.
36. O'Keeffe GS, Clarke-Pearson K. The impact of social media on children, adolescents, and families. Pediatrics. 2011;127(4):800–4.
37. Dowdell EB, Burgess AW, Flores JR. Original research: online social networking patterns among adolescents, young adults, and sexual offenders. Am J Nursing. 2011;111(7):28–36.
38. Mitchell KJ, Finkelhor D, Jones LM, Wolak J. Prevalence and characteristics of youth sexting: a national study. Pediatrics. 2012;129(1):13–20.
39. Lenhart A, Smith A, Anderson M. Teens, technology and romantic relationships. 2015.
40. Eliot M, Cornell D, Gregory A, Fan X. Supportive school climate and student willingness to seek help for bullying and threats of violence. J Sch Psychol. 2010;48(6):533–53.
41. Della Cioppa V, O'Neil A, Craig W. Learning from traditional bullying interventions: a review of research on cyberbullying and best practice. Aggress Violent Behav. 2015;23:61–8.
42. Del Rey R, Casas JA, Ortega R. The impacts of the CONRED program on different cyberbulling roles. Aggress Behav. 2016;42(2):123–35.
43. Freeman BW, Thompson C, Jaques C. Forensic aspects and assessment of school bullying. Psychiatr Clin N Am. 2012;35(4):877–900.
44. Elledge LC, Williford A, Boulton AJ, DePaolis KJ, Little TD, Salmivalli C. Individual and contextual predictors of cyberbullying: the influence of children's provictim attitudes and teachers' ability to intervene. J Youth Adolesc. 2013;42(5):698–710.
45. Ortega-Ruiz R, Del Rey R, Casas JA. Knowing, building and living together on internet and social networks: the ConRed cyberbullying prevention program. Int J Conflict Violence. 2012;6(2):302–12.

46. Williford A, Elledge LC, Boulton AJ, DePaolis KJ, Little TD, Salmivalli C. Effects of the KiVa antibullying program on cyberbullying and cyber-victimization frequency among Finnish youth. J Clin Child Adolesc Psychol. 2013;42(6):820–33.
47. Agatston PW, Kowalski R, Limber S. Students' perspectives on cyber bullying. J Adolesc Health. 2007;41(6):S59–60.
48. Bowman G. Newsround survey reveals majority of 10 to 12 year-olds are on social media. BBC online; 2016 Sep 2 [cited 2017 Apr 23]. http://www.bbc.co.uk/mediacentre/latestnews/2016/newsround-survey-social-media.

8 Media Multitasking and Mental Health

Nancy A. Cheever, Kristin Peviani, and Larry D. Rosen

The rapid pace of technological growth has produced dramatic shifts in sociocultural norms surrounding media use. Advances in communication technology have made it increasingly common for individuals and households to possess multiple portable and fixed media sources, impacting the way they interface with media. We are always "connected" and most often with more than one device at a time. According to a study of technology ownership conducted in 2015, 68% of Americans have smartphones, 45% have tablet computers, and about 90% of American adolescents have access to smartphones [1]. About three quarters of all media are consumed on mobile devices, and people spend an average of 6 h per day using their devices [2]. A national survey of 8–18-year-olds back in 2010 found that 20% of the media they consume is on mobile devices [3], and for 29% of the time young people use media, they are using more than one medium at the same time. Larger screens, longer battery life, device portability, and greater accessibility to multiple devices [4] make it easier than ever to "media multitask" or tune into multiple streams of media at a time [3].

Multitasking refers to performing more than one physical or cognitive task at a time. Media multitasking is performing media and technology-related tasks together and includes texting, talking on the phone, using a smartphone, watching television, sending and receiving email, and so on. The term multitasking is a bit of a misnomer, given that people of all ages are relatively ineffective multitaskers, and the mere attempt to simultaneously balance our attention between competing stimuli leads to less efficient information processing [5]. Further, the consensus among psychologists is that it is impossible to simultaneously combine tasks involving a heavy cognitive load [6], such as media multitasking. Therefore, we refer to this activity as task switching or rapidly switching from one task to the next. We use these terms interchangeably throughout this chapter since multitasking is more commonly used. Talking on the telephone and checking email, texting and writing a term paper, playing video games, and watching television—these are just a few of the task combinations that overload adolescents' mental processes and result in loss of time and reduced outcome quality.

N.A. Cheever (✉)
Department of Communications, California State University, Dominguez Hills, Carson, CA, USA
e-mail: ncheever@csudh.edu

K. Peviani
Department of Psychology, Virginia Tech, Blacksburg, VA, USA
e-mail: kpev33@vt.edu

L.D. Rosen
Department of Psychology, California State University, Dominguez Hills, Carson, CA, USA
e-mail: lrosen@csudh.edu

M.A. Moreno, A. Radovic (eds.), *Technology and Adolescent Mental Health*,
https://doi.org/10.1007/978-3-319-69638-6_8

Individual Differences in Multitasking

Individual differences confound the ease in which tasks are performed, and some task combinations are intrinsically easier to perform than others, such as listening to music and checking email. The complexity and familiarity of the task will alter the amount of mental strain the multitasking will cause. Further, personality correlates are an important indicator of media multitasking ability [7]. People who possess high levels of energy, sociability, and self-reliance, for instance, "have the positive energy and outlook needed to take on multiple tasks at the same time. Individuals who prefer more organization and detail-orientation are likely to feel less comfortable in roles requiring multitasking" ([7], p. 67).

Research shows that youth in particular suffer negative consequences when attempting to multitask with media including poor academic performance, poor social skills, diminished capacity to focus, and increased anxiety [8]. It is estimated that task switching with media among youth occurs every few minutes, and technological distractions such as social media, text messages, email, and notification alerts are the main sources of this behavior. Because technology has become a ubiquitous tool in young people's lives [8], adolescents tend to feel more comfortable task switching. As a result, teens and young adults task switch more frequently than older adults and often perform better and more efficiently than older people [9]. However, extreme multitaskers—those who perform the most combined tasks—do not perform tasks more efficiently than young people who multitask less frequently [10].

In 2009 we published a study looking at the multitasking ability and difficulty ratings of three generations [11]. We queried 1319 American adults and adolescents to determine what tasks they combine and how often and how difficult they rated each of the task pairs. The tasks included media- and technology-related tasks and tasks that do not require media such as eating and talking face-to-face. The youngest generation reported performing the most task pairs and all three generations found the same task pairings difficult. For instance, eating and listening to music were reported to be quite easy to do simultaneously, while playing video games and reading were rated as the most difficult tasks to combine.

In summary, because most American households are "media multitasking environments" [12]—with most having a television in every room and each member owning a smartphone or cell phone, video game consoles, digital music players, computers, laptops, and now hands-free-voice-controlled devices that can do almost anything—it is nearly impossible for young people to avoid media and technology and therefore are susceptible to mental health disorders associated with media multitasking. Specifically this chapter will examine the association of teens' media-rich lives and their general development, as well as symptoms of depression, anxiety, and sleep disorders.

Multitasking and Adolescent Development

The use of technology can lead to enhanced communication and monitoring between parents and their adolescent children as well as social relationships between teens and their peer groups. Further, adolescents without access to mobile devices report they are at a social disadvantage, relative to their peers [13]. In order to understand how media multitasking is impacting adolescent development, it is necessary to understand what motivates adolescent media multitasking.

It is quite possible that the preference for multitasking is generalizable for adolescents [14], such that the tendency to multitask might be exhibited across social, work, and school contexts. Younger generations rate themselves especially proficient at multitasking and task switch with media more frequently than older generations [11, 12], and those possessing greater strengths in multitasking might actually multitask less frequently [15]. This discrepancy between perceived and actual media multitasking ability and behaviors could be in part due to developmental differences associated with brain functioning. The dorsolateral prefrontal cortex, involved in selective attention and task management [16], is also involved in self-monitoring [17] and facilitates more efficient multitasking by filtering distractors in the presence of competing stimuli. Thus, maturational differences in brain network connectivity and function may place adolescents at a disadvantage not only when it comes to inhibiting distractions for multitasking [18] but also when it comes to their perceived self-awareness of the impact media multitasking has on their well-being or cognitive and emotional self-evaluations [19].

Socioemotional Functioning and Multitasking

The changing landscape of social engagement from real life to virtual socialization has altered the way adolescents engage with others and conduct themselves virtually. The nature of online socialization may facilitate disinhibition behind the screen [20], exhibited by less inhibited social exchanges online which can have deleterious effects on social skill development and peer relationships [21]. These close interpersonal relationships with peers are fundamental to adolescent well-being and set the stage for romantic relationships [22]. Taken together, the nuances of adolescent brain development make adolescents especially vulnerable to the pitfalls of media multitasking and could lead to deficits in social functioning.

Cognitive Development and Functioning

Up to about age 5, human children and chimpanzees have the about same ability to focus and shift attention as needed. As children grow and their brains develop more fully, humans are able to multitask and process information much more efficiently than our genetically similar primates [23]. Hebbian theory posits that neurons that fire together, wire together [24], and during adolescence, the brain undergoes extensive pruning, discarding unused neurons, and leaving behind a network of strengthened connections. This process helps facilitate the acquisition of new information and the formation of lasting preferences and behaviors. In the context of media use, the preference for multitasking could be rewiring the brain [25, 26] by strengthening neural pathways related to scanning and shifting attention and neglecting the pathways related to social awareness and emotional intelligence [27].

The relationship between the adolescent brain and multitasking behavior consequences can be seen in the academic performance and studying habits of teens. We conducted an observational study of middle school, high school, and college students showing how easily young people are distracted by technology when studying at home [28]. More than 250 students were observed in their natural environment. Observers recorded minute-by-minute activities over a 15-min period and found that participants averaged less than 6 min on their main task before being distracted by technology such as checking their social media and texting with friends. Having the television on at least once while studying significantly reduced the amount of time they spent studying.

If media multitasking is impairing adolescents' cognitive abilities and evaluations, then why do they do it? The answer is complex and may be that media multitasking may obfuscate their objective evaluation of its impact by effectively rewarding them for doing it. Take, for example, a well-intentioned adolescent who sets out to complete a homework assignment while listening to music with their cell phone at their side. They may not even set out to media multitask. Their goal is to complete their homework assignment, but their cell phone vibrates as a result of an incoming text from a friend. Five minutes of text messages, a Snapchat, and an Instagram post later and the adolescent is back to where they started. But now, their train of thought is derailed. They are thinking about the exchange and not the assignment at hand. It then takes a few minutes to recapture where they were in the assignment. This is one example of how multitasking may produce secondary gratifications associated with relaxation or improved emotional state, regardless of the gratifications obtained through the primary task (in this case, the homework assignment). This powerful emotional reinforcement may lead to positive associations between homework and media multitasking and prevent discontinuation of subsequent media multitasking regardless of whether it is distracting or negatively impacts learning [29]. The negative impact of media multitasking on well-being may be especially pronounced for adolescents who possess greater time management skills [30]. This association could be due to greater self-monitoring and goal setting associated with time management and greater disappointment when they do not meet their goals and expectations.

Media Multitasking and Depression

The National Survey on Drug Use and Health 2015 report on the prevalence of major depressive disorder among American adolescents found that 12.5% of 12–17-year-olds had major depressive disorder [31], with symptoms reflected by changes in functioning due to depressed mood or loss of interest and impaired work or social functioning [32]. Associations between media use during adolescence and later depression during young adulthood [33] suggest that greater exposure to media may lead to depressive symptoms during adulthood. Although these findings did not parse out whether media were consumed independently or simultaneously via media multitasking, their associations may be especially problematic for heavy media multitaskers who consume more media by multitasking. Additional research on the associations between media multitasking and depression in college-aged adults suggests that media multitasking contributes to depression above and beyond the total amount of time spent consuming media [34]. These findings demonstrate that media multitasking may contribute additional risk for depression, beyond what can be explained by the total amount of media exposure. Future research is needed to clarify whether the risks associated with media multitasking or depression found in college-aged adults extends to adolescents.

The theoretical associations between media multitasking and adolescent depression could be explained by the behavioral theory of depression, which posits that avoidance contributes to depressive symptoms by limiting experiences that could otherwise be beneficial to psychological health [35]. Accordingly, media multitasking could be used in a compensatory manner to avoid or escape stressful situations and reduce discomfort [36]. This experiential avoidance of aversive stimuli involves altering unpleasant experiences to alleviate negative emotions and has been linked with psychopathology [37]. Avoidance strategies that include behavioral diversion have been associated with poor psychological health outcomes, particularly in the presence of acute stressors [38]. Heavy multitaskers may possess a bias toward high impulsivity and sensation seeking [15] which could drive successive increases in media multitasking despite problems associated with its use. In this way, media multitasking can be considered a form of behavioral diversion for adolescents to avoid unpleasant affective or emotional states and quickly escape stress. The immediate reinforcement and accessibility of media multitasking from almost anywhere make it a quick and easy escape from situations that produce discomfort, while the salience and frequency of associated rewards may obscure the ability to perceive its negative impact on psychological health.

However, there exists a trade-off between the almost instantaneous gratification and security associated with media multitasking and real-world interactions that could potentially strengthen coping skills and buffer against depression. These skills are crucial for adolescents to learn as they become independent from their families and more reliant on social networks. Media multitasking may also come at the cost of engagement in face-to-face social interactions [14], which help protect against depression and anxiety. These are just some of the ways that media multitasking may interfere with adolescent socioemotional development and contribute to depression.

Body Image

Despite the brevity of exposure to media while media multitasking, the impressions of the media can still be lasting and seem to be determined more by individual differences than by the amount of time spent immersed in content. For adolescent girls who identify strongly with the idealized images in the media they consume, even brief exposure to television and music videos can result in body dissatisfaction [39]. In a study of the effects of media consumption by type on teenage girls' body dissatisfaction, the adolescents' identification with the model in the media predicted the impact of media on body image, not the amount of time spent viewing media. Long-term implications of negative body image during adolescence include depression during adulthood. One longitudinal study found that self-esteem during adolescence predicted depression 20 years later [40].

While it cannot be determined whether media multitasking contributes to or is a symptom of depression, the associations raise concern about the impact of our changing technological landscape on the well-being and socioemotional health of generations immersed in media who see it as a fundamental part of their lives. The rapid pace of technological advancement and shifts in how adolescents interact with and use media pose challenges to researchers interested in studying the impacts on psychopathology and well-being.

Adolescents lead the way in adopting mobile technology as their primary mode of accessing the Internet [41]. Thus, media multitasking might be a double-edged sword, increasing media consumption through quantity and type and replacing opportunities that could protect adolescents from psychopathology and enhance well-being.

Media Multitasking and Anxiety

Brianna is a 14-year-old high school freshman who relies heavily on her smartphone to communicate with her friends. The device never leaves her side, even when she is sleeping. While she showers she keeps the device on the bathroom counter with the volume set to high so she doesn't miss a text or alert from her favorite social media site. In addition to communicating with friends, Brianna is an avid video gamer and loves to watch television and listen to music. During the school year, most days are filled with all of these activities, often performed simultaneously. Brianna's smartphone use was less prevalent in middle school because of a strict policy precluding these devices in the classroom. However in the summer between middle school and high school, Brianna increased her media and technology use and developed the common habit of using her smartphone while eating dinner with her family, checking her social media while shopping, and using it constantly while out with friends.

That summer, Brianna's family went to a mountain cabin for a 3-week vacation. As Brianna stepped through the door her first words were: "What's the Wi-Fi password?" Brianna's mom replied: "I'm sorry, honey, they don't have Wi-Fi here." "You took us to a cabin with NO Wi-Fi?" Brianna exclaimed, and she immediately became agitated, quickly went to a bedroom, and began to sob. Over the next 3 days, Brianna sulked and cried and even attempted to hitch a ride from a local boy on a motorcycle to the nearest Wi-Fi-enabled coffee shop. She became increasingly agitated; her heart would race, and internally her mind was swirling with negative thoughts: "What are my friends doing?" "What are they posting?" "What will they think of me when I don't post or like anything?" "They will think I'm dead." Her racing thoughts kept her up at night and permeated her dreams. Brianna's mother suggested other activities, but since her media multitasking had become so habitual, Brianna was experiencing heavy anxiety symptomatology. As the days progressed, Brianna started engaging in non-mediated activities with the family. During the second week of vacation, Brianna's symptoms became less severe, and by the time they returned from vacation, she was able to function for longer periods of time without checking her smartphone.

Approximately one quarter of all American adolescents experience symptoms of an anxiety disorder, and 6% of 13–18-year-olds experience severe anxiety [42]. Girls are more likely than boys to experience anxiety in their teenage years (30% and 20%, respectively) and that anxiety tends to be related to social situations; 5.5% of teens suffer some sort of social phobia. In addition, 6% of girls experience some form of post-traumatic stress disorders—panic disorders are less prevalent in adolescence, with less than 3% of the US population of teens experiencing these issues [42]. Characteristics of media multitasking-induced anxiety include (1) fear of missing out (FoMO), when they cannot check their social media, alerts, or text messages; (2) obsessive-compulsive disorder (OCD), in which adolescents obsessively check their devices even when they haven't received a text or alert; (3) generalized anxiety from being overwhelmed by media multitasking; and (4) social anxiety, marked by rapid heartbeat, racing thoughts, and excessive sweating in social situations.

In order to get a clearer picture of the impact of media multitasking on adolescent anxiety, we need to examine motivational and behavioral differences in consumption. Differences in motivation for media use could distinguish between adaptive media consumption and maladaptive use associated with psychopathology [43]. Uses and gratifications theory suggests that we selectively consume media to fulfill our needs for information, identification, entertainment, socialization, and escape [44]. Accordingly, media multitasking is frequently used to escape from boredom, stress, or discomfort, and different psychological outcomes have been connected to different types of escape. Research examining the consequences of multitasking associated with differing motivational drives suggest that when it is used for entertainment to escape boredom, it is not significantly associated with anxiety [43]. In fact, it may even be beneficial in helping teens achieve greater social connectivity with others [45] even when they are not physically present [46]. However, adolescents who use media multitasking as a way of coping with stress may be at greater risk for anxiety and depression. For teens who struggle with stress and anxiety, clinging to media in the face of discomfort may be maladaptive because despite the immediate relief it provides, it can prevent them from learning adaptive coping strategies that aid in resolution. Adaptive coping styles provide relief for individuals dealing with stress through resolution rather than escape or avoidance and over time lead to better health and less psychopathology. Becker [39] found that media multitasking—but not overall media use—was a predictor of social anxiety. Media multitasking is also used to lessen social anxiety in some users. Young people who reported they were socially anxious, but not lonely, spent the least amount of time online compared to adolescents who were both socially anxious and lonely or lonely and not socially anxious. Further, the authors found that lonely teens use the Internet and social media as a coping mechanism more than non-lonely teens [47].

We discovered generational differences in anxiety levels for all technology use measured except personal email [48]. Across all media platforms, younger generations were more anxious than older ones, and the most anxiety was prompted by being unable to check text messages, cell phone calls, email, and social networks, in that order. Further generational differences were found in the amount of technology used, with the younger generations checking their devices far more frequently than older generations. The authors found that the younger generations checked their social networks and text messages very often, while the older generations checked older technologies such as email and voicemail. The authors concluded that the anxiety felt about not checking text messages may cause three quarters of the young people queried to check their text messages more than once per hour. And while half of all teens possess awareness about the addictive nature of their relationships with their smartphones [49], heavy users still become anxious when they cannot use it.

In an experiment that measured anxiety levels using the state portion of the State-Trait Anxiety Inventory (STAI) in college students who were restricted from using their smartphones in a room void of stimuli (no clocks, no media, no interaction, etc.), we found that being unable to use their devices caused moderate and heavy smartphone users to feel significantly more anxious over time, regardless of whether or not they had their devices with them [50]. We concluded that in addition to experiencing FoMO from not checking in with their social media and text messages, participants experienced a form of separation anxiety from their devices. When faced with a situation in which all stimuli were removed, those who used their smartphones the most were most anxious.

Young adults who use multiple social media platforms are more likely than those who use fewer to possess anxiety symptomatology. In a survey of 1787 young adults, researchers measured anxiety symptoms using the Patient-Reported Outcomes Measurement Information System (PROMIS) and also assessed the participants' use of multiple social media platforms with an adapted Pew Internet Research scale [51]. Statistical models that show the likelihood of an event happening were used to understand the associations between multiple social media platform use and mental health outcomes. The researchers found that people who use more social media platforms had significantly higher likelihood of having increased anxiety symptoms.

Clinical Considerations

A major factor in determining whether media multitasking is associated with adaptive or maladaptive outcomes seems to be the motivation for use and its impact on social development. If media multitasking is facilitating teens' avoidance of stressful situations, it may be limiting opportunities for them to learn adaptive coping styles which would help them better handle stress in the future. By implementing strategies surrounding media multitasking and use, teens can achieve greater balance and improve associated adaptive outcomes.

Previous studies support that it may be prudent for clinicians to ask people with anxiety disorders about their social media use and explain how the media may contribute to their condition [51]. Cognitive behavioral therapy can be helpful for teens who experience media multitasking-induced anxiety. Taking both short and sometimes even longer breaks from technology, as Brianna was forced to do, is perhaps the most effective way to assuage these symptoms.

Sleep Disorders

We spend up to one third of our lives sleeping, and if we are rested the process of sleep is fairly patterned and defined. As we drift off to sleep, our brains enter into the first of four stages of what is known as NREM or non-rapid eye movement sleep [52, 53]. Each stage deepens sleep until at the end of stage 4, the brain enters REM—rapid eye movement—sleep, which is where most dreaming takes place. Each stage is important to mental and physical health as the brain performs a host of housekeeping chores called "synaptic rejuvenation"—synaptic for the junctions of nerve cells and rejuvenation for processes known as pruning and consolidation. Pruning is where the brain removes unimportant connections created during the day, and consolidation is where the brain practices and solidifies important information learned during the day. In addition, the brain, in concert with the spinal column and spinal fluid, also flushes out a variety of toxins that remain from the day's thinking which, if left in the brain, would make the brain sluggish and make it more difficult to retain new material [54]. Without a good night's sleep, we accumulate a "sleep debt" which must eventually be repaid by either napping or sleeping longer. Even so, a bad night's sleep means that synaptic rejuvenation and brain flushing does not occur effectively, and we are left with a brain that can't remember what it learned the day before and has trouble concentrating on new material [55, 56]. A review of sleep physiology is outside the scope of this chapter. The interested reader can find further information on this from additional sources [54, 55, 57, 58].

During adolescence, circadian rhythms shift and teens feel more awake later at night, which then reduces daily alertness due to lack of sleep and an accumulating sleep debt. The US National Heart, Lung, and Blood Institute and the National Sleep Foundation have examined sleep research and advise that adolescents need 9–10 h of sleep a night [59, 60]. Studies have shown that the average adolescent sleeps 6.5 h per school night [61] leading to an ever-increasing sleep debt that they attempt to repay by sleeping in on the weekends. Doing the math this means that an adolescent would have to add roughly 12 h of extra weekend sleep or several naps during the week to catch up.

Numerous studies have shown that nearly every technology use close to bedtime has negative consequences for adolescents, and almost nine in ten adolescents have at least one device in their sleep environment [62]. Further studies have shown that the typical adolescent does not simply use a single device at night but is more likely to multitask with several devices. Studies have shown that multitasking is responsible for a longer time to fall asleep and less total sleep [61, 62] as well as a greater chance of falling asleep in school the following day [14, 55]. A comprehensive study of the impact of sleep on Americans found that the use of more interactive devices and the more multitasking with those devices resulted in more difficulty falling asleep and feelings of unrefreshing sleep [59]. The research is clear: Nighttime users and multitaskers of most "handheld devices"—particularly those that deal with connections with other people such as social media and texting—sleep less, have more difficulty falling asleep, get poorer-quality sleep, exhibit more frequent early awakenings, and have excessive daytime sleepiness [61–67].

The impact of lack of sleep among adolescents is profound and serious. One study that examined 27,939 adolescents found that each lost hour of sleep was associated with a 38% increase in the chances of feeling sad and hopeless, a 42% increase in the chances of seriously considering suicide, a 58% increase in the odds of a suicide attempt, and a 23% increase in the chance of future substance use [68]. Studies in the USA [69–71] and other countries [72] validate that sleep problems may be responsible for the relationship between the use of technology and emotional health. For example, a meta-analysis of studies examining the relationship between sleep and depression among adolescents found that depressed teens had more sleep problems including an increase in lighter stage 1 sleep and a decrease in the deeper sleep that is responsible for synaptic rejuvenation [63]. Additional research suggests that shortened sleep may be related to increases in BMI and pose a risk for the adolescent becoming overweight or obese [73, 74]. Finally, one study where adolescents completed cognitive control and risk-taking tasks while having their brains scanned found that poor-quality sleep was associated with reduced activity in the parts of the brain that involve decision-making and risk-taking, making poor sleepers more prone to making bad decisions about taking risks [75].

Sleep problems also lead directly to academic problems. A study looking at the impact of a single night's sleep loss found reductions in reaction time, recall, and judgment [76], while another study found that a loss of 8 h of sleep over a few nights produced reduced alertness and memory deficits [77]. Other studies have shown similar impacts on mental performance even up to 6–8 years following sleep assessment [69, 78].

Experts have focused attention on protective factors for adolescents to avoid sleep problems related to media and technology use and hence avoid resultant mental and emotional issues. The consensus is that good sleep hygiene is defined as including the following [78, 79]:

- A suggested cutoff time for using devices at least 1–2 h prior to bedtime
- No device use in the bedroom at all
- A charging station for devices outside the bedroom
- Replacing 1 h of daily screen time with 1 h of physical activity during the day (which helps increase nighttime sleep [64, 65])
- Parents modeling good nighttime technology use behaviors

As one systematic review of all studies concerning sleep among school-aged children and adolescents concluded, "Youth should be advised to limit or reduce screen time exposure, especially before or during bedtime hours to minimize any harmful effects of screen time on sleep and well-being" ([80], p. 56).

Concluding Thoughts

Today's adolescents spend their days squeezing 24 h of media use into 6 or 7 h by constantly diverting their focus from one medium to the next and often having two, three, or more screens competing for their attention. This era of media multitasking has led young people to adopt this practice, even though research shows doing so may not lead to more efficiency or better task performance [10]. As Carrier and his colleagues concluded, "While multitasking is rampant in young people due to the technologies that are being used, on the whole, this multitasking madness does not appear to lead to an across-the-board improvement of multitasking skill" ([10], p. 386). Instead, as we have discussed in this chapter, adolescents who media multitask or rapidly task switch may incur negative costs to their mental health. Intentional breaks from technology tend to assuage the symptoms of these potential problems, and cognitive behavioral therapy is appropriate for adolescents with clinical psychopathological symptoms. One promising direction for adolescent media coping strategies lies in mindfulness and meditative practice [81]. The inundation of technology from multiple sources can be combatted through attention to consumption and selective disengagement from time to time. Merely paying attention to how and what adolescents themselves pay attention to can help them achieve greater balance and self-awareness. An experimental study on the efficacy of meditation found that meditation training facilitated fewer task switches, greater task orientation, and improved memory [81]. Cultivating mindfulness surrounding media use could strengthen adolescents' interactions with media so that it is beneficial to their psychological health and well-being. Using applications that assuage anxiety and the impulse to check social media may be a helpful suggestion as well.

We recommend that clinicians screen for multitasking and discuss links between multitasking and concerns such as academic performance, sleep deprivation, and increased anxiety with patients. For patients who struggle with multitasking or exhibit symptoms associated with these behaviors, consider recommending counseling, particularly with someone with expertise in mindfulness or other mindful resources especially those specific to adolescents [82].

References

1. Anderson M. Technology device ownership: 2015. Pew Research Center, October, 2015, http://www.pewinternet.org/2015/10/29/technology-device-ownership-2015.
2. eMarketer. 2017. https://www.emarketer.com/Article/Growth-of-Time-Spent-on-Mobile-Devices-Slows/1013072.
3. Rideout VJ, Foehr UG, Roberts DF. Generation M²: media in the lives of 8-to 18-year-olds. Menlo Park: Henry J. Kaiser Family Foundation; 2010.
4. Kononova A, Chiang Y-H. Why do we multitask with media? Predictors of media multitasking among internet users in the United States and Taiwan. Comput Hum Behav. 2015;50:31–41. https://doi.org/10.1016/j.chb.2015.03.052.
5. Posner MI. Hierarchical distributed networks in the neuropsychology of selective attention. In: Cognitive neuropsychology and neurolinguistics: advances in models of cognitive function and impairment. Hillsdale, NJ: Lawrence Erlbaum Associates; 1990. p. 187–210.
6. American Psychological Association. Multitasking: Switching costs, 2016. http://www.apa.org/research/action/multitask.aspx.
7. Mesmer-Magnus J, Viswesvaran C, Bruk-Lee V, Sanderson K, Sinha N. Personality correlates of preference for multitasking in the workplace. J Organ Psychol. 2014;14(1):67–76.
8. Carrier LM, Rosen LD, Cheever NA, Lim A. Causes, effects, and practicalities of everyday multitasking. Dev Rev. 2015;3(23):35.
9. Butler KM, Weywadt C. Age differences in voluntary task switching. Psychol Aging. 2013;28(4):1024–31. https://doi.org/10.1037/a0034937.
10. Carrier LM, Kersten M, Rosen LR. Searching for generation M: does multitasking practice improve multitasking skill? In: Rosen LR, Cheever NA, Carrier LM, editors. The Wiley handbook of psychology, technology and society. Hoboken, NJ: Wiley-Blackwell. p. 373–87.
11. Carrier LM, Cheever NA, Rosen LD, Benitez S, Chang J. Multitasking across generations: Multitasking choices and difficulty ratings in three generations of Americans. Comput Hum Behav. 2009;25(2):483–9. https://doi.org/10.1016/j.chb.2008.10.012.
12. Brasel SA, Gips J. Media multitasking behavior: concurrent television and computer usage. Cyberpsychol Behav Soc Network. 2011;14(9):527–34. https://doi.org/10.1089/cyber.2010.0350.
13. Blair BL, Fletcher AC. "The only 13-year-old on planet earth without a cell phone": meanings of cell phones in early adolescents' everyday lives. J Adolesc Res. 2011;26(2):155–77.
14. Pea R, Nass C, Meheula L, Rance M, Kumar A, Bamford H, et al. Media use, face-to-face communication, media multitasking, and social well-being among 8- to 12-year-old girls. Dev Psychol. 2012;48(2):327–36. https://doi.org/10.1037/a0027030.

15. Sanbonmatsu DM, Strayer DL, Medeiros-Ward N, Watson JM. Who multi-tasks and why? Multi-tasking ability, perceived multi-tasking ability, impulsivity, and sensation seeking. PLoS One. 2013;8(1):e54402. https://doi.org/10.1371/journal.pone.0054402.
16. Smith EE, Jonides J. Storage and executive processes in the frontal lobes. Science. 1999;283(5408):1657–61.
17. Raz A, Buhle J. Typologies of attentional networks. Nat Rev Neurosci. 2006;7(5):367–79.
18. Ophir E, Nass C, Wagner AD. Cognitive control in media multitaskers. Proc Nat Acad Sci. 2009;106(37):15583–7. https://doi.org/10.1073/pnas.0903620106.
19. Diener E, Oishi S, Lucas RE. Personality, culture, and subjective well-being: Emotional and cognitive evaluations of life. Ann Rev Psychol. 2003;54(1):403–25. https://doi.org/10.1146/annurev.psych.54.101601.14505.
20. Lapidot-Lefler N, Barak A. Effects of anonymity, invisibility, and lack of eye-contact on toxic online disinhibition. Comput Hum Behav. 2012;28(2):434–43. https://doi.org/10.1016/j.chb.2011.10.014.
21. Suler J. The online disinhibition effect. Cyberpsychol Behav. 2004;7(3):321–6.
22. Connolly J, Furman W, Konarski R. The role of peers in the emergence of heterosexual romantic relationships in adolescence. Child Dev. 2000;71(5):1395–408.
23. Herrmann E, Tomasello M. Focusing and shifting attention in human children (Homo sapiens) and chimpanzees (Pan troglodytes). J Compar Psychol. 2015;129(3):268–74. https://doi.org/10.1037/a0039384.
24. Hebb DO. The organization of behavior: a neuropsychological theory. New York: Wiley; 1949.
25. Richtel M. Attached to technology and paying a price. The New York Times 2010 Jun 6;6.
26. Rosen LD, Carrier LM, Cheever NA. Rewired: understanding the iGeneration and the way they learn. New York: Palgrave-MacMillan.
27. Carr N. Author Nicholas Carr: the web shatters focus, Rewires Brains Wired Magazine 2010 May 24;24.
28. Rosen LD, Carrier LM, Cheever NA. Facebook and texting made me do it: media-induced task-switching while studying. Comput Hum Behav. 2013;29:948–58.
29. Foerde K, Knowlton BJ, Poldrack RA. Modulation of competing memory systems by distraction. Proc Nat Acad Sci. 2006;103(31):11778–83. https://doi.org/10.1073/pnas.0602659103.
30. Yang X, Xu X, Zhu L. Media multitasking and psychological wellbeing in Chinese adolescents: time management as a moderator. Comput Hum Behav. 2015;53:216–22. https://doi.org/10.1016/j.chb.2015.06.034.
31. National Institute of Mental Health. Major depression among adolescents. 2015. https://www.nimh.nih.gov/health/statistics/prevalence/major-depression-among-adolescents.shtml. Accessed 9 Mar 2017.
32. Pratt LA, Brody DJ. Depression in the U.S. household population, 2009–2012. NCHS data brief, no 172. Hyattsville, MD: National Center for Health Statistics. p. 2014.
33. Primack BA, Shensa A, Escobar-Viera CG, Barrett EL, Sidani JE, Colditz JB, James AE. Use of multiple social media platforms and symptoms of depression and anxiety: a nationally-representative study among U.S. young adults. Comput Hum Behav. 2017;69:1e9.
34. Becker MW, Alzahabi R, Hopwood CJ. Media multitasking is associated with symptoms of depression and social anxiety. Cyberpsychol Behav Soc Network. 2012;16:132–5. https://doi.org/10.1089/cyber.2012.0291.
35. American Psychiatric Association. Diagnostic and statistical manual of mental disorders (DSM–5). 5th ed. Arlington, VA: APA; 2013.
36. Carvalho JP, Hopko DR. Behavioral theory of depression: Reinforcement as a mediating variable between avoidance and depression. J Behav Ther Exp Psychiatry. 2011;42(2):154–62. https://doi.org/10.1016/j.jbtep.2010.10.001.
37. Kardefelt-Winther D. A conceptual and methodological critique of internet addiction research: towards a model of compensatory internet use. Comput Hum Behav. 2014;31:351–4. https://doi.org/10.1016/j.chb.2013.10.059.
38. Chawla N, Ostafin B. Experiential avoidance as a functional dimensional approach to psychopathology: an empirical review. J Clin Psychol. 2007;63(9):871–90. https://doi.org/10.1002/jclp.20400.
39. Bell BT, Dittmar H. Does media type matter? The role of identification in adolescent girls' media consumption and the impact of different thin-ideal media on body image. Sex Roles. 2011;65(7–8):478–90. https://doi.org/10.1007/s11199-011-9964-x.
40. Steiger AE, Allemand M, Robins RW, Fend HA. Low and decreasing self-esteem during adolescence predict adult depression two decades later. J Pers Soc Psychol. 2014;106(2):325–38. https://doi.org/10.1037/a0035133.
41. Pew Internet. Teens and Technology 2013. 2013. http://www.pewinternet.org/2013/03/13/teens-and-technology-2013. Accessed 9 Mar 2017.
42. National Institutes for Health. Prevalence of anxiety disorders among children. 2017. https://www.nimh.nih.gov/health/statistics/prevalence/any-anxiety-disorder-among-children.shtml.
43. Panova T, Lleras A. Avoidance or boredom: negative mental health outcomes associated with use of information and communication technologies depend on users' motivations. Comput Hum Behav. 2016;58:249–58. https://doi.org/10.1016/j.chb.2015.12.062.
44. Katz E, Blumler JG, Gurevitch M. The uses and gratifications approach to mass communication. Beverly Hills: Sage; 1974.
45. Xu S, Wang Z. (Joyce), David P. Media multitasking and well-being of university students. Comput Hum Behav. 2016;55:242–50. https://doi.org/10.1016/j.chb.2015.08.040.

46. CAGJ H, WA IJ, Markopoulos P, de Ruyter B. Social presence and group attraction: exploring the effects of awareness systems in the home. Cognition Technol Work. 2004;6(1):41–4. https://doi.org/10.1007/s10111-003-0141-z.
47. Bonetti L, Campbell MA, Gilmore L. The relationship of loneliness and social anxiety with children's and adolescents' online communication. Cyberpsychol Behav Soc Netw. 2010;13:279–85.
48. Rosen LD, Whaling K, Rab S, Carrier LM, Cheever NA. Is Facebook creating "iDisorders"? The link between clinical symptoms of psychiatric disorders and technology use, attitudes and anxiety. Comput Hum Behav. 2013;29(3):1243–54.
49. Wallace K. Half of teens think they're addicted to their smartphones. CNN. 29 July 2016. http://www.cnn.com/2016/05/03/health/teens-cell-phone-addiction-parents/.
50. Cheever NA, Rosen LD, Carrier LM, Chavez A. Out of sight is not out of mind: the impact of restricting wireless mobile device use on anxiety among low, moderate and high users. Comput Hum Behav. 2015;37:290–7.
51. Primack BA, Swanier B, Georgiopoulos AM, Land SR, Fine MJ. Association between media use in adolescence and depression in young adulthood. Arch Gen Psychiatry. 2009;66(2):181. https://doi.org/10.1001/archgenpsychiatry.2008.532.
52. Dement W, Kleitman N. Cyclic variations in EEG during sleep and their relation to eye movements, body motility, and dreaming. Electroencephalogr Clin Neurophysiol. 1957;9(4):673–90.
53. Colten HR, Altevogt BM, editors. Sleep disorders and sleep deprivation: an unmet public health problem. Washington, DC: National Academies Press; 2006.
54. Lewis PA. The secret world of sleep: the surprising science of the mind at rest. New York: Macmillan; 2013.
55. Phillips B, Gelula R. Sleep-wake cycle: its physiology and impact on health. Retrieeved October. 2006;22:2007.
56. Harvard Health Publications. Repaying your sleep debt. August 2007. http://www.health.harvard.edu/staying-healthy/repaying-your-sleep-debt.
57. Sparks SD. Blue light may impair students' sleep, studies say. Educ Week. 2015;33(14):20–1.
58. Kim M/Washington Post. Blue light from electronics disturbs sleep, especially for teenagers[internet]; 2014. https://www.washingtonpost.com/national/health-science/blue-light-from-electronics-disturbs-sleep-especially-for-teenagers/2014/08/29/3edd2726-27a7-11e4-958c-268a320a60ce_story.html?utm_term=.01e106877e48.
59. Gradisar M, Wolfson AR, Harvey AG, Hale L, Rosenberg R, Czeisler CA. The sleep and technology use of Americans: findings from the National Sleep Foundation's 2011 sleep in America poll. J Clin Sleep Med. 2013;9(12):1291–9.
60. U.S. Department of Health and Human Services/National Heart, Lung and Blood Institute. Your guide to healthy sleep [internet]. NIH publication 11-5271. 2005 Nov. Revised 2011 Aug. https://www.nhlbi.nih.gov/files/docs/public/sleep/healthy_sleep.pdf.
61. Calamaro CJ, Mason TBA, Ratcliffe SJ. Adolescents living the 24/7 lifestyle: effects of caffeine and technology on sleep duration and daytime functioning. Pediatrics. 2009;123(6):e1005–10.
62. Hysing M, Pallesen S, Stormark KM, Jakobsen R, Lundervold AJ, Sivertsen B. Sleep and use of electronic devices in adolescence: results from a large population-based study. BMJ Open. 2015;5(1):e006748.
63. Carter B, Rees P, Hale L, Bhattacharjee D, Paradkar MS. Association between portable screen-based media device access or use and sleep outcomes: a systematic review and meta-analysis. JAMA Pediatr. 2016;170(12):1202–8.
64. Cain N, Gradisar M. Electronic media use and sleep in school-aged children and adolescents: a review. Sleep Med. 2010;11(8):735–42.
65. Falbe J, Davison KK, Franckle RL, Ganter C, Gortmaker SL, Smith L, Land T, Taveras EM. Sleep duration, restfulness, and screens in the sleep environment. Pediatrics. 2015;135(2):e367–75.
66. Arora T, Broglia E, Thomas GN, Taheri S. Associations between specific technologies and adolescent sleep quantity, sleep quality, and parasomnias. Sleep Med. 2014;15(2):240–7.
67. King DL, Gradisar M, Drummond A, Lovato N, Wessel J, Micic G, Douglas P, Delfabbro P. The impact of prolonged violent video-gaming on adolescent sleep: an experimental study. J Sleep Res. 2013;22(2):137–43.
68. Winsler A, Deutsch A, Vorona RD, Payne PA, Szklo-Coxe M. Sleepless in Fairfax: the difference one more hour of sleep can make for teen hopelessness, suicidal ideation, and substance use. J Youth Adolesc. 2015;44(2):362–78.
69. Asarnow LD, McGlinchey E, Harvey AG. The effects of bedtime and sleep duration on academic and emotional outcomes in a nationally representative sample of adolescents. J Adolesc Health. 2014;54(3):350–6.
70. Lovato N, Gradisar M. A meta-analysis and model of the relationship between sleep and depression in adolescents: recommendations for future research and clinical practice. Sleep Med Rev. 2014;18(6):521–9.
71. Lemola S, Perkinson-Gloor N, Brand S, Dewald-Kaufmann JF, Grob A. Adolescents' electronic media use at night, sleep disturbance, and depressive symptoms in the smartphone age. J Youth Adolesc. 2015;44(2):405–18.
72. Nuutinen T, Roos E, Ray C, Villberg J, Välimaa R, Rasmussen M, Holstein B, Godeau E, Beck F, Léger D, Tynjälä J. Computer use, sleep duration and health symptoms: a cross-sectional study of 15-year olds in three countries. Int J Public Health. 2014;59(4):619–28.
73. Arora T, Hussain S, Lam KH, Yao GL, Thomas GN, Taheri S. Exploring the complex pathways among

specific types of technology, self-reported sleep duration and body mass index in UK adolescents. Int J Obes. 2013;37(9):1254–60.
74. Guidolin M, Gradisar M. Is shortened sleep duration a risk factor for overweight and obesity during adolescence? A review of the empirical literature. Sleep Med. 2012;13(7):779–86.
75. Telzer EH, Fuligni AJ, Lieberman MD, Galván A. The effects of poor quality sleep on brain function and risk taking in adolescence. NeuroImage. 2013;71:275–83.
76. National Sleep Foundation. Backgrounder: why sleep matters. http://www.sleepfoundation.org/hottopics/index.php?secid=15&id=293.
77. National Sleep Foundation. Sleep-wake cycle: Its physiology and impact on health. 2006. https://sleepfoundation.org/sites/default/files/SleepWakeCycle.pdf.
78. Burke SM. The impact of media use on sleep in adolescents. J Pediatr Nurs. 2016;5(31):556–8.
79. Bartel KA, Gradisar M, Williamson P. Protective and risk factors for adolescent sleep: a meta-analytic review. Sleep Med Rev. 2015;21:72–85.
80. Hale L, Guan S. Screen time and sleep among school-aged children and adolescents: a systematic literature review. Sleep Med Rev. 2015;21:50–8.
81. Levy DM, Wobbrock JO, Kaszniak AW, Ostergren M. The effects of mindfulness meditation training on multitasking in a high-stress information environment. In Proceedings of Graphics Interface 2012, 2012 May 28 (pp. 45–52). Canadian Information Processing Society.
82. Vo D. Mindfulness for teens. http://mindfulnessforteens.com/dzung-vo/dr-dzung-vo/.

9 Internet Gaming Disorder

Jeffrey N. Rokkum, Jorge A. Blanco-Herrera, Manuela E. Faulhaber, and Douglas A. Gentile

What follows is a real case of Internet Gaming Disorder (IGD). Xi Wang's first day in a Chinese Internet addiction treatment center for IGD came as a surprise [1]. The night before, his parents had him drugged and institutionalized. Xi Wang's parents had no idea how to handle their son's behavior nor did they know anything about video games. They just knew they were losing their son. He had grown apathetic to his health, school, friends, and family. They had also heard reports of teenagers dying of blood clots, starvation, and dehydration at Internet cafes, the same ones Xi Wang had lied about attending when he should have been at his friend's house or in school. In the past, his parents tried punishing him, bribing him, and even hiding his computer cables, but all of these measures proved unsuccessful. Ultimately, institutionalization was their last resort.

The Wangs are not alone in their experience: news reports of severe video game addiction include stories about seizures, childhood neglect, and deaths after marathon game playing sessions [2–4]. This coverage has contributed to public concerns about the potentially pathological effects of excessive video game play. Although most cases are not life-threatening, they have drawn attention which has driven an increase in video gaming and Internet addiction research over the past 10 years.

J.N. Rokkum (✉) • J.A. Blanco-Herrera
M.E. Faulhaber • D.A. Gentile
Iowa State University, Ames, IA, USA
e-mail: rokkum@iastate.edu; jorgeb@iastate.edu; manufa@iastate.edu; dgentile@iastate.edu

Most researchers have defined IGD based on damage to psychological functioning, social support, school performance, family relationships, and occupational performance [5]. Even though Xi Wang reported more than 10 h of video game playing a day, he denied having a problem. He described himself as enjoying the virtual world more than the physical world. He did not get any sense of happiness from the world around him and found the games and Internet to be a source of happiness. He suspected his behavior would not be labeled problematic if he had played the same amount of hours but kept up his grades and followed the social norms of what a "good boy" is supposed to be. Even as he suffered nausea, physical pain, restlessness, fatigue, and insomnia from Internet withdrawal, Wang claimed that the definition of IGD would result in 80% of the population suffering from IGD.

Symptoms

Work on IGD has led to the inclusion of pathological gaming as a potential formal disorder in the *Diagnostic and Statistical Manual of Mental Disorders, 5th Edition* [6]. The American Psychiatric Association (APA) tasked 12 experts and more than 20 outside advisors to review over

M.A. Moreno, A. Radovic (eds.), *Technology and Adolescent Mental Health*,
https://doi.org/10.1007/978-3-319-69638-6_9

240 publications concerning pathologic Internet and video game use. Their conclusion, based on the evidence they reviewed, was sufficient to warrant inclusion of IGD in the research appendix of the DSM-5 to encourage future research on the prevalence, etiology, risk factors, clinical course, and treatment of IGD [6]. This section aims to provide an overview of IGD as described by the DSM-5.

The DSM-5 appendix has nine criteria to identify individuals with IGD. Five or more of these criteria must be met within a 1-year period to diagnose IGD. To meet the criteria, a patient must show dysfunction or impairment in their lives from their symptoms. Symptoms include a preoccupation with Internet gaming, withdrawal, tolerance, unsuccessful reduction in gaming behaviors or cessation of attempts to stop gaming, disinterest in other hobbies, escapism, excessive use despite problems, deception of game playing habits, and the jeopardizing of significant relationships or life opportunities [6].

Preoccupation

Preoccupation is the tendency for individuals to think excessively about playing video games in non-game situations. Constant intrusive thoughts about and preoccupation with video games cause individuals to have difficulty focusing on anything besides video games. In practical terms, such preoccupation leads to missed deadlines, overlooked details, and inattention to other life domains. Preoccupation must cause dysfunction. A lifeguard and a professional gamer may spend the same amount of time thinking about video games, but it may only be dysfunctional preoccupation for the lifeguard.

Preoccupation can be assessed with scales where people rate their agreement with statements such as "I [often] think about playing League of Legends when I am not using a computer" [7]. Prevalence of this symptom in the general population ranges from 5 to 25% [8–13].

Withdrawal

Withdrawal symptoms are unpleasant physical effects and/or negative emotions that occur when an individual stops or reduces their video game playing. Withdrawal is more than just craving or compulsions to play again. It is normal to want more of a fun and engaging activity. It is dysfunctional when withdrawal leads to uncontrollable physical feelings, emotions, behaviors, and moods. Both withdrawal and tolerance (described below) are consequences of physiological and psychological dependence, similar to biologically based addiction, which can result in anxiety, uncontrollable physical tics, depression, or more.

Functional magnetic resonance imaging studies have shown that addicted gamers have similar brain activity to substance abusers when it comes to cravings associated with their addictions [14]. A recent experimental study found that addicted gamers have stronger and more extreme emotional reactions in response to games than nonaddicted gamers, similar to how alcoholics have strong reactions when seeing a shot glass, a reaction known as cue reactivity [15]. Further suggesting their similarity, treatments designed to help those with substance abuse were effective in addicted gamers, reducing their cravings and brain activation in response to game cues [16]. Prevalence of withdrawal symptoms in the general population ranges between 2 and 22% [8–12, 17].

Unsuccessful Reduction or Cessation Attempts

One of the core symptoms for any type of addiction is difficulty controlling, reducing, or ceasing their addictive habits. Given that video games are designed to be as compelling as possible, unsuccessful cessation attempts are not surprising. Many online games depend on a loyal player base. As such habitual game play or occasional failure to reduce game play is normal. However, these unsuccessful events are dysfunctional when gamers are unable to inhibit their playing behavior after realizing they have a problematic relationship with games. Gamer addicts often describe life as "dark" or "boring" without games in their lives [18].

Many games are designed to motivate play through a combination of variable reward schedules, instant feedback rewards, enveloping narratives, a sense of personal development, social opportunities, and social costs [19]. Because they are designed to elicit compulsive, habitual playing behavior, not playing games can become a personal and a social struggle. Wang and Zhu [20] note that players often feel "all [their] closest friends today are playing games." As such, when players try to reduce their own gaming habits, they find "it's hard to find new friends." Prevalence of unsuccessful reduction attempts in the general population ranges between 2 and 36% [8–10, 12, 17].

Escapism

Escapism is the use of games to avoid daily stressors or negative emotions. While relying on entertainment for escapism is normal, escapism becomes a clinical concern when it becomes the individual's main coping strategy for responding to stressors. Wan and Chiou [18] found that addicted gamers tend to turn to games to avoid discomfort, in comparison with nonaddicted people who typically play games seeking satisfaction [21].

Escapism delays productive resolution of stressors' causes. While useful when it comes to unsolvable stressors, escapism can lead to escalation of solvable stressors. For example, a student can avoid finishing a dreaded school project by playing games, but the school project remains undone, their grades suffer, and the next school project becomes more dreadful. In contrast, a child can use escapism in games to avoid the pain of chemotherapy. Escapism is normal but dysfunctional in its excessiveness when it comes to IGD. Prevalence of escapism in the general population ranges from 8 to 30% [8–13, 17].

Excessive Gaming Despite Problems

Excessive gaming despite problems is closely tied to disinterest in other hobbies and the inability to cease game playing habits. That is, despite noticing that the gaming is causing problems in other areas of life, the person is unable to make the changes needed to reduce those problems. For example, a vicious cycle could occur when habitual gaming is itself the source of strained social relationships, financial concerns, or deteriorating health, and the addicted gamer retreats further into games to cope with the stress. Nearly 20% of massively multiplayer online role-playing games (MMORPG) players report that their video game playing had negatively affected their relationships with their non-playing partners [22].

Peng and Liu [23] note that video game dependency (defined as "psychological discomfort experienced by online gamers when they are unable to play online games as they wish"), but not weekly play time, is highly associated with problems in physical health, personal life, and professional/academic opportunities. Prevalence of excessive gaming despite problems in the general population is between 9 and 29% [8, 10, 12].

Deception with Regard to Gaming Habits

Similar to other addictions, loved ones' concerns about the problematic behavior can be met with deception from the addicted person with regard to the scope of their behavior. The addicted gamer may underreport the time or money they spend on gaming, may misrepresent their intentions for not participating in other activities, or may simply avoid admitting to the addictive behavior. This deception need not be intentionally malicious. An addicted gamer may not be aware of how much they spend on gaming, may have different intentions but be compelled to game when they otherwise would have done something else, or may be afraid to admit to themselves that their gaming habits are a problem. Nonetheless, deception is damaging for social relationships and trust and is therefore dysfunctional. Prevalence of deception of gaming habits in the general population is between 5 and 14% [8, 9, 11, 12, 17].

Jeopardizing Significant Relationships or Life Opportunities

When video games become a person's main priority, they may jeopardize significant relationships and life opportunities. Playing games can become more important than other people, career development, or important life goals. Overall, video game players received poorer grades in school, skipped school more often, got poorer sleep, and performed worse on the Scholastic

Aptitude Test when compared to those who did not play video games or played less [9, 23]. Gentile [17] reports that 23% of video game players skipped their homework to play and 20% perform poorly on subsequent homework or tests because of playing. Critically, Internet Gaming Disorder predicted poorer school performance even after controlling for time spent playing video games [17]. Students addicted to gaming had lower grades than nonaddicted students, even when they played the same amount of hours. Prevalence of jeopardizing important life opportunities in the general population ranges from 5 to 48% [8, 10–12, 17].

Loss of Interest in Previous Hobbies

Disinterest in previous hobbies results from gaming becoming a dominating force in the social and recreational life of the gamer. This may not always be negative. Video game play can be preferable than going outside in crime-struck neighborhoods or could replace riskier habits like drinking, smoking, or gambling. A dysfunctional loss of interest in previous hobbies results in discontinuing beneficial activities.

Addicted gamers demonstrate significant reductions in previously favored activities, spending less time or showing less interest in volunteering, playing sports, socializing with friends, or any other previously preferred activities in lieu of video game play. Prevalence of disinterest in previous hobbies in the general population ranges between 7 and 14.4% [9, 10].

Tolerance

Tolerance is the need for increasing amounts of something one is addicted to in order to achieve the same level of satisfaction. For gamers, tolerance results in needing more frequent and longer play sessions to feel similar levels of happiness, excitement, or fulfillment in their game playing habits. Prevalence of tolerance symptoms in the general population ranges between 6.7 and 9.8% [8, 9, 11, 12].

Prevalence

IGD has a prevalence rate between 2 and 10% among video game players [6]. However, the DSM-5 notes that "the literature suffers … from lack of a standard definition from which to derive prevalence data" [6]. Although this is technically correct, it may be less important than it appears at first. Despite using different definitional criteria, most studies in fact use very similar types of questions and yield similar results. For example, Fisher [11] reported 6% of children met four of nine criteria for IGD. A study of American youth 8–18 found that 8.5% of players met 6 of 11 criteria for addictive behavior [17]. Choo et al. [9] found that 9% of players met five of 10 criteria for addictive behavior. Thomas and Martin [13] reported approximately 5% of players met four of nine criteria for addictive behavior. In another recent study, 8% of individuals met 7 out of 14 criteria for addictive behavior [24]. Many of these studies use similar criteria to those now established by the DSM-5. Studies that most closely mirror the DSM-5 criteria and classification range between 3 and 9% prevalence rates.

Etiology and Comorbidities

Few studies have examined the etiology, comorbidities, and course of development of IGD. One study measured the IGD-style gaming symptoms of more than 3000 Singaporean elementary and secondary school children over a 2-year period [25]. Out of the approximately 9% of children who met the criterion for clinical significance at the beginning of the study (based on DSM-5 dichotomous criteria), 84% remained at that level 2 years later. Individuals with IGD also had greater levels of depression, poorer grades, worse relationships with parents, and increased aggressive tendencies. These comorbidities increased for those who reached IGD status during the study and decreased for those who dropped below the IGD threshold during the study. Similar results were found in a longitudinal study using a continuous scale measurement approach [26]. Additionally, Choo et al. [9] provided evidence for the divergent validity of IGD by showing that pathological video game players scored no differently from non-pathological players on measures of intelligence or socioeconomic status.

Li, Liau, and Khoo [27] asked participants to respond to a total of ten yes/no/sometimes items about pathological gaming adapted from the DSM-IV-TR criteria for pathological gambling. Researchers examined the relations among discrepancies between individuals' ideal and actual selves, depression, and subsequent pathological game play. Individuals who felt that their ideal self was different from their actual self experienced increased feelings of depression when compared to their peers. This depression led to increased levels of self-reported escapism and the heightened escapism led to an increase in pathological video game use. Escapism and discrepancies between actual and ideal self also had direct effects on pathological gaming—indicating a complex, multi-causal etiology.

These studies indicate that IGD is not simply a symptom of other disorders, such as depression, but does undergo changes based upon any other pathologies. These comorbidities may make treatment more difficult.

Treatment

Research into the efficient treatment of IGD is still in its infancy [28], although some studies have reported successful treatments [29]. These studies usually modify strategies shown to be successful in other types of addictions to target video game playing habits. Of note, bupropion (antidepressant and smoking cessation aid) treatment and cognitive behavioral therapy (CBT) have been shown to have short-term benefits [16, 30]. Bupropion treatment reduced cravings to play and video game cue-induced activity in the dorsolateral prefrontal cortex. This suggests that IGD can be treated in a manner similar to substance abuse or dependence. That said, critics have argued that the majority of studies into IGD treatment have failed to provide long-term follow-up reports after treatment and that there are not any strong randomized controlled studies yet. Since there is inadequate evidence to assess relapse and remission rates following IGD treatments, researchers should be cautious in interpreting their initial success. If the reliability and the validity of the IGD diagnosis are improved, an optimal treatment can be designed and utilized.

Conclusion

Since IGD is now in the DSM-5 as an emerging diagnosis, more research can be done to display inconsistencies in the classification of IGD. The American Psychiatric Association's DSM-5 behavioral addiction work group investigated the literature on several potential behavioral addictions, such as Internet, shopping, exercise, work, video gaming, as well as excessive eating and sexual behaviors [31]. The researchers concluded that the literature was too limited on all topics other than gaming, particularly when connected to the Internet, and thus only Internet Gaming Disorder was recommended for inclusion in the DSM-5.

Are Pathological Gaming and Internet Distinct?

The literature tends to cluster into two study foci—video games or the Internet more broadly. At one level of analysis, this is simply a distinction made by how questionnaires are worded. At another, however, it may signify different disorders. If Internet Gaming Disorder and Pathological Internet Use (PIU) are distinct disorders, what evidence would be needed to differentiate them? No matter the conceptualization, all addictions are based on the assumption that they are only clinically relevant if they cause dysfunction.

Preoccupation for PIU would be the excessive thinking about using the Internet or a preoccupation with the Internet that would lead to difficulties focusing on normal tasks. Chen, Wang, and Su (2003) cross over into the withdrawal domain with their criteria for PIU. Withdrawal for PIU would be near identical as it is for IGD, people would undergo unpleasant physical effects and/or negative emotions when attempting to cease or lower their Internet use. A requirement for Internet use to be problematic would be the inability to reduce usage overall, even after realizing the detriment it has. Davis, Flett, and Besser [32] mention social rejection as a drive for PIU, which leads to utilizing the Internet for escaping from the stressors of daily life. This becomes a problem when the only way that people are able to cope is through using the Internet.

Given the current state of the literature, we believe it is most parsimonious to consider PIU and IGD to be two different morphologies of a similar underlying technology addiction. This is similar to how people can be addicted to gambling despite doing almost nothing that looks the same—one puts money in a slot and pulls a lever, whereas another researches horses and jockeys. Nonetheless, we would diagnose both gambling addicts the same way, we would look for similar symptoms and outcomes, and treatment would share many characteristics. Thus, despite morphological differences, they are not distinct slot machine and horse racing addictions. Similarly, the vast majority of the research on video game or Internet addiction tend to show similar patterns of dysfunctional symptoms, similar outcomes, and similar responses to treatment.

That said, it is certainly possible that future research may find important distinctions between them. Within the past 5 years, work groups have been formed and given the task to further examine different disorders. More specifically, the "substance use disorder" (SUD) work group investigated different addictions, such as video gaming, shopping, exercise, work, as well as excessive eating and sexual behaviors [31]. The researchers concluded that the literature found on all other topics, besides video gaming, was limited, which resulted in the exclusion from Section III. Although there is no space to go into detail here, it is useful to consider what evidence would indicate that IGD and PIU were distinct taxons?

One might assume that they were distinct if the populations did not overlap much, that there would be limited comorbidity of IGD and PIU. Yet, there is no strong evidence of this. Only a small subset of slot machine addicts are also addicted to roulette or horse racing, but these are not distinctly different types of addiction. Therefore, we should not expect a majority of people addicted to video games to also be addicted to the Internet. IGD can also be viewed as dissimilar to PIU due to the distinctions and similarities with Internet use, gambling, and video gaming with the use of visual and auditory rewards [33].

One might also assume that if different scales are used to measure symptoms that they should be considered distinct issues. Yet, our experience with multiple video game addiction scales is that the disorder is robust to measurement differences. That is, we find essentially the same results no matter how we define or measure it. The good (?) news is that we can trust that the underlying problem seems to be real. The bad news is that it becomes more difficult to know what the specific characteristics are that might differentiate IGD and PIU.

Our current thinking is that we would be convinced that PIU is distinct from IGD if at least several of the following conditions were met:

- There are clearly different risk factors for who becomes addicted to the Internet or to games.
- There are clearly different protective factors between PIU and IGD.
- The etiologies and course of the pathologies were clearly distinct.
- There are different patterns of comorbidity with other mental health problems.
- The outcomes of each were clearly distinct.
- The treatments for one did not work for the other.

At present, there is not enough research to answer most of these questions, although the research on outcomes seems to show very similar outcomes for both (e.g., depression, anxiety, poor school performance, etc.). Therefore, given the dearth of clear evidence for most of these questions and the presence of similar outcomes, we argue that the argument over whether these are importantly different disorders is premature. It is, however, an important question that should motivate future research.

Clinical Implications

At our university, we have many first-year freshmen fail out at some point during their first year. Anecdotally, it seems that many of them have trouble with gaming, perhaps because they are away from home with no one checking up on them to see if they are going to class, they are in dorm rooms with other gamers, and they have 24-h high-speed Internet at their disposal. They may stay up all night gaming and skip classes. As their grades slip, they use games to help cope with the feelings of anxiety about failing. If they succeed in going to our student counseling service, they typically present with a complaint about failing grades. The therapist hears this and therefore asks grade-relevant questions in the clinical interview. These include, we expect, questions about their study habits, note-taking, class attendance, sleep, etc. The clinician does not ask about video games because the patient did not present with a complaint about gaming. The patient does not talk about video games, because to the patient, they are part of the solution, not the problem. That is, no one talks about what is likely to be an important part of the problem. One clinical implication, therefore, is that media habits should be part of standard intake questions. At a minimum, it would be useful to know how much time patients spend with electronic screens *not* for work or school purposes. We will note, however, that there is no magic number at which gaming or Internet appears to be clinically important. We recommend that children be limited to perhaps 1–2 h a day of total screen time (as the American Academy of Pediatrics used to recommend).We also recommend that screen time not be measured with a single item. In our experience, if you ask people how much time they play video games or watch TV a day or a week, they underestimate by more than half. If you ask them instead how much time they usually play from 6 am to noon, noon to 6 pm, 6 pm to midnight, and midnight to 6 am, separately for weekdays and weekends, then (in our experience) you get numbers that are more in line with the national averages. This can be done separately for games, for Internet, and for television (or other devices/uses) to get a detailed picture of screen time. It is important, however, to measure the use that is not for school or work, as these are functional uses and should not be used as a screen for potentially dysfunctional uses.

Screening: What tests should clinicians use in what ages (preferably validated instruments)?

For IGD we recommend using "The Internet Gaming Disorder Scale" [7] which is a scale that fits within the suggested APA guidelines for screening.

Conclusion

We feel that research on IGD (and also PIU) has been moving in the right direction. We are moving away from arguing over how to define and measure it and are starting to ask the more useful questions about risk and protective factors, etiology, comorbidity, and treatment. Asking these questions will also help to answer definitional and measurement questions.

As an example, we currently consider IGD (and PIU) to be likely to be a type of impulse control disorder. If this is correct, then treatments that are effective for those should work on these issues. This view is not universally accepted, however, and research that answers this question would be relevant for definitions and measurement.

Despite many questions still to be answered, the early research appears to be strong enough to warrant continuing to ask the questions and to treat seriously patients who present with concerns about gaming.

References

1. RTD. China's Digital Detox. A life reboot for internet gaming addicts [Internet]. YouTube. YouTube; 2016. https://www.youtube.com/watch?v=WtQevsY3OYw.
2. Chuang Y-C. Massively multiplayer online role-playing game-induced seizures: a neglected health problem in internet addiction. Cyberpsychol Behav. 2006;9(4):451–6.
3. Salmon A. CNN [Internet]. CNN. Cable News Network; 2010. http://edition.cnn.com/2010/WORLD/asiapcf/05/28/south.korea.virtual.baby/.

4. www.smh.com.au [Internet]. Chinese gamer dies after 'marathon' session—Games—Technology. http://www.smh.com.au/news/games/chinese-gamer-dies-after-marathon-session/2007/03/01/1172338774317.html.
5. Sim T, Gentile DA, Bricolo F, Serpelloni G, Gulamoydeen F. A conceptual review of research on the pathological use of computers, video games, and the internet. Int J Ment Heal Addict. 2012;10(5):748–69.
6. American Psychiatric Association. Diagnostic and statistical manual of mental disorders: DSM-5. Washington, DC: American Psychiatric Association; 2013.
7. Lemmens JS, Valkenburg PM, Gentile DA. The internet gaming disorder scale. Psychol Assess. 2015;27(2):567–82.
8. Bioulac SCA, Arfi L, Bouvard MP. Attention deficit/hyperactivity disorder and video games: a comparative study of hyperactive and control children. Eur Psychiatry. 2008;23(2):134–41.
9. Choo H, Gentile DA, Sim T, Li DD, Khoo A, Liau AK. Pathological video-gaming among Singaporean youth. Ann Acad Med Singapore. 2010;39(11):822–9.
10. Desai RA, Krishnan-Sarin S, Cavallo D, Potenza MN. Video-gaming among high school students: health correlates, gender differences, and problematic gaming. Pediatrics. 2010;126(6):e1414–24.
11. Fisher S. Identifying video game addiction in children and adolescents. Addict Behav. 1994;19(5):545–53.
12. Salguero RAT, Morán RMB. Measuring problem video game playing in adolescents. Addiction. 2002; 97(12):1601–6.
13. Thomas N, Martin FH. Video-arcade game, computer game and internet activities of Australian students: participation habits and prevalence of addiction. Aust J Psychol. 2010;62(2):59–66.
14. Ko C-H, Liu G-C, Hsiao S, Yen J-Y, Yang M-J, Lin W-C, et al. Brain activities associated with gaming urge of online gaming addiction. J Psychiatr Res. 2009;43(7): 739–47.
15. Groves C, Gentile D, Tapscott R, Lynch P. Testing the predictive validity and construct of pathological video game use. Behav Sci. 2015;5(4):602–25.
16. Han DH, Hwang JW, Renshaw PF. Bupropion sustained release treatment decreases craving for video games and cue-induced brain activity in patients with internet video game addiction. Exp Clin Psychopharmacol. 2010;18(4):297–304.
17. Gentile D. Pathological video-game use among youth ages 8 to 18: a National Study. Psychol Sci. 2009;20(5): 594–602.
18. Wan C-S, Chiou W-B. Psychological motives and online games addiction: a test of flow theory and humanistic needs theory for Taiwanese adolescents. Cyberpsychol Behav. 2006;9(3):317–24.
19. Granic I, Lobel A, Engels RC. The benefits of playing video games. Am Psychol. 2014;69(1):66.
20. Wang L, Zhu S. Online game addiction among university students. 2011. [Master's thesis]. Available from DiVA—Academic Archive Online database.
21. Wan C-S, Chiou W-B. Why are adolescents addicted to online gaming? An interview study in Taiwan. Cyberpsychol Behav. 2006;9(6):762–6.
22. Cole H, Griffiths MD. Social interactions in massively multiplayer online role-playing gamers. Cyberpsychol Behav. 2007;10(4):575–83.
23. Peng W, Liu M. Online gaming dependency: a preliminary study in China. Cyberpsychol Behav Soc Netw. 2010;13(3):329–33.
24. Hilgard J, Engelhardt CR, Bartholow BD. Individual differences in motives, preferences, and pathology in video games: the gaming attitudes, motives, and experiences scales (GAMES). Front Psychol. 2013;4:608.
25. Gentile DA, Choo H, Liau A, Sim T, Li D, Fung D, et al. Pathological video game use among youths: a two-year longitudinal study. Pediatrics. 2011;127(2).
26. Lam LT, Peng ZW. Effect of pathological use of the internet on adolescent mental health: a prospective study. Arch Pediatr Adolesc Med. 2010;164(10):901–6.
27. Li D, Liau A, Khoo A. Examining the influence of actual-ideal self-discrepancies, depression, and escapism, on pathological gaming among massively multiplayer online adolescent gamers. Cyberpsychol Behav Soc Netw. 2011;14(9):535–9.
28. King DL, Delfabbro PH. Internet gaming disorder treatment: a review of definitions of diagnosis and treatment outcome. J Clin Psychol. 2014;70(10):42–55.
29. Winkler A, Dörsing B, Rief W, Shen Y, Glombiewski JA. Treatment of internet addiction: a meta-analysis. Clin Psychol Rev. 2013;33(2):317–29.
30. Young KS. Cognitive behavior therapy with internet addicts: treatment outcomes and implications. Cyberpsychol Behav. 2007;10(5):671–9.
31. Petry NM, O'brien CP. Internet gaming disorder and the DSM-5. Addiction. 2013;108(7):1186–7.
32. Davis RA, Flett GL, Besser A. Validation of a new scale for measuring problematic internet use: implications for pre-employment screening. Cyberpsychol Behav. 2002;5(4):331–45.
33. Yau YH, Crowley MJ, Mayes LC, Potenza MN. Are internet use and video-game-playing addictive behaviors? Biological, clinical and public health implications for youths and adults. Minerva Psichiatr. 2012;53(3):153–70.

Check for updates

10 When Does Internet and Smartphone Use Become a Problem?

Nancy A. Cheever, Megan A. Moreno, and Larry D. Rosen

Fernando is a 14-year-old high school freshman who grew up with electronic screens in front of his face. His parents used an iPad to soothe him as a toddler and bought him his first smartphone at age 6. His elementary and middle school teachers prevented Fernando from using his device in the classroom; however, computer use was part of the curriculum. When not in school, Fernando used the smartphone to communicate with his parents—who both worked full-time—and with friends who also had a device. At night he kept his smartphone in his bed, along with a laptop and his video game controller, which was connected to a television that was on all night every night. Fernando was constantly connected and by the age of 11 was spending every minute of the day while not at school playing video games, surfing the Internet, posting and commenting on social media, listening to music, and texting and video chatting with friends. By the time Fernando turned 14, his parents noticed a drastic change in his mood—the once cheery boy had morphed into a moody, withdrawn, and anxiety-ridden teenager—and his grades had dropped considerably. All Fernando was interested in was his electronic devices, and when his parents attempted to put restrictions on their use, Fernando became increasingly agitated. His parents sought help from a therapist who diagnosed Fernando with an Internet addiction and encouraged his parents to remove all electronic devices—except the television—from the home for a period of time to slowly halt his addictive behavior and teach him to engage in more productive activities.

Did Fernando truly have a clinical disorder or was this a normal part of adolescence? How did his therapist know this was a disorder and not an emotional or developmental problem? These are the questions researchers attempt to answer as they investigate the ways in which these ubiquitous tools impact adolescents' mental health. This chapter will explore the various constructs and definitions of the negative mental health outcomes of Internet and smartphone use and examine the wide array of research devoted to identifying, understanding, and labeling this phenomenon.

N.A. Cheever (✉)
Department of Communications, California State University, Dominguez Hills, Carson, CA, USA
e-mail: ncheever@csudh.edu

M.A. Moreno
Department of Pediatrics, University of Wisconsin-Madison, Madison, WI, USA
e-mail: mamoreno@pediatrics.wisc.edu

L.D. Rosen
Department of Psychology, California State University, Dominguez Hills, Carson, CA, USA
e-mail: lrosen@csudh.edu

M.A. Moreno, A. Radovic (eds.), *Technology and Adolescent Mental Health*,
https://doi.org/10.1007/978-3-319-69638-6_10

allow for improved diagnosis and symptom monitoring without relying on patient self-report, such as those using technology tools.

The main characteristic of most mental health problems is the chronic and longitudinal aspect of the illness that requires continuous monitoring and treatment. Mental illness is often accompanied with physiological and behavioral changes in the patient's life that span over a period of time. However, traditional methods of treatment are limited to regular or occasional visits to the clinic and therapy sessions where the medical professional gets an update of the patient's status by asking questions and filling out psychiatric questionnaires. The practitioner must rely on the patient's explanation, memory, and subjective measurements (which are often biased depending on the patient's condition, memory, and willingness to share) to acquire the patient's health status and to adjust treatment accordingly (e.g., changing medication). As such, treatments for mental health problems often lack objective measurements and personalization that are aligned with the patients' lifestyle.

Advances in technology now make it possible to continuously and effectively monitor physiological, social, and sleep behaviors outside of the clinical environment, offering the potential of early detection, management, and treatment of mental health problems. Early detection could be used to stage an earlier intervention, thus preventing relapse and shortening the total time patients suffer from mental illnesses.

The following describes three major application areas where technology could offer significant benefits in mental healthcare, namely, *detection and diagnosis*, *monitoring and treatment management*, and *patient self-monitoring*. As much of this research has focused on adult populations, the focus of this chapter will be in describing methods in which technology can be used to measure depressive symptoms, with a discussion on specific utility in adolescents at the end. The chapter will discuss how the technology can be used to monitor mental health conditions rather than when and why monitoring should happen.

Detection and Diagnosis

The onset of mental illness is associated with a change from normal life patterns and behavior, and therefore, an understanding of a person's state of being before the illness is required for accurate diagnosis. Most mental health problems share some key behavioral indicators including change in activity, sleep, social interactions, and physical and cognitive responses. Technology can be used to detect if there is a behavior change that may indicate a person is transitioning from a healthy mental state to a risk state. The baseline for normal behavior can be acquired from traces of technology use, e.g., patterns of web surfing, smartphone usage, and social communications on the phone before the start of a mental condition. Such digital traces are already being tracked and collected. For example, web browsers keep a history of visited websites, and each person on average has at least 6 months of call and SMS logs as well as e-mail communications and social media use. This data can be analyzed to detect the onset or progress of mental illnesses.

The Big Black Dog (BBD) is an example of such applications that was designed to detect the onset of depression by identifying behavior change in people with major depression via longitudinal monitoring of the phone and technology use in adults [16]. The BBD app runs in the background of the phone and collects data related to movement, communication, and technology use to generate a baseline of normal behavior. A relapse or an onset of depression is detected when a change in behavior is continuously observed for at least 2 weeks (which is the time window for clinical diagnosis of depression).

Clinical Monitoring and Treatment Management

As mentioned, the longitudinal aspect of mental disorders makes it challenging for practitioners to track the development and progress of the illness outside of the clinical environment. Current treatment of mental illnesses is based on pharmacological and psychotherapeutic techniques, which are often characterized by low compliance from patients. Intelligent health and behavior monitoring systems can help practitioners more effectively track and monitor the reactions patients have to different therapies and medical treatments. The system can provide significantly more fine-grained behavior data as well as models and visualizations of this data, thus providing insights on the illness beyond what can be done today. Practitioners could use the models and visualizations during treatment to assess how well a treatment is working. This is important as many drug and psychotherapies fail to have a beneficial effect.

The wide usage of personal devices such as smartphones, wearable devices (e.g., [17]), and laptops as well as social media and web provides opportunities for tracking and monitoring behavioral and health status of patients on a daily basis. Smartphones, with embedded sensors, expand the ability to track symptoms, provide feedback, and deliver interventions as part of clinical treatment. As more people adopt today's technology, treatment protocols in mental health involving technology are becoming increasingly acceptable. This adaptation allows healthcare workers to remotely monitor patients' conditions and adjust their treatments accordingly in a timely manner. MONARCA (Figs. 11.1 and 11.2) is an example of such an application that provides multimodal sensing and monitoring of bipolar disorder by both therapists and patients themselves. MONARCA [18–20] incorporates self-reporting, automatic manic-depressed episode prediction, and professional management of bipolar disorder to enable communication and continuous monitoring of the condition. A study of the MONARCA application showed the feasibility of self-monitoring by combining sensor data with self-reports [18]. Both patients and practitioners appreciated the insights the MONARCA system provides through processing and visualizing data collected on patients' mobile phones.

Patient Self-Monitoring

In addition to medical treatment, patients' adherence to the treatment and their awareness of their condition is crucial in controlling the illness. Self-monitoring is especially important in mental illness, e.g., bipolar disorder, where treatment requires patient engagement in treatment and awareness of change in mood and behavior. Self-tracking of symptoms and behavior can help patients control and better understand their condition. It can also help reveal how patients' explicit actions impact their illness.

A relatively new research field called Personal Informatics [21, 22] or Quantified Self [23, 24] studies the use of technology to collect and reflect on personal information. Smartphone technology has extensively been used for health

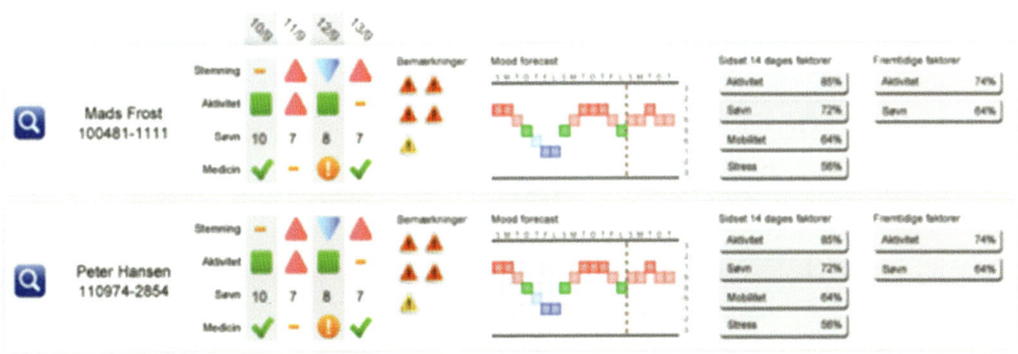

Fig. 11.1 Web portal for practitioners in the MONARCA project [18] provides an overview of the state of each bipolar patient. When a patient is at risk of a manic or depressed episode for consecutive days (according to the forecast), the practitioner contacts the patient or caregivers to check the status of the patient and acquire more information. The patient names are fake in the figure

and well-being monitoring and feedback. Numerous self-tracking applications in the App Store and Play Store (e.g., [25]) allow users to use their smartphone to track and monitor different aspects of their life including health, fitness, behavior, emotions, and habits. These applications gather data from different sources and visualize it in a personal dashboard. Examples of such applications include Health Mashups [26], UbiFitGarden [27], Bewell [28] (Fig. 11.3), Health Buddy [29], Mobile Mood Diary [30], MONARCA [18, 20] (Fig. 11.2), and Mobilyze! [31]. Other applications collect more general-purpose data that can be used for different purposes including health monitoring. AWARE [32] is an example of such an application that is able to collect data from the rich set of built-in sensors in smartphones and wearable devices including accelerometers, location (GPS, WiFi, signal strength), light, and microphone as well as sensors for tracking heart rate, skin temperature, and galvanic skin response (Fig. 11.4). AWARE can securely collect and transfer/synchronize data to the central server.

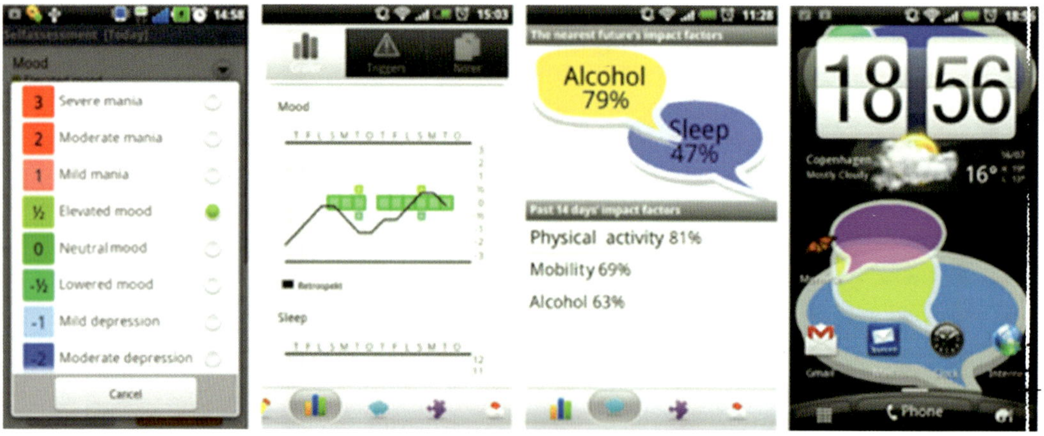

Fig. 11.2 The ambient display on patient's phone in the MONARCA app [18] shows impact factors related to mood in bipolar patients. Both self-reports and sensor data are processed to provide an overview of the patient's mental state for self-monitoring

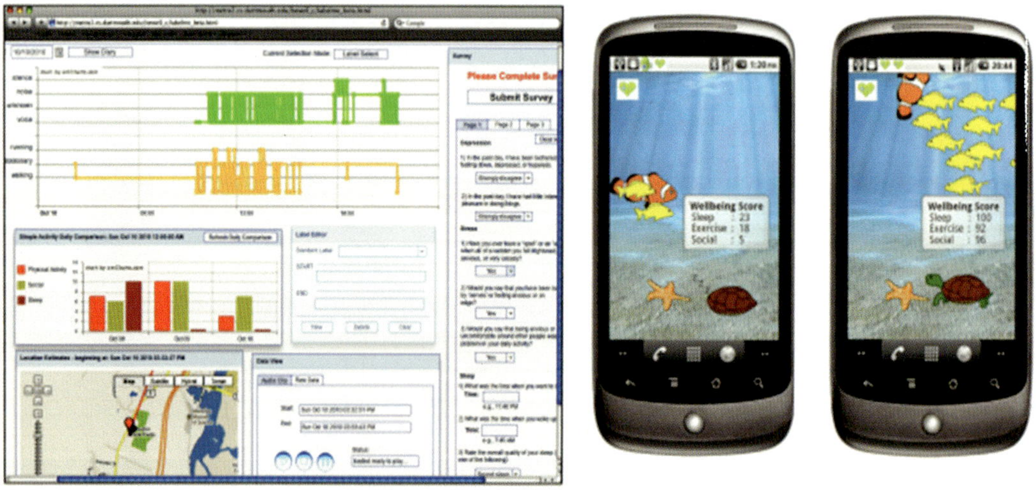

Fig. 11.3 Web portal and ambient display in the Bewell app [28] show the status of physical, social, and sleep in individuals. The three different animals in the animated aquatic ecosystem each represent a behavior aspect that is affected by change in well-being

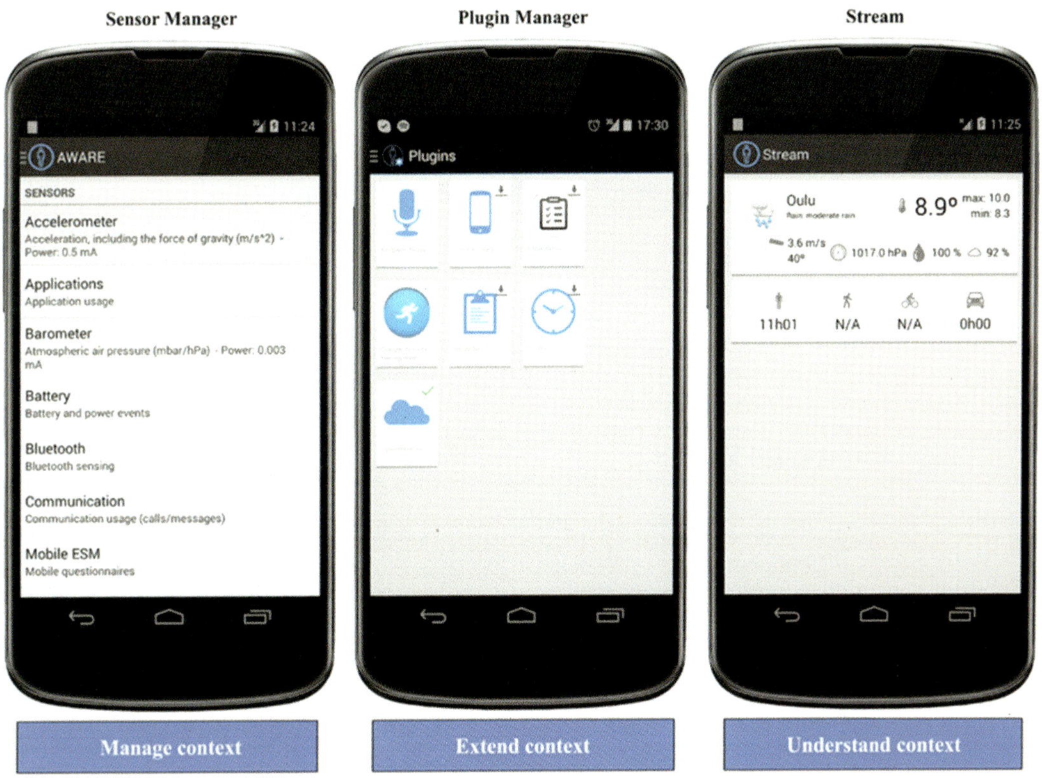

Fig. 11.4 AWARE mobile client with capability to collect data from phone channels, wearable devices, and online sources such as weather websites [32]

Health community websites and online tools are other ways for people to share experience; record their mood, sleep, medication taken, and life events; as well as seek support and help. Websites such as curetogether.com, patientslikeme.com, and mentalhelp.net allow users to log an enormous range of conditions, symptoms, and feelings and to see visualizations and statistical analyses of patient's progress over time. Technology-based self-tracking has shown good receptivity and adherence by individuals with mental health conditions, e.g., bipolar disorder [33–35].

The rest of the chapter focuses on describing how technology can be used in identifying the symptoms of depression.

Identifying Symptoms of Depression Using Technology

Depression is a mood disorder that can take many different forms, including major depressive disorder, bipolar disorder, and substance-induced mood disorder. Depression can also be a major symptom of other disorders such as post-traumatic stress disorder (PTSD). This section describes the common symptoms of depression followed by technological advances that can help with detection of those symptoms. According to the DSM-V, a manual used to diagnose mental disorders, major depressive disorder occurs when a person has at least five of the following physical, behavioral, and cognitive symptoms at the same time for at least 2 weeks:

- A depressed mood during most of the day (in adolescents can be an irritable mood)
- Fatigue or loss of energy almost every day
- Feelings of worthlessness or guilt almost every day
- Impaired concentration, indecisiveness
- Insomnia (inability to sleep) or hypersomnia (excessive sleeping) almost every day

- Markedly diminished interest or pleasure in almost all activities nearly every day
- Recurring thoughts of death or suicide (not just fearing death)
- A sense of restlessness or being slowed down
- Significant weight loss or weight gain

The following sections describe how technology can be used to identify each of those symptoms from nonverbal (physiological and behavioral) and verbal signals.

Physiological and Brain Signals

Nonverbal cues including physiological and behavioral signals provide a rich data source for identifying symptoms of depression. Researchers have investigated brain signals [36], heart rate [37], blood pressure [38], voice prosody [39, 40], and facial expression [39] as proxies for psychophysiological information. For example, heart rate variability (HRV), which is the change in the inter-beat interval of the heart, has been shown to indicate levels of stress (both physical and mental) and fatigue [41, 42] as well as physical activity [43].

Although EEGs, heart rate trackers, and skin conductors provide means to collect physiological data, they are cumbersome to wear, often difficult to use, and typically limited to being used in clinics. With smartphones, laptops, and wearable devices, it is possible to acquire physiological and behavioral expressions related to inner emotional and mental state in a less cumbersome way by collecting the physiological signals and traces of technology use.

The following describes technology to extract information from nonverbal communications such as voice quality, facial expressions, and interactions with technology.

Vocal Prosody

Vocal prosody can strongly convey a person's psychological and emotional state [44]. These features are especially valuable in detecting depression where disruption in emotion expression, communication, and self-regulation are key factors [45–47]. There has been extensive work in the link between vocal prosody features and emotion (e.g., [48–51]). Vocal prosody consists of acoustic features extracted from speech and includes pitch or vocal fundamental frequency (F0), loudness or intensity, and timing "which is perceived as speech rate, rhythm, and patterning in normal conversation. Related features include jitter and shimmer (cycle-to-cycle variation in frequency and intensity), energy distribution among formants, and cepstral features" [52].

As depression causes psychomotor retardation (including slowness, insensitivity to positive and negative stimuli, and attenuated interest in other people), acoustic features such as decreased intensity, irregular timing, and decreased F0 variability can be useful indicators of depression. Acoustic features have also been used to detect stress with more than 76% accuracy [53].

Since acoustic processing methods are prone to privacy concerns, the audio signals can be locally processed and features can be extracted in real time. This in turn requires usage of the least computationally expensive processing methods to compensate the battery demand in, e.g., smartphones.

More sophisticated methods can be used to extract more information from a person's voice. This, e.g., includes speech analysis algorithms [53–58] to do voice segmentation and to extract pitch information to characterize the psychological state of patients with depression.

Facial Expressions

Facial expression is an important and observable modality that can reflect internal state. Common depression symptoms such as extreme sadness and depressed mood, lack of interest and indifference, and tiredness are often revealed in the face. Image processing techniques provide the opportunity to infer facial expressions from captured images, and studies have demonstrated that emotions and pain can be detected from those images (e.g., [59–61], [62]). Mobile and personal devices are equipped with cameras capable of capturing the facial images momentarily and easily. This data is a useful source of information to identify the emotional and mental state of people with depression. Some facial expressions have a high level of consistency and repetition that help distinguish different emotions using image processing methods and techniques.

Despite the usefulness of facial expression in detecting depression, acquiring this data in the everyday life of patients (out of lab and uncontrolled) is challenging. Smartphone cameras can be used for collecting facial expression [47]; however, real-time capturing of facial images is affected by situations such as light conditions, motions, rotations, and image quality. In addition, to preserve privacy, local processing might be preferred which adds power and computational constraints (in case a smartphone or another personal device is used for data collection). Another challenge occurs when patients themselves collect their facial images (to capture the moments they feel, e.g., sad). The patients' conditions and compliance has also an impact on the time the image is captured. For example, if the patient feels extremely sad or suicidal, the last thing they can care about is to capture their facial expression. Additionally, the effect of acting for the camera also generates a further confound, though in most cases, acted and natural emotions can be automatically differentiable. However, most of those challenges can be addressed with enough data collection, namely, having multiple instances of each expression over a period of time and analyzing the data to infer the state of the patient. The widespread use of smartphone cameras and the tendency of taking frequent selfies in especially young adults provide opportunity to collect a rich set of facial expressions from individuals in different emotional and mental states and use it to help diagnose potential development of depression.

The accuracy of computational models to recognize facial expressions depends on the number of training samples collected from patients. However, as mentioned previously, data collection from people with depression is affected by their condition and status of illness. A solution to the lack of enough facial expressions from individual patients is to use the available datasets that contain real-world classified samples of facial images (e.g., AM-FED dataset) [63] along with software that can facilitate image analysis (e.g., Affdex) and use them as baseline to further build a model and incorporate it in a system that is used for classifying the facial expression of each patient in real time. Using this approach, Suk et al. demonstrated the successful classification of seven affective states on mobile devices [64].

Reaction Time and Physical Responses

Some emotional and mental states impact the body and physical responses to the external stimuli. For example, fatigue has been shown to affect reaction time in individuals [65]. Fatigue is a common symptom of depression and typically classified into two general types, mental fatigue that affects an individual's cognitive processes and physical fatigue that affects an individual's ability to maintain physical actions. Mental fatigue impacts task motivation [66] and results in a loss of efficiency and lower productivity [67]. Studies have shown that reaction time is adversely affected by both physical and mental fatigue [65] suggesting we may see slower reaction times in depressed people. Measuring the reaction time is often done using a simple reaction time (SRT) test developed by Galton in 1889 where a person's response to a simple stimulus is recorded (Galton, 1889). This early test is also used as the basis for the choice reaction time (CRT) test, which records the time it takes a person to choose a correct response from a number of alternatives.

Today's technology makes it possible to acquire data to help detect such physical responses as a result of the mental and emotional state. For instance, widespread availability of touch-based devices and increase in the usage of instant messaging apps (e.g., WhatsApp) have opened new possibilities of inferring the reaction time from touch interactions and keystroke dynamics (Fig. 11.5).

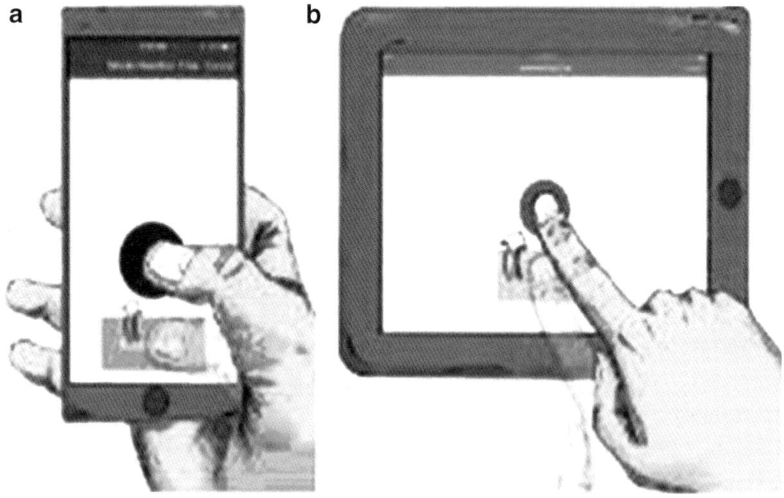

Fig. 11.5 A mobile app for acquiring the reaction time, with permission from [110]. (**a**) mobile phone version. (**b**) tablet version

Numerous studies have used typing and touch interactions to infer emotions and mental state. For example, Gao et al. used multiple finger-stroke-related features to identify different emotional states during a touch-based game play [68]. Wac et al. detected stress conditions by analyzing multiple features of swipe, scroll, and text input interactions in a smartphone [69]. Kim et al. [70] proposed an emotion recognition framework analyzing touch behavior during touch interaction using 12 attributes from 3 onboard sensors.

Keystroke dynamics has been shown to be an effective modality for automatic detection of person's affective states [71]. A person's typing pattern on a computer or keyboard is a useful and easy-to-get source of data that can reveal the physical, emotional, and cognitive state of the person [72]. Typing attributes such as typing speed, duration of typing, speed of typing, use of special characters, mistakes while typing denoted by the use of delete key, delay between typing each letter, and use of emoticons are among the most informative features.

Similar to typing activity, useful features related to touch such as pressure, speed of touch, scroll, swipe, and the number of switches between screens or apps (e.g., on tablet or smartphone) can reveal cues about the psychological state of the person including stress, fatigue, and different emotions. The consistency in emotions will indicate the overall normal or depressed mood of the person on a daily basis. These measures can also be acquired during games.

Social Behavior

Change in social relationships and communication between people with strong ties is a strong indicator of developing depression. For example, in a study of behavior change in people with major depression using the Big Black Dog (BBD) application, an increase in the number of outgoing calls in female participants was a predictor of worsening in the status of depression [16].

Social isolation, which is a mental health classification for describing people with weak social integration, poor social networks, and few ongoing relationships with strong social ties, has been linked with an increased likelihood for major depression [73] and increased risk of suicide [74]. Social behavior can be used as a proxy for social support and social isolation. For example, dramatic changes in the quantity of social interaction and the places people spend their time is indicative of social isolation. Detection of change in social relationships, however, requires having a baseline of people's normal behavior and network. Smartphone and social media communication logs provide the possibility to acquire this baseline as most people on average have at least 6 months of social media and call and messaging logs. Studies have used communication logs from smartphones and from people's online social networking services to model social interactions and interpersonal relationships. One study [75] applied machine learning techniques to contact lists, call logs, and SMS logs to classify the social facet (family, work, social) of a contact. By extracting features such as communication intensity, communication regularity, temporal tendency, and choice of communication channels, they could classify the life facet of participants at around 90% accuracy based on these factors. Another work used the same dataset from above to create computational models of social tie strength (people's self-reported feelings of closeness to one another) and achieved about 75% accuracy in classifying contacts as high, medium, or low tie strength.

Additional tools that collect logs of e-mail activity and activity on the social networking service (e.g., Facebook) can also be developed to capture the social behavior. For both e-mail and Facebook, the actions of sending/posting/commenting, receiving/viewing, and replying/commenting on communications can be logged, modeled, and compared to normal behavior before development of illness as evidence of changes in social patterns.

Location data can also help understand certain aspects of people's social relationships with others. For example, past work [76, 77] has developed the concept of place entropy, which characterizes the number of unique people seen at a place. Places with high entropy tend to be public places, such as coffee shops, stores, and restaurants, whereas places with low entropy tend to be residential. By analyzing the places that people go, and by also linking it to addresses in their contact list, we can gain more insight into a person's social behaviors. The WiFi ID, GSM signal strength, and GPS are useful in determining location information at various levels of accuracy.

Numerous applications have used location data to extract different information about individuals' behavior and daily life. For example, data from apps such as Locaccino, a mobile app for sharing one's current location with friends, can be used to characterize the social quality of different places that people spend time at [77] and to predict friendships between people based on co-location patterns [76]. Location data can also be used to learn routine activities and to characterize people's social behaviors and develop ways of modeling and visualizing changes over time.

Physical Activity and Mobility

Symptoms such as fatigue, sense of slowness, and decreased interest in daily activities can be detected from changes in physical activity and mobility patterns. Canzian and Musolei [78] show significant correlations between various measures of mobility derived from location traces with depressive mood. The findings in [20, 79] demonstrate correlations between activity levels and psychiatric evaluation scores for mania and depression in bipolar disorder.

Both activity and mobility patterns can be extracted fairly accurately using current smartphone and wearable technology [80–82]. These devices are capable of counting steps, tracking exercise and aerobic activities, and movement patterns. Smartphones and wearable devices can track the states of stationary (sitting), walking, running, biking, or in vehicle. In addition, the location information captured by the phone's GPS or derived from WiFi signals is often used to infer the locational context in which the activities were taking place (e.g., gym). Other sensors such as barometer combined with accelerometer and gyroscope can identify the degree of incline of a particular route taken and speed to detect, e.g., hiking or climbing.

Weight monitoring can also be utilized by detection of gait change through a phone's accelerometer. Current technology for weight tracking is limited to diary apps to monitor food consumption and body weight measured by a scale. Smart scales provide the capability of logging weight measures into a mobile app. However, these approaches require compliance and continuous self-monitoring which is pruned to discontinuity and missing measures as the patients' condition changes or worsens. Mobile phone accelerometer has shown to detect changes in gait in cases of alcohol use [83].

Sleep Duration and Quality

Depression has been strongly linked to sleep quality. Past work has found that sleep disorders are correlated with depression, and many patients experience excessive sleepiness or insomnia when in a depressed state [84]. In addition, an emerging pattern of disrupted sleep has been found to predict the onset of recurrence [85].

Detection of sleep disruption is important in the diagnosis of depression. Healthcare practitioners typically diagnose sleep disruptions by having patients fill out paper-based instruments. The Pittsburgh Sleep Quality Index [86] is one of the most widely used instruments for sleep.

Polysomnography is the gold standard for assessing sleep, which combines an all-night electroencephalogram with measures of muscle tone and eye movements. However, polysomnography is only suited for laboratory settings as it requires professional staff, special equipment, and setup. Actigraphy (used in, e.g., Fitbit and Microsoft Band) is another successful approach in detecting sleep using movements captured by the accelerometer in, e.g., wearable devices. Actigraphy has been surprisingly accurate and is widely used in clinical settings to measure basic sleep information, such as sleep duration, number of waking, and sleep efficiency (i.e., percent of total sleep time) [87].

In addition to sensors, a number of smartphone apps help users manually track their sleep, for example, Tylenol PM Sleep Tracker [88], YawnLog [89], and Wellness Diary [90]. Other apps try to automate sleep logging. Examples include apps that use sound [91, 92] and accelerometers to track movement in bed [93, 94]. These apps require the phone to be placed on the bed. Bai et al. designed a system to predict sleep quality based on mobility, activity, and social interaction of the previous day [95].

Toss 'N' Turn (TNT) [96] is an automated sleep monitoring that only requires keeping the phone in the bedroom but not necessarily on the bed. This works well as people increasingly are using their smartphones as alarm clocks [97]. TNT (Fig. 11.6) is less focused on detecting precise sleep start and end times and more focused on inferring disruptions associated with insomnia or unusually long sleep sessions which are indicators of depression. TNT was designed to support complex sleep situations including people who sleep with others in the same room (romantic partner, baby, roommate, or pet) and people who sleep with lights, music, or white noise generators turned on. The app captures accelerometer, sound level (only amplitude for privacy reasons), proximity, and light. It also captures whether the phone's screen is on or off, what applications are running, location data (to know time zone as well and if the person is at home or not), and the local sunrise and sunset times. The app uses this data to infer sleep duration and quality with 84% accuracy in sleep quality.

Location data can be useful for sleep time and quality detection, allowing us to understand if the person is at home or elsewhere, as well as looking up sunrise and sunset data, two features that can

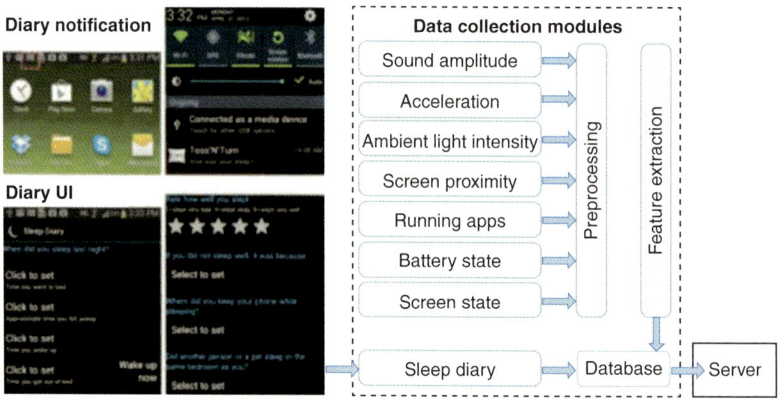

Fig. 11.6 Overview of Toss 'N' Turn [96]. The app shows a notification for a daily sleep diary, collects sensor data, and uploads the data every day to a server

be used for inferring sleep efficiency. Sound also provides clues about the sleep stages (awake-asleep), but it is the most sensitive piece of data to collect. To protect privacy, only the sound level and not actual sound can be collected. The logs of smartphone usage, including timestamps for screen on/off and a usage log with timestamps for all apps are also useful sources of information for sleep duration and quality detection.

Patterns of Technology Use

Technology is extensively used in everyday life of individuals especially the younger population. Traces of technology use provide a tacit yet useful source of data for identifying the psychological state of individuals. Patterns of usage correlate with lifestyle and state of well-being, and change in those patterns can be indicative of change in mental state. For example, if a person is using their phone significantly less or making fewer phone calls than usual, it might reveal the tendency toward social isolation and feeling of indifference, or frequent switching between apps may indicate lack of concentration. Smartphone logs including timestamps for screen on/off (indicating how frequently the phone was used), the types of apps a person has installed on the phone as well as their frequency and duration of usage, number of calls and text messages, and the patterns of using instant messaging apps, e.g., WhatsApp and Snapchat, are among feature attributes that provide useful clues about the mental state of the person. This data can help reveal if people are generally using their phone more or less, if they have a change in the apps they are using, or if there is a change in the time of day when they are using their phone. As depression is associated with change in the normal behavior, these feature attributes can help detect the symptoms of depression. Results of a study for detecting behavior change in people with depression demonstrated an inverse relationship between the CESD score and outgoing calls in male patients (fewer calls when more depressed), and a direct relationship between the CESD score and outgoing calls in female patients, i.e., more and longer outgoing calls when more depressed [16].

An observation of Internet traffic patterns among 216 students also showed that students with depressive symptoms used internet significantly more than those without symptoms [98, 99]. Information about traffic flow that the university customarily collects for troubleshooting network connections and such was used as data source for the analysis. The analysis showed that participants with depressive symptoms tended to engage in very high e-mail usage which is in line with another research by the psychologists Janet Morahan-Martin and Phyllis Schumacher demonstrating the correlation between frequent checking of e-mail and high levels of anxiety, which itself correlates with depressive symptoms [99]. It may also be indicative of social isolation and avoiding face-to-face interaction with other people. The Internet usage of depressed people also showed a so-called high flow duration entropy as a sign of frequent switching between Internet applications such as e-mail, chat rooms, social media, and games. This frequent switching may indicate difficulty concentrating. Another feature indicative of depressive symptoms included increased amounts of video watching, gaming, and chatting which again relates to isolation and avoidance of face-to-face social interaction.

Verbal Expressions

People with depression or other mental health issues may seek social support in their networks through social media and instant messaging tools. The text analysis and natural language processing methods provide means to analyze communications and thoughts of a person and use it to measure possible symptoms of depression. De Choudhury et al. used messages on Twitter to detect depression [100]. They analyzed 1 year of tweets from people who had experienced an episode of depression and measured behavioral attributes relating to social engagement, emotion, language and linguistic styles, ego network, and mentions of antidepressant medications. They find that social media contains useful signals for characterizing the onset of depression in individuals.

Important indicators included a decrease in social activity, raised negative affect, highly clustered ego networks, heightened relational and medicinal concerns, and greater expression of religious involvement.

Another research examined differences in language usage among depressed and non-depressed college students, and the findings demonstrated that depressed people used negative words more often than non-depressed people. The study also showed more frequent use of the word "I" in depressed people [101].

Self-Reports as Signals

As mentioned previously, most diagnosis and treatment of mental illness rely on patients' self-reporting of the crisis episodes often after they occurred. These self-reports are subject to bias due to patients' condition and subjective assessments. Although some emotional, mental, and physical cues can objectively be collected from personal devices and sensors, they are more complicated to be recognized with the existing out-of-the-lab instruments. Recent research studies have addressed this issue by using ecological momentary assessment (EMA) or experience sampling method (ESM) to collect subjective data from patients in different intervals (e.g., daily or weekly) via triggering a very short survey or diary/journal on their mobile phones. This subjective data is often used as the ground truth for further diagnosis and analysis of patients' status. The EMA data may include information about sleep quality, medication intake, alcohol intake, smoking, and the standard instrumental questions (e.g., CES-D for depression [102]) to acquire the patient's mental state and well-being. Depending on the type of data, these self-reports will have varying frequencies. For example, sleep quality should be acquired once every day, while it is enough for CES-D questions to be asked every week. A growing number of studies have begun using technology to deliver EMAs as part of psychological monitoring, for instance, to track interpersonal processes [103] or depression [104]. Photographic affect meter (PAM), developed at Cornell University, is another form of ESM where users choose among photos one that best describes their affective state (Fig. 11.7). PAM has been successfully used in several health studies and is integrated into AWARE data collection framework [32] (Table 11.1).

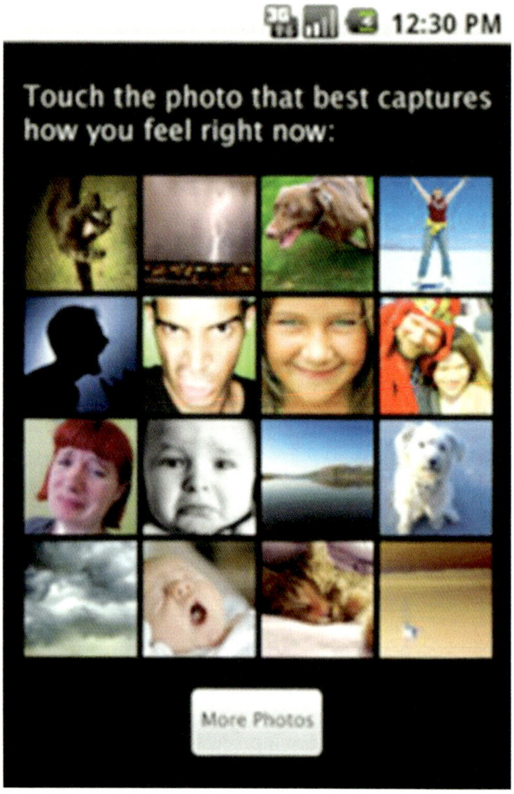
12:30 PM
Touch the photo that best captures how you feel right now:
More Photos

Fig. 11.7 PAM for measuring affect through the choice of a photo that describes one's affective state [111]

Technological Challenges in Data Collection and Interpretation

Although rapid advances in technology provide means to track and collect fine-grained physiological, psychological, and behavioral signals, a variety of factors affect data quality and data interpretation which in some cases have a major impact on the outcome. On one hand, more fine-grained, more frequent, and continuous sampling is ideal to capture all aspects of a patients' life, and on the other hand, technological boundaries such as battery life (in, e.g., smartphones and wearable devices), privacy concerns (e.g., tracking location

Table 11.1 Summary of signals for identifying symptoms related to depression

Type of signal	Technology and tools	Features	Symptoms to identify
Physiological (heart rate, galvanic skin response, skin temperature, blood pressure) and brain signals	Heart rate trackers, blood pressure tracker, skin conductors, wearable devices (e.g., Fitbit, band, smartphone), MRI, FMRI, EEG	Heart rate intensity, heart rate variability, brain waves	Fatigue, stress and anxiety, lack of concentration, depressed mood, negative emotions, cognitive impairment
Vocal prosody	Microphone (e.g., in smartphones and laptop)	Pitch, intensity, speech rate and rhythm, variation in frequency and intensity, energy distribution among formants, and cepstral features	Slowness in activities, lack of interest in other people and daily activities, and a feeling of indifference
Facial expressions	Camera (e.g., in smartphones or laptop)	Image processing, classification of facial images	Extreme sadness and depressed mood, lack of interest and indifference, and tiredness
Reaction time and physical responses	Personal devices (e.g., smartphone and laptop), skin conductors	Simple reaction time test, choice reaction time test, touch interactions (e.g., pressure, speed of touch, scroll, swipe, and the number of switches between screens or apps), and keystroke dynamics (e.g., typing speed, duration of typing, speed of typing, use of special characters, mistakes while typing denoted by the use of delete key, delay between typing each letter, and use of emoticons)	Fatigue, stress and anxiety, lack of concentration, depressed mood, negative emotions, cognitive impairment
Social behavior	Microphone, location tracking, call logs, messages, social media	Changes in quantity of social interaction, social media activity (number and time of posts, likes, comments, time, frequency, and duration of visits), frequent places people spend their time, time and duration of stay (e.g., bar vs. home), communication intensity (e.g., number and duration of calls and messages), communication regularity, temporal tendency, and choice of communication channel (e.g., call vs. text) and social ties from contact lists	Social isolation, lack of interest and indifference, stress and anxiety
Physical activity and mobility	Location tracking, accelerometer (e.g., in smartphones and wearable devices)	Travel distance, amount of active time vs. sedentary, amount of time staying at a place (e.g., home or work), gait detection	Slowness in activities, lack of interest and indifference, social isolation, weight change
Sleep duration and quality	Accelerometer, microphone, EEG, MRI, FMRI, smartphone, laptop use and web surfing patterns	Time, duration, and frequency of phone usage during night hours, type of apps, time and duration of computer/internet use, noise amplitude, magnitude of movement	Insomnia or hypersomnia

(continued)

Table 11.1 (continued)

Type of signal	Technology and tools	Features	Symptoms to identify
Patterns of technology use	Social media and web, personal devices (e.g., smartphone, laptop, wearables)	Time, duration, and frequency of phone usage, type of apps, time and duration of computer/internet use	Social isolation, lack of concentration, lack of interest in daily activities and indifference
Social media and communication content	Social media, text messages, e-mail	Heightened relational and medicinal concerns, greater expression of religious involvement, type and frequency of words being used (e.g., negative vs. positive, use of word I)	Depressed mood, thoughts of suicide, negative emotions and sadness, stress and anxiety
Self-reports	Smartphone, web portal	Frequency of self-reports, missing reports, self-report scores	Depressed mood, thoughts of suicide, negative emotions and sadness, stress and anxiety

and voice), and novelty effect limit our abilities to take full advantage of the available resources and technology. It is, therefore, recommended to find markers in the signals that are discriminative enough and can be acquired with a higher quality as a trade-off for lower sampling frequency.

Continuous data collection has to be seamless without affecting a patients' regular usage of technology and lifestyle. For example, too fine-grained location data and high sampling frequency has a draining effect on a smartphone battery, which will become a source of disengagement with the technology in a short time. The sampling rate and accuracy requirements should be adjusted to better manage usage of the battery while minimizing the loss of information. New versions of location-tracking applications adjust the sampling frequency based on the change in movements and distance detected from the phone's accelerometer. This approach has been proposed in several research studies [105, 106] and been integrated in smartphone APIs.

Using Technology for Monitoring Mental Health in Adolescents

Self-reports and behavioral therapy may not have the same effect in adolescents as in adults due to adolescents' reluctance to disclose emotions and mental issues. The widespread use of technology among adolescents, however, allows for objective measurements as well as improved diagnosis and symptom monitoring in this vulnerable population. In adolescents, smartphone use is ubiquitous and nondiscriminatory across race, ethnicity, and socioeconomic status. Using a mobile phone to detect and monitor depressive symptoms offers an opportunity, which may be feasible and generalizable in the adolescent population.

Recent research studies have focused on using mobile technology for mental health monitoring in young adults (e.g., [107, 108]). For example, a randomized controlled trial used the mobiletype program [108], a mental health assessment and management mobile phone application to examine the benefits of using mobile applications to monitor mental health status in adolescents and young adults aged 14–24. The users reported their mood, stress, coping strategies, activities, eating, sleeping, exercise patterns, and alcohol and cannabis use on a daily basis for 2–4 weeks, and this information was shared with general practitioners via a secure website for medical review. The results showed using mobiletype application significantly increased emotional self-awareness among young adults compared to the control group. This application, however, relies on self-reports and is bound to subjective bias and lack of objectivity.

StudentLife study [109], on the other hand, tried to assess mental health in college students via objective behavior tracking on mobile phones. Activities, sleep, conversations, and mobility patterns showed negative correlations with depression score among 48 college students during one semester at Dartmouth College. Another study [98], which was previously discussed in this chapter, showed the reverse relationship between Internet use and depression in college students. A third study demonstrated the negative language use in depressed college students on social media [101]. These results provide evidence for the feasibility of tracking technology in monitoring health status in adolescents. As such, a system such as MONARCA [19] that incorporates the full feedback loop between patients, caregivers, and practitioners can be adapted to monitor the progress of mental health conditions in adolescents.

A typical scenario can be described as follows:

Jim, a 15-year-old boy, has been diagnosed with bipolar disorder. He installs the mental health assessment app on his phone that tracks his phone usage, activities, locations, social communications, facial expression, and voice quality while preserving his privacy. Jim also fills out a short diary everyday to answer questions about his condition and to track his warning signs. Jim enters sleeping in the living room as a sign of manic episode. This information is shared with Jim's doctor and therapist. The app tracks Jim's sleep quality and the place he sleeps. When a change in Jim's sleep location is detected for consecutive days, the app sends a warning sign to Jim as well as a notification to his therapist and parents. Jim or his parents schedule a visit to the therapist. During the session, the therapist reviews the history of Jim's medication and his daily behavior patterns over the past 2 weeks to discuss the change with Jim and his parents.

References

1. NMIH. http://www.mentalhealthamerica.net/issues/state-mental-health-america. Retrieved June 2017.
2. Coyne JC, Schwenk TL, Fechner-Bates S. Nondetection of depression by primary care physicians reconsidered. Gen Hosp Psychiatry. 1995;17(1):3–12.
3. Jencks SF. Recognition of mental distress and diagnosis of mental disorder in primary care. JAMA. 1985;253:13.
4. Halfin A. Depression: the benefits of early and appropriate treatment. Am J Manag Care. 2007; 13:4.
5. Kupfer DJ, Frank E, Perel JM. The advantage of early treatment intervention in recurrent depression. Arch Gen Psychiatry. 1989;46(9):771–5.
6. Avenevoli S, Swendsen J, He JP, Burstein M, Merikangas KR. Major depression in the national comorbidity survey-adolescent supplement: prevalence, correlates, and treatment. J Am Acad Child Adolesc Psychiatry. 2015;54(1):37–44e32.
7. Torio CM, Encinosa W, Berdahl T, McCormick MC, Simpson LA. Annual report on health care for children and youth in the United States: national estimates of cost, utilization and expenditures for children with mental health conditions. Acad Pediatr. 2015;15(1):19–35.
8. Substance Abuse and Mental Health Services Administration. The NSDUH Report: major depressive episode and treatment among adolescents: 2009. Rockville, MD, April 28, 2011.
9. Wang PS, Berglund PA, Olfson M, Kessler RC. Delays in initial treatment contact after first onset of a mental disorder. Health Serv Res. 2004;39(2): 393–415.
10. March J, Silva S, Petrycki S, et al. Fluoxetine, cognitive-behavioral therapy, and their combination for adolescents with depression: treatment for adolescents with depression study (TADS) randomized controlled trial. JAMA. 2004;292(7):807–20.
11. Merikangas KR, He JP, Rapoport J, Vitiello B, Olfson M. Medication use in US youth with mental disorders. JAMA Pediatr. 2013;167(2):141–8.
12. O'Connor BC, Lewandowski RE, Rodriguez S, et al. Usual care for adolescent depression from symptom identification through treatment initiation. JAMA Pediatr. 2016;170(4):373–80.
13. Keenan-Miller D, Hammen CL, Brennan PA. Health outcomes related to early adolescent depression. J Adolesc Health. 2007;41(3):256–62.
14. Hengehold T, Boyd S, Liddy-Hicks S, Bridge J, Grupp-Phelan J. Non-responders for a suicide screen are important. San Francisco, CA: Pediatric Academic Societies; 2017.
15. Richardson LP, McCauley E, McCarty CA, et al. Predictors of persistence after a positive depression screen among adolescents. Pediatrics. 2012; 130(6):e1541–8.
16. Doryab A, et al. Detection of behavior change in people with depression. AAAI Workshop: Modern Artificial Intelligence for Health Analytics. 2014.
17. FitBit. http://www.fitbit.com.
18. Frost M, Doryab A, Faurholt-Jepsen M, Kessing LV, Bardram JE. Supporting disease insight through data analysis: refinements of the monarca self-assessment system. In: Proceedings of the 2013 ACM international joint conference on pervasive and ubiquitous computing, UbiComp '13. New York: ACM; 2013. p. 133–42. https://doi.org/10.1145/2493432.2493507.

19. Bardram JE, Frost M, Szanto K, Marcu G. The monarca self-assessment system: a persuasive personal monitoring system for bipolar patients. In: Proceedings of the 2nd ACM SIGHIT international health informatics symposium, IHI '12. New York: ACM; 2012. p. 21–30. https://doi.org/10.1145/2110363.2110370.
20. Doryab A, et al. Impact factor analysis: combining prediction with parameter ranking to reveal the impact of behavior on health outcome. Pers Ubiquit Comput. 2015;19(2):355–65.
21. Li I, Dey A, Forlizzi J. A stage-based model of personal informatics systems. In: Proceedings of the SIGCHI conference on human factors in computing systems, CHI '10. New York: ACM; 2010. p. 557–66. https://doi.org/10.1145/1753326.1753409.
22. Rooksby J, Rost M, Morrison A, Chalmers MC. Personal tracking as lived informatics. In: Proceedings of the 32Nd annual ACM conference on human factors in computing systems, CHI '14. New York: ACM; 2014. p. 1163–72. https://doi.org/10.1145/2556288.2557039.
23. Choe EK, Lee NB, Lee B, Pratt W, Kientz JA. Understanding quantified-selfers' practices in collecting and exploring personal data. In: Proceedings of the SIGCHI conference on human factors in computing systems, CHI '14. ACM, New York, pp. 1143–1152. 2014. https://doi.org/10.1145/2556288.2557372.
24. Quantifiedself. http://quantifiedself.com/.
25. Healthkit. https://www.apple.com/ios/ios8/health/.
26. Bentley F, Tollmar K, Stephenson P, Levy L, Jones B, Robertson S, Price E, Catrambone R, Wilson J (2013) Health mashups: presenting statistical patterns between wellbeing data and context in natural language to promote behavior change. ACM Trans Comput Hum Interact 20(5):30:1–30:27 doi:https://doi.org/10.1145/2503823.
27. Consolvo S, McDonald DW, Toscos T, Chen MY, Froehlich J, Harrison B, Klasnja P, LaMarca A, LeGrand L, Libby R, Smith I, Landay JA. Activity sensing in the wild: a field trial of ubifit garden. In: Proceedings of ACM CHI 2008, CHI '08. New York: ACM; 2008. p. 1797–806. https://doi.org/10.1145/1357054.1357335.
28. Lane ND, Choudhury T, Campbell A, Mohammod M, Lin M, Yang X, Doryab A, Lu H, Ali S, Berke E. BeWell: a smartphone application to monitor, model and promote wellbeing. In: Proceedings of the 5th international ICST conference on pervasive computing technologies for healthcare (Pervasive Health 2011), Pervasive health 2011. IEEE Press. 2011.
29. Kasckow J, Zickmund S, Rotondi A, Mrkva A, Gurklis J, Chinman M, Fox L, Loganathan M, Hanusa B, Haas G. Development of telehealth dialogues for monitoring suicidal patients with schizophrenia: consumer feedback. Community Mental Health J. 2014;50(3):339–42. https://doi.org/10.1007/s10597-012-9589-8.
30. Matthews M, Doherty G, Sharry J, Fitzpatrick C. Mobile phone mood charting for adolescents. Br J Guid Counsel. 2008;36(2):113–29.
31. Burns M, Begale M, Duffecy J, Gergle D, Karr C, Giangrande E, Mohr D. Harnessing context sensing to develop a mobile intervention for depression. J Med Internet Res. 2011;13(3):e55. https://doi.org/10.2196/jmir.1838.
32. Ferreira D, Kostakos V, Dey AK. AWARE: mobile context instrumentation framework. Front ICT. 2015; 2(6):1–9. https://doi.org/10.3389/fict.2015.00006.
33. Bauer M, Grof P, Gyulai L, Rasgon N, Glenn T, Whybrow PC. Using technology to improve longitudinal studies: self-reporting with ChronoRecord in bipolar disorder. Bipolar Disord. 2004;6:67–74.
34. Bopp JM, Miklowitz DJ, Goodwin GM, Stevens W, Rendell JM, Geddes JR. The longitudinal course of bipolar disorder as revealed through weekly text messaging: a feasibility study. Bipolar Disord. 2010;12:327–34.
35. Schärer LO, Hartweg V, Valerius G, Graf M, Hoern M, Biedermann C, Walser S, Boensch A, Dittmann S, Forsthoff A, Hummel B, Grunze H, Walden J. Life charts on a palmtop computer: first results of a feasibility study with an electronic diary for bipolar patients. Bipolar Disord. 2002;4(Suppl. 1):107–8.
36. Stewart JL, Bismark AW, Towers DN, Coan JA, Allen JJB. Resting frontal EEG asymmetry as an endophenotype for depression risk: sex-specific patterns of frontal brain asymmetry. J Abnorm Psychol. 2010;119(3):502.
37. Yeragani VK, Radha Krishna Rao KA, Ramesh Smitha M, Pohl RB, Balon R, Srinivasan K. Diminished chaos of heart rate time series in patients with major depression. Biological Psychiatry. 2002;51(9):733–44. https://doi.org/10.1016/S0006-3223(01)01347-6.
38. Shinn EH, Poston WSC, Kimball KT, Jeor STS, Foreyt JP. Blood pressure and symptoms of depression and anxiety: a prospective study. Am J Hypertens. 2001;14(7):660–4. https://doi.org/10.1016/S0895-7061(01)01304-8.
39. Cohn JF, Kruez TS, Matthews I, Yang Y, Nguyen HM, Padilla MT, Zhou F, De la Torre F. Detecting depression from facial actions and vocal prosody. Affective Computing and Intelligent Interaction and Workshops, 2009. ACII 2009. 3rd International Conference on, vol. 1, no. 2, pp. 10–12, Sept. 2009. https://doi.org/10.1109/ACII.2009.5349358.
40. France DJ, Shiavi RG, Silverman S, Silverman M, Wilkes DM. Acoustical properties of speech as indicators of depression and suicidal risk. Biomed Eng IEEE Trans. 2000;47(7):829–37. https://doi.org/10.1109/10.846676.
41. Hjortskov N, Rissén D, Blangsted AK, Fallentin N, Lundberg U, Søgaard K. The effect of mental stress on heart rate variability and blood pressure during computer work. Eur J Appl Physiol. 2004;92(1):84–9.
42. Chandola T, Britton A, Brunner E, Hemingway H, Malik M, Kumari M, Badrick E, Kivimaki M, Marmot M. Work stress and coronary heart disease: what are the mechanisms? Eur Heart J. 2008;29(5):640.

43. Kaur S, Bhalla B, Bajaj SK, Sanyal S, Babbar R. Effect of physical and mental stress on heart rate variability in type-A and type-B personalities. Indian J Appl Basic Med Sci. 2014;15(20):59–70.
44. Weninger F, Wollmer M, Schuller B. Emotion recognition in ¨ naturalistic speech and language—a survey. Emotion Recog, A Pattern Anal Approach, pp. 237–267, 2014.
45. American Psychiatric Association. Diagnostic and statistical manual of mental disorders. Washington, DC: American Psychiatric Association; 1994.
46. Cohn JF, Campbell SB. Influence of maternal depression on infant affect regulation. In: Cicchetti D, Toth SL, editors. Developmental perspectives on depression. Rochester: University of Rochester Press; 1992. p. 103–30.
47. Yang Y, Fairbairn C, Cohn JF. Detecting depression severity from vocal prosody. IEEE Trans Affective Comput. 2013;4(2):142–50.
48. Zlochower AJ, Cohn JF. Vocal timing in face-to-face interaction of clinically depressed and nondepressed mothers and their 4-month-old infants. Infant Behav Dev. 1996;19:373–6.
49. Schuller B, Batliner A, Steidl S, Seppi D. Recognising realistic emotions and affect in speech: State of the art and lessons learnt from the first challenge. Speech Commun. 2010;53(9–10):10621087.
50. Juslin PN, Laukka P. Communication of emotions in vocal expression and music performance: different channels, same code? Psychological Bulletin, 129:770–814, 2003. .Patientslikeme: http://www.patientslikeme.com/.
51. Frick RW. Communicating emotion: the role of prosodic features. Psychol Bull. 1985;97(3):412–29.
52. Yang X, You CW, Lu H, Lin M, Lane ND, Campbell AT. Visage: a face interpretation engine for smartphone applications. In: Uhler D, Mehta K, Wong JL, editors. Mobile Computing, Applications, and Services. MobiCASE 2012, Lecture notes of the Institute for Computer Sciences, Social Informatics and Telecommunications Engineering, vol. 110. Berlin: Springer; 2013.
53. Lu H, Frauendorfer D, Rabbi M, Mast MS, Chittaranjan GT, Campbell AT, Gatica-Perez D, Choudhury T. StressSense: detecting stress in unconstrained acoustic environments using smartphones. Paper presented at the Proceedings of the 2012 ACM conference on ubiquitous computing, Pittsburgh, PA. 2012, September.
54. Saon G, Thomas S, Soltau H, Ganapathy S, Kingsbury B. The IBM speech activity detection system for the DARPA RATS program. In: Proceeding of INTERSPEECH, 2013, pp. 3497–3501.
55. Hansen JH, Kim W, Rahurkar M, Ruzanski E, Meyerhoff J. Robust emotional stressed speech detection using weighted frequency subbands. EURASIP J Adv Signal Process. 2011;1:1–10.
56. Grimm M, Kroschel K, Mower E, Narayanan S. Primitives-based evaluation and estimation of emotions in speech. Speech Commun. 2007;49(10):787–800.
57. Thomas S, Saon G, Van Segbroeck M, Narayanan SS. Improvements to the IBM speech activity detection system for the DARPA RATS program. In: Proceeding of IEEE International Conference on Acoustics, Speech and Signal Lession. 2015. pp. 4500–4504.
58. Vanello N, Guidi A, Gentili C, Werner S, Bertschy G, Valenza G, Lanata A, Scilingo EP. Speech analysis for mood state characterization in bipolar patients. Paper presented at the Engineering in Medicine and Biology Society (EMBC), 2012 Annual international conference of the IEEE, San Diego, CA. 2012, August–September.
59. Dhall A, Joshi J, Sikka K, Goecke R, Sebe N. The more the merrier: Analysing the affect of a group of people in images. Proc IEEE Int Conf Automat Face Gesture Recog. 2015;12:1–8.
60. Prkachin KM. The consistency of facial expressions of pain—a comparison across modalities. Pain. 1992;51(3):297–306.
61. Monwar M, Rezaei S. Pain recognition using artificial neural network. In: Proceeding of IEEE International Symposium on Signal Processing and Information Technology. 2006. pp. 28–33.
62. Ashraf AB, Lucey S, Cohn JF, Chen T, Ambadar Z, Prkachin KM, Solomon PE. The painful face—pain expression recognition using active appearance models. Image Vis Comput. 2009;27:1788–96.
63. McDuff D, El Kaliouby R, Senechal T, Demirdjian D, Picard R. Automatic measurement of ad preferences from facial responses gathered over the internet. Image Vis Comput. 2014;32(10):630–40.
64. Suk M, Prabhakaran B. Real-time mobile facial expression recognition system—a case study. In Proceeding of IEEE Conference on Computer Vision and Pattern Recognition (CVPR) Workshops: IEEE. 2014. pp. 132–137.
65. Brisswalter J, Arcelin R, Audiffren M, Delignieres D. Influence of physical exercise on simple reaction time: effect of physical fitness. Percept Mot Skills. 1997;85(1997):1019–27.
66. van der Linden D, Frese M, Meijman TF. Mental fatigue and the control of cognitive processes: effects on perseveration and planning. Acta Psychologica. 2003;113(1):45–65.
67. Murata A, Uetake A, Takasawa Y. Evaluation of mental fatigue using feature parameter extracted from event-related potential. Int J Ind Ergon. 2005;35(8):761–70.
68. Gao Y, Bianchi-Berthouze N, Meng H. What does touch tell us about emotions in touchscreen-based gameplay? ACM Trans on Computer Human Interactions 19, 4 (Dec. 2012). 2012.
69. Wac K, Ciman M, Gaggi O. iSenseStress: assessing stress through human-smartphone interaction analysis. In 9th international conference on pervasive computing technologies for Healthcare-PervasiveHealth. 8–p. 2015.
70. Kim H-J, Choi YS. Exploring emotional preference for smartphone applications. In: IEEE Consumer Communications and Networking Conference (CCNC). 2012.

71. Kolakowska A. A review of emotion recognition methods based on keystroke dynamics and mouse movements. In human system interaction (HSI), 2013 the 6th international conference on. IEEE, pp. 548–555. 2013.
72. Epp C, Lippold M, Mandryk RL. Identifying emotional states using keystroke dynamics. In: Proceedings of the SIGCHI Conference on Human Factors in Computing Systems. ACM, pp. 715–724. 2011.
73. Barnett PA, Gotlib IH. Psychosocial functioning and depression: distinguishing among antecedents, concomitants, and consequences. Psychol Bull. 1988;104(1):97–126.
74. Berkman LF, Glass T, Brissette I, Seeman TE. From social integration to health: Durkheim in the new millennium. Soc Sci Med. 2000;51(6):843–57.
75. Min JK, Wiese J, Hong JI, Zimmerman J. Mining smartphone data to classify life-facets of social relationships, CSCW '13. 2013. pp. 285–294.
76. Cranshaw J, Toch E, Hong JI, Kittur A, Sadeh N. Bridging the gap between physical location and online social networks. In: Proc. Ubicomp '10, pp. 119–128. 2010.
77. Toch E, Cranshaw J, Drielsma PH, Tsai JY, Kelley PG, Springfield J, Cranor LF, Hong JI, Sadeh N. Empirical models of privacy in location sharing. In: Ubicomp 2010. 2010.
78. Canzian L, Musolesi M. Trajectories of depression: unobtrusive monitoring of depressive states by means of smartphone mobility traces analysis. In Proceedings of the 2015 ACM International Joint Conference on Pervasive and Ubiquitous Computing, ACM, pp. 1293–1304. 2015.
79. Osmani V, Maxhuni A, Grünerbl A, Lukowicz P, Haring C, Mayora O. Monitoring activity of patients with bipolar disorder using smart phones. In: Proceedings of International Conference on Advances in Mobile Computing & Multimedia. ACM. 2013. p. 85.
80. Bort-Roig J, Gilson ND, Puig-Ribera A, Contreras RS, Trost SG. Measuring and influencing physical activity with smartphone technology: a systematic review. Sports Med. 2014;44(5):671–86.
81. Case MA, Burwick HA, Volpp KG, Patel MS. Accuracy of smartphone applications and wearable devices for tracking physical activity data. JAMA. 2015;313(6):625–6.
82. Lane ND, Miluzzo E, Lu H, Peebles D, Choudhury T, Campbell AT. A survey of mobile phone sensing. IEEE Commun Mag. 2010;48(9):140–50.
83. Kao H-LC, et al. Phone-based gait analysis to detect alcohol usage. In: Proceedings of the 2012 ACM conference on ubiquitous computing. ACM, 2012.
84. Livingston G, Blizard B, Mann A. Does sleep disturbance predict depression in elderly people? A study in inner London. Br J Gen Pract. 1993;43:376.
85. Perlis ML, Giles DE, Buysse DJ, Tu X. Self-reported sleep disturbance as a prodromal symptom in recurrent depression. J Affect Disord. 1997;42:2–3.
86. Buysse DJ, Reynolds CF, Monk TH, Berman SR, Kupfer DJ. The Pittsburgh sleep quality index (PSQI): a new instrument for psychiatric research and practice. Psychiatry Res. 1989;28(2):193–213.
87. Ancoli-Israel S, Cole R, Alessi C, Chambers M, Moorcroft W, Pollak CP. The role of actigraphy in the study of sleep and circadian rhythms. Sleep. 2003;26(3):342–92.
88. Tylenol PM Sleep Tracker. http://www.tylenol.com/pain-sleeplessness/sleeptracker
89. YawnLog. http://beta.yawnlog.com.
90. Mattila E, Pärkkä J, Hermersdorf M, Kaasinen J, Vainio J, Samposalo K, Merilahti J, Kolari J, Kulju M, Lappalainen R, Korhonen I. Mobile diary for wellness management—results on usage and usability in two user studies. IEEE Trans Inform Technol Biomedicine. 2008;12(4):501–12.
91. Krejcar O, Jirka J, Janckulik D. Use of mobile phones as intelligent sensors for sound input analysis and sleep state detection. Sensors. 2011;11(6):6037–55.
92. Lawson SW, Jamison-Powell S, Garbett AT, Linehan C, Kucharczyk E, Verbaan S, Rowland DA, Morgan K. Validating a mobile phone application for the everyday, unobtrusive, objective measurement of sleep. In: Proceeding of CHI '13, pp. 2497–2506. 2013.
93. Sleep Cycle. http://www.sleepcycle.com.
94. Sleepbot. http://mysleepbot.com.
95. Bai Y, Xu B, Ma Y, Sun G, Zhao Y. Will you have a good sleep tonight?: sleep quality prediction with mobile phone. In: Proceeding of BodyNets '12, pp. 124–130. 2012.
96. Min J-K, et al. Toss'n'turn: smartphone as sleep and sleep quality detector. In: Proceedings of the SIGCHI Conference on Human Factors in Computing Systems. ACM, 2014.
97. Lenhart A, Ling R, Campbell S, Purcell K. Teens and Mobile Phones. Pew Internet and American Life Project. 2010. http://www.pewinternet.org/~/media/Files/Reports/2010/PIP-Teens-and-Mobile-2010.pdf. Accessed 27 May 2013.
98. Katikalapudi R, et al. Associating internet usage with depressive behavior among college students. IEEE Technol Soc Mag. 2012;31(4):73–80.
99. NYTimes. How Depressives Surf the Web. http://www.nytimes.com/2012/06/17/opinion/sunday/how-depressed-people-use-the-internet.html. Retrieved June 2017.
100. De Choudhury M, Gamon M, Counts S, Horvitz E. Predicting depression via social media. In: Proceeding of ICWSM '13. 2013.
101. Rude S, Gortner E-M, Pennebaker J. Language use of depressed and depression-vulnerable college students. Cognit Emot. 2004;18(8):1121–33.

102. Radloff LS. The CES-D scale a self-report depression scale for research in the general population. Appl Psychol Meas. 1977;1(3):385–401.
103. Roche MJ, Pincus AL, Rebar AL, Conroy DE, Ram N. Enriching psychological assessment using a person-specific analysis of interpersonal processes in daily life. Assessment. 2014;21:515–28.
104. Wichers M, Simons CJP, Kramer IMA, Hartmann JA, Lothmann C, Myin-Germeys I, van Bemmel AL, Peeters F, Delespaul P, van Os J. Momentary assessment technology as a tool to help patients with depression help themselves. Acta Psychiatr Scand. 2011;124:262–72.
105. Amini S, Lindqvist J, Hong JI, Lin J, Toch E, Sadeh N. Caché: caching location-enhanced content to improve user privacy. In Proceeding of Mobisys '11, pp. 197–210. 2011.
106. Lin J, Xiang G, Hong J, Sadeh N. Modeling people's place naming preferences in location sharing. In Proceedings of Ubicomp, 2010. 2010.
107. Merry SN, et al. The effectiveness of SPARX, a computerised self help intervention for adolescents seeking help for depression: randomised controlled non-inferiority trial. BMJ. 2012;344:e2598.
108. Reid SC, et al. A mobile phone application for the assessment and management of youth mental health problems in primary care: a randomised controlled trial. BMC Family Pract. 2011;12(1):131.
109. Wang R, Chen F, Chen Z, Li T, Harari G, Tignor S, Zhou X, Ben-Zeev D, Campbell AT. StudentLife: Assessing Mental Health, Academic Performance and Behavioral Trends of College Students using Smartphones. In Proceedings of the ACM Conference on Ubiquitous Computing. 2014.
110. Burke D, Linder S, Hirsch J, Dey T, Kana D, Ringenbach S, Schindler D, Alberts J. Characterizing information processing with a mobile device: measurement of simple and choice reaction time. Assessment. 2017;24(7):885–95.
111. Pollak JP, Adams P, Gay G. PAM: a photographic affect meter for frequent, in situ measurement of affect. In: The proceedings of the ACM conference on human factors in computing systems (CHI 2011) Vancouver, BC, Canada, May 5–12. 2011. pp. 725–734.

12 Social Media Data for Online Adolescent Suicide Risk Identification: Considerations for Integration Within Platforms, Clinics, and Schools

Molly Adrian and Aaron R. Lyon

Suicide is a significant and preventable public health problem across the lifespan. During adolescence, suicide is rare yet a leading cause of death that increases dramatically in incidence during this developmental period [1–3]. Despite efforts to address the devastating impact of adolescent death by suicide, rates increased from 1999 to 2014 [4]. The National Vital Health Statistics data demonstrated the increase in suicide was observed for all age groups under 75 years old, with young adolescent girls (aged 10–14) demonstrating the largest increase (200%) in the 15-year period observed. Considering the full spectrum of suicidal behaviors from suicidal ideation, suicide attempts, and death by suicide, the scope of the problem during adolescence is significant. Data suggest that 17% of US high school-aged adolescents seriously consider suicide, and nearly 9% will make an attempt in a given year [5]. Suicide prevention strategies must include the adolescent age group, and developmentally targeted interventions should be considered.

M. Adrian, Ph.D. (✉) • A.R. Lyon
Department of Psychiatry and Behavioral Sciences, University of Washington, Seattle, WA, USA
e-mail: adriam@uw.edu

Current Suicide Prevention Strategies

Data underscore the critical need for innovative approaches to aid effective suicide prevention strategies [6]. Estimates of the eight most frequently utilized suicide prevention strategies (coordinated after care, means restriction, media guidelines, public awareness, gatekeeper training, practitioner training, screening, and psychosocial treatment) indicate that the combined impact of all evidence-based approaches if widely implemented would only lead to a reduction of about 20% of suicide deaths [7]. Our brief review of current suicide prevention strategies will be limited to gatekeeper, practitioner training, and screening, as we see the opportunities for detection of suicide risk through social media to be directly connected to the issues related to accurate and timely identification of suicide risk.

Gatekeeper Training

Gatekeeper training is a suicide prevention strategy that aims to train specific groups of people who have high visibility in the community to identify individuals at risk for suicide and refer them to appropriate supports [8]. Gatekeepers for adolescent suicide prevention are often school

M.A. Moreno, A. Radovic (eds.), *Technology and Adolescent Mental Health*,
https://doi.org/10.1007/978-3-319-69638-6_12

personnel. Gatekeeper training is theorized to impact four main factors—knowledge about suicide, beliefs and attitudes about prevention, reluctance/stigma, and self-efficacy to intervene—that influence an individual's decision to intervene with a person at risk of suicide [9]. Research to date suggests that gatekeeper training can improve knowledge and beliefs about suicide intervention; however, actual intervention behavior and whether subsequent connection reduced suicide attempts and death are understudied. In a notable exception to this dearth of literature, recent evaluations of the Garrett Lee Smith legislation [10] indicate that efforts to train gatekeepers to identify individuals at risk for suicide and connect at-risk individuals to services can be effective in reducing suicide attempts [11] and death by suicide [12]. Another important finding from this series of studies is that gatekeeper training efforts must be *ongoing* to yield reductions in suicide-related outcomes, as 1 year post-implementation suicide attempt and death rates returned to pre-implementation levels.

Practitioner Training

Practitioner training is a suicide prevention strategy that highlights the healthcare system's role in identifying and assessing suicide risk. Suicide risk is under-recognized and undertreated across healthcare settings [13]. The data informing the importance of practitioner training is that general practitioners are often the first point of contact in the healthcare system for concern about mental health and suicide risk, and ½ of individuals who die by suicide have been seen in the past 30 days within a healthcare system [14]. Frontline medical practitioner (e.g., primary care physicians) training is estimated to have the largest individual impact on reducing suicide death through the identification and treatment of depression and suicidal behaviors [6, 7, 15]. In addition to general practitioner training, mental health professionals also need increased training regarding assessment and treatment of suicidal adolescents. Almost all mental health professionals encounter patients who are suicidal [16], and insufficient or absent assessment is reported as a root cause in over 80% of suicide deaths that occur in healthcare systems [13].

Screening

Screening aims to identify high-risk individuals and connect them with treatment. In a community setting, screening discriminates adolescents with a high probability of suicide from the bulk of adolescents who do not have suicide risk [17]. Screening can be done in several settings, including schools, health clinics, emergency departments, or detention settings, and are done so to detect whether any actionable risk is present at the current moment [18]. An ideal screening instrument is easily administered, highly sensitive, and specific to suicide risk identification. In ideal circumstances, screening is conducted universally, using standardized and validated measures with specific decision rules regarding risk identification and management. Unfortunately, the current state of screening for suicide risk for youth illustrates that there are brief, psychometrically sound measures for screening [19]; however, standard screening is infrequently conducted in primary care, emergency departments, or schools [20, 21]. Although identifying students at risk is critical to effective suicide prevention, additional identification approaches are clearly necessary for the potential of suicide prevention efforts to be fully realized. To be most effective, these approaches should capitalize on existing data that can support risk monitoring on an ongoing basis, resulting in gradual and continuous identification of at-risk youth.

These three approaches highlight that detection of increased risk for suicide remains a significant challenge. Over the last two decades, research has elucidated many of the developmental, cognitive, diagnostic, and family environmental factors that contribute to risk for adolescent suicide and self-injury. Although effective suicide prevention hinges on identification of high-risk individuals, the extant literature indicates that one cannot accurately assess an individual's risk for engaging in self-injury [22]. Past suicide attempts and non-suicidal self-injury have the most predictive power in future risk for suicide; however, fewer than 35% of individuals repeat self-injury [23, 24]. Further, past behavior does not provide critical information for first self-injuries nor does it designate *when* a person is at highest risk. Systematic and repeated risk assessments for predisposing, precipitating, and acute risk and protective factors may be the most efficacious method of identifying when high-risk individuals are at increased risk [25]; yet, there is insufficient evidence to demonstrate that current assessment approaches constitute an accurate and feasible preventative strategy [16, 26]. Current risk assessment procedures do not have adequate predictive power [26, 27]. This, combined with the fact that errors in assessment are root causes of suicide events [13], indicates that innovate strategies that improve risk assessment in healthcare settings would substantially advance the field of suicide prevention. Current practices rely on clinical judgment, in which errors are widespread and inevitable, particularly when under pressure to be lifesaving [26, 28]. Individuals who consider suicide may deny, conceal, or not be aware of their suicidality, with data indicating up to 78% of patients who die by suicide do not verbalize intent to healthcare providers prior to killing themselves [29]. Current suicide risk assessments have been criticized for their overreliance on suicidal ideation, which has poor predictive abilities and may not reflect true risk [30]. This state of the science and art of suicide risk assessment leaves practitioners responsible for making decisions about risk, but without strategies for making reliable and valid judgments [30]. Despite some clear successes in identifying and reducing suicide risk, the extant research suggests practical concerns that reduce the scalability and sustainment of traditional suicide prevention strategies. A data-based approach to help inform risk status would be of great value with potential to prevent injury and death.

Social Media Data Provides an Opportunity to Improve Suicide Risk Identification

Social media (SM) can be leveraged to improve suicide risk surveillance. Online signals appear to correspond with individual behavior and intentions, with emerging data indicating that online information may provide an opportunity for increase detection and surveillance and ultimately prevention of suicide. Patient-generated data, combined with advances in predictive analytics (i.e., techniques using data mining and machine learning), may provide the information needed to drive improvement in suicide risk prediction by applying machine learning algorithms to big data sets such as social media (SM) content.

As discussed in Chap. 2, SM has quickly spread among the US population independent of education, race/ethnicity, or healthcare access [31]. SM has transformed communications by providing interactive and moment-to-moment disclosures of personal information to large associated networks of people. SM is a core communication strategy for teens, and some adolescents disclose information that may indicate increased risk for self-injury on SM profiles [32]. Over 97% of teens are online and devote significant amounts of time to digital communications [33]. SM has become a fundamental channel for adolescents to communicate, obtain, and share information, with 81% of teens utilizing some kind of SM and 24% indicating "almost constant" use [33–35]. Because of the broad access and scalable quality of strategies which capitalize on SM data, prevention researchers have suggested that SM be utilized to reduce health-risk behaviors with adolescent populations [36]. Information provided on SM also appears to be a meaningful and valid indicator of teen depression [34]. Preliminary work suggests that even minor amounts of SM behavior (i.e., Facebook "likes") can successfully predict an individual's personal—and private—attributes with high degree of accuracy for user's religion, political views, relationship status, and substance use (65–82% accuracy; [37]). Many teens display

Finally, drawing from the field of implementation science, which focuses on promoting the use of research evidence in practice to improve service quality [68, 69], research should also directly evaluate the extent to which social media monitoring is fully integrated into real-world service settings. This often includes assessing a variety of implementation outcomes, such as appropriateness (i.e., contextual fit), reach (i.e., penetration into a service system), cost, or sustainment (i.e., continued use over time) [70]. Given that the impact of social media monitoring on individual outcomes is largely unknown, this research may be best accomplished in the context of hybrid effectiveness-implementation trials that simultaneously evaluate impact on service recipients and installation of the innovation in a service system [71]. "Type 1" hybrid trials, which emphasize the evaluation of the effectiveness of new innovations (i.e., social media monitoring), may currently be most appropriate. These designs are well suited to experimentally test impact on service recipient outcomes to establish an evidence base while collecting more descriptive information about the context in which implementation occurs. Regarding the latter, appropriate questions much include what factors of the organizational context are associated with uptake of social media monitoring innovations, which types of personnel are most critical to have involved in different roles (e.g., monitoring the system and attending to high-risk youth), or the costs associated with its maintenance under routine conditions.

Settings to Integrate Social Media Data for Improved Risk Identification

Machine learning is a rapidly growing segment of healthcare and one that will be an increasingly central part of the research and practice landscape for decades to come [72]. New applications of machine learning technologies that leverage social media data for suicide risk identification are likely to expand substantially during this period. As discussed above, these may include the development of prediction technologies that are freestanding and leverage social media data (e.g., via API), that are fully integrated into social media platforms, or that represent independent social media platforms, dedicated to suicide risk detection and intervention (e.g., [73]). Moreover, novel applications in contexts that support ready access to adolescents for follow-up or intervention—such as outpatient clinical settings and schools—provide excellent opportunities to ensure human involvement, safety, and effectiveness.

Clinical Applications

Current applications of SM monitoring for adolescents tend to exist largely outside of standard clinical service workflows. Nevertheless, there is tremendous opportunity to integrate these new technologies for the purposes of ongoing evaluation and intervention planning for youth who are already engaged in services. Such research could build on the rapidly expanding literature on the use of digital measurement feedback systems (MFS; [74]) to support the use of measurement-based care in clinical service delivery [75]. Although approximately 50 MFS exist in mental and behavioral health [76, 77], none of these currently incorporate real-time monitoring of social media data to gauge risk status. If social media monitoring was integrated into outpatient clinicians' clinical workflows via a MFS, it could provide an efficient information source to clinicians serving populations at high risk for suicide. In particular, the passive nature of social media evaluation to drive treatment decisions removes one of the most commonly cited barriers to the implementation of measurement-based care, which is the potential burden placed on clinicians to administer or interpret assessment measures during their clinical sessions.

Clinical applications also extend to ways in which parents monitor youth SM use. Parents frequently report that tracking adolescent technology use is frequently a struggle and source of relationship distress, driven in part by their own unfamiliarity with technology platforms [78]. Automated monitoring of online behavior may help to lessen parents' perceived burden and decrease opportunities for unnecessary conflicts. There is potential for increased passive parental monitoring, with the utilization of an SM data aggregation application. This may allow for connection and information regarding their teen's status and potentially improve the quality of the parent-teen relationship.

Case Example

Nadia is a 15-year-old who was referred to psychiatric outpatient clinic after an emergency department evaluation due to a suicide attempt via medication overdose. In addition to a 1-year history of suicidal ideation, Nadia has significant symptoms of depression and anxiety and engages in non-suicidal self-injury on a weekly basis when she is overwhelmed. At her first clinic visit, Nadia consents to treatment including using the online opt-in for the Durkheim Project Application—which enables the aggregation of posts and status updates from Twitter and Facebook. The clinician logs into the clinician dashboard, where one can view the overall risk ratings and key information driving the risk rating. The clinician notes a change in risk rating from low to moderate on Sunday evening prior to their visit on Tuesday. The therapist uses this information to prioritize suicide risk assessment and key targets of the session. At their second visit, the clinician sets the agenda with Nadia, including the risk rating to facilitate suicide risk assessment as well as chain analysis around the increase risk rating. After setting the agenda, the clinician and Nadia discuss the week's events using the DPA system to facilitate recall around events that make prompt self-injury urges. Nadia notes she became frustrated and overwhelmed with her schoolwork and posted on Twitter "I can't focus on this project as all I can do is cry and think of my pain. I need to do something to escape this pain." The therapist and Nadia use this example to identify precipitating events leading to urges to self-injury. They proceed with a solutions analysis to use alternative strategies to reduce distress and manage self-injury urges.

School-Based Applications

In schools, social media monitoring may have the most opportunity for impact as a method for universal screening for suicide risk. Although schools represent the most common setting for initial identification of and intervention for a wide variety of mental health problems [79], schools struggle to identify many at-risk students, particularly those with internalizing problems (e.g., depression and anxiety) who are at heightened risk for suicide or non-suicidal self-injury [21, 80, 81]. Traditional approaches to the identification of student problems in schools are typically non-systematic, often relying on referrals from school professionals [82, 83], and tend to underemphasize internalizing concerns [84]. Identified issues that impact the extent to which effective screening programs may be systematically implemented in schools include problems with scheduling, staffing, and acceptability [21, 85]. Additional concerns include questions about the usability and practicality of screening tools, such as the cultural and contextual appropriateness of specific measures, general concerns about reliability and validity of screening measures and implications regarding false positives and negatives, legal and ethical issues related to parental consent and confidentiality, as well as fear of stigmatizing students (Table 12.1; [86, 87]). Given this, it is perhaps unsurprising that studies indicate only 15% of schools conduct any sort of school-wide health screening [88] and only 2% carry out universal screening for emotional and behavioral problems [89]. Smaller still is the percentage of schools that routinely screen their students for suicide risk. Furthermore, when screening does occur, it is mostly likely to happen once during a school year (e.g., in the fall; [90]). Given the episodic nature of mental health problems and suicide risk, such approaches are likely to miss the substantial number of students whose risk status changes over the course of the year [91, 92]. Simultaneously, screening at a single time point in the year yields a tidal wave of at-risk students, which is likely to overwhelm service system capacity [93]. Programs that capitalize on existing data that can support risk monitoring on an ongoing basis should allow for low-cost, gradual, and continuous identification of youth.

Table 12.1 Barriers to identifying suicide risk in high schools and technological solutions using online data for identification

Limitations of traditional screening approaches	Technological strategies for reducing limitation
Screening tool	
Relies on explicit report suicidal ideation	Does not rely on suicidal ideation
False positives	Continuously refines accuracy with supervised and semi-supervised artificial intelligence to increase positive and negative predictive power
Differential cultural relevance	Developed with attention to cultural factors
Administration process	
Single screening time point: Misses students previously or not yet at risk; delays in identification	Occurs continuously; identifies students as risk emerges. Mobile and internet based platform increases uptake and accessibility
Single screening time point: Rapid influx of students for immediate follow-up overwhelms service capacity	Follow up is indicated over the course of monitoring. Identification does not occur all at once
Missed instructional time	Does not require instructional time

Summary

There is an opportunity to capitalized on "big data" and the strengths of machine learning to improve healthcare for individuals—an approach that is broad in its reach and scale. Evaluation of the efficacy of indicated prevention work based on SM is a necessary approach to reach teens as current paradigms have not affected SI rates [6]. To date, individually focused work to improve surveillance within a healthcare system utilizing strategies through the Zero Suicide toolkit (www.zerosuicide.sprc.org) shows promise, but additional strategies to monitor and engage adolescent would be of tremendous value to identify those at highest risk for future self-injury.

Future research should evaluate the impact of social media monitoring approaches (including in the context of hybrid effectiveness-implementation trials), promote their integration into novel and accessible service contexts (e.g., schools), and refine their associated algorithms, digital packaging, and implementation strategies. Such work is likely to carry significant public health value by supporting low-resource and scalable strategy for monitoring suicide risk to build safe and efficient prevention programs with maximum potential for reach (Fig. 12.2). Strategic monitoring of SM has the potential to have a considerable impact on

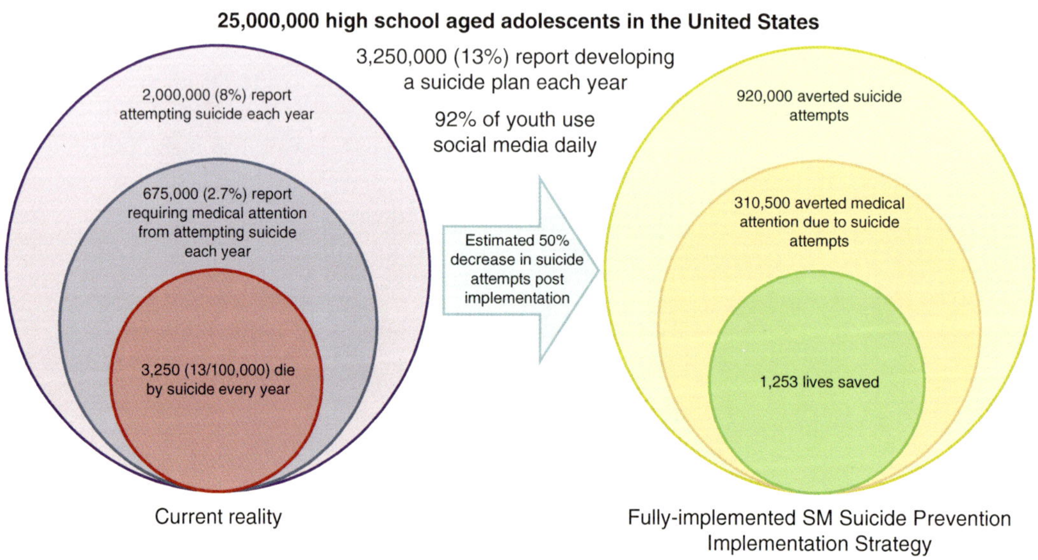

Fig. 12.2 The estimated impact of strategic monitoring of suicide risk on adolescent suicide deaths

improving and integrating systems' surveillance of suicide events by identifying individuals during times of high risk and connecting to supports. We believe this approach is needed to decrease adolescent suicide rates.

References

1. Crosby AE, Ortega L, Stevens MR, Centers for Disease Control and Prevention (CDC). Suicides-United States, 1999–2007. Morb Mortal Wkly Rep. 2011;60:56.
2. Nock MK. Why do people hurt themselves? New insights into the nature and functions of self-injury. Curr Dir Psychol Sci. 2009;18(2):78–83.
3. Whitlock J, Eckenrode J, Silverman D. Self-injurious behaviors in a college population. Pediatrics. 2006; 117(6):1939–48.
4. Curtin S, Warner M, Hedegaard H. Increase in Suicide in the United States, 1999–2014. NCHS Data Brief. 2016;(241):1–8.
5. Lowry R, Crosby AE, Brener ND, Kann L. Suicidal thoughts and attempts among U.S. high school students: trends and associated health-risk behaviors, 1991–2011. J Adolesc Health. 2014;54(1):100–8.
6. Christensen H, Cuijpers P, Reynolds CF. Changing the direction of suicide prevention research: a necessity for true population impact. JAMA Psychiat. 2016;73(5):435–6.
7. Krysinska K, Batterham PJ, Tye M, Shand F, Calear AL, Cockayne N, et al. Best strategies for reducing the suicide rate in Australia. Aust N Z J Psychiatry. 2016;50(2):115–8.
8. Goldsmith SK, Pellmar TC, Kleinman AM, Bunney WE, editors. Reducing suicide: a national imperative [Internet]. National Academies Press; 2002 [cited 2017 Jan 13]. https://books.google.com/books?hl=en&lr=&id=9xGdAgAAQBAJ&oi=fnd&pg=PT17&dq=Reducing+Suicide:+A+National+Imperative.&ots=mRHF6lpIjD&sig=gBYeJMJxXA7YVmWtsM_pr5HauI4.
9. Burnette C, Ramchand R, Ayer L. Gatekeeper training for suicide prevention: A theoretical model and review of the empirical literature [Internet]. DTIC Document; 2015 [cited 2017 Jan 13]. http://oai.dtic.mil/oai/oai?verb=getRecord&metadataPrefix=html&identifier=ADA615291.
10. Dodd AP. Garrett Lee Smith Memorial Act. 108–355 Oct 21, 2004. p. 2008.
11. Garraza LG, Walrath C, Goldston DB, Reid H, McKeon R. Effect of the Garrett Lee Smith memorial suicide prevention program on suicide attempts among youths. JAMA Psychiat. 2015;72(11):1143–9.
12. Walrath C, Garraza LG, Reid H, Goldston DB, McKeon R. Impact of the Garrett Lee Smith youth suicide prevention program on suicide mortality. Am J Public Health. 2015;105(5):986–93.
13. Joint Commission. Sentinel event data root causes by event type 2004–2013. Sect. Standards on Accreditation of Healthcare Organizations. 2014.
14. Luoma JB, Martin CE, Pearson JL. Contact with mental health and primary care providers before suicide: a review of the evidence. Am J Psychiatry. 2002;159(6):909–16.
15. Mann JJ, Apter A, Bertolote J, Beautrais A, Currier D, Haas A, et al. Suicide prevention strategies: a systematic review. JAMA. 2005;294(16):2064–74.
16. Schmitz WM, Allen MH, Feldman BN, Gutin NJ, Jahn DR, Kleespies PM, et al. Preventing suicide through improved training in suicide risk assessment and care: an American Association of Suicidology Task Force Report Addressing Serious Gaps in U.S. Mental Health Training. Suicide Life Threat Behav. 2012;42(3):292–304.
17. Jekel JF, Katz DL, Elmore JG. Sample size, randomization and probability study. In: Epidemiology, biostatistics and preventive medicine. 2nd ed. Amsterdam, The Netherlands: Elsevier Health Sciences; 2001. p. 194–209.
18. Boudreaux ED, Horowitz LM. Suicide risk screening and assessment: designing instruments with dissemination in mind. Am J Prev Med. 2014;47(3, Supplement 2):S163–9.
19. Horowitz LM, Bridge JA, Teach SJ, Ballard E, Klima J, Rosenstein DL, et al. Ask suicide-screening questions (ASQ): a brief instrument for the pediatric emergency department. Arch Pediatr Adolesc Med. 2012;166(12):1170–6.
20. Horowitz LM, Ballard ED. Suicide screening in schools, primary care and emergency departments. Curr Opin Pediatr. 2009;21(5):620.
21. Hallfors D, Brodish PH, Khatapoush S, Sanchez V, Cho H, Steckler A. Feasibility of screening adolescents for suicide risk in "real-world" high school settings. Am J Public Health. 2006;96(2):282–7.
22. Gould MS, Marrocco FA, Kleinman M, Thomas JG, Mostkoff K, Cote J, et al. Evaluating iatrogenic risk of youth suicide screening programs: a randomized controlled trial. JAMA. 2005;293(13):1635–43.
23. Borges G, Angst J, Nock MK, Ruscio AM, Kessler RC. Risk factors for the incidence and persistence of suicide-related outcomes: a 10-year follow-up study using the National Comorbidity Surveys. J Affect Disord. 2008;105(1–3):25–33.
24. Pokorny AD. Prediction of suicide in psychiatric patients: report of a prospective study. Arch Gen Psychiatry. 1983;40(3):249–57.
25. Wintersteen MB. Standardized screening for suicidal adolescents in primary care. Pediatrics. 2010; 125(5):938–44.
26. Silverman MM, Berman AL. Suicide risk assessment and risk formulation part I: a focus on suicide ideation in assessing suicide risk. Suicide Life Threat Behav. 2014;44(4):420–31.
27. Simon RI. Imminent suicide: the illusion of short-term prediction. Suicide Life Threat Behav. 2006;36(3): 296–301.

28. Berman AL, Silverman MM. Suicide risk assessment and risk formulation part II: suicide risk formulation and the determination of levels of risk. Suicide Life Threat Behav. 2014;44(4):432–43.
29. Kovacs M, Beck AT, Weissman A. The communication of suicidal intent: a reexamination. Arch Gen Psychiatry. 1976;33(2):198–201.
30. Fowler JC. Suicide risk assessment in clinical practice: pragmatic guidelines for imperfect assessments. Psychotherapy. 2012;49(1):81–90.
31. Chou W-YS, Hunt YM, Beckjord EB, Moser RP, Hesse BW. Social media use in the United States: implications for health communication. J Med Internet Res. 2009;11(4):e48.
32. Bridge JA, Goldstein TR, Brent DA. Adolescent suicide and suicidal behavior. J Child Psychol Psychiatry. 2006;47(3–4):372–94.
33. Kluger AN, DeNisi A. The effects of feedback interventions on performance: a historical review, a meta-analysis, and a preliminary feedback intervention theory. Psychol Bull. 1996;119(2):254–84.
34. Moreno MA, Christakis DA, Egan KG, Jelenchick LA, Cox E, Young H, et al. A pilot evaluation of associations between displayed depression references on Facebook and self-reported depression using a clinical scale. J Behav Health Serv Res. 2011;39(3):295–304.
35. Lenhart A, Page D. Teens, social media & technology overview 2015, vol. 9. Washington, DC: Pew Research Center; 2015.
36. Whitlock JL, Powers JL, Eckenrode J. The virtual cutting edge: the internet and adolescent self-injury. Dev Psychol. 2006;42(3):407–17.
37. Kosinski M, Stillwell D, Graepel T. Private traits and attributes are predictable from digital records of human behavior. Proc Natl Acad Sci. 2013;110(15):5802–5.
38. Egan KG, Moreno MA. Prevalence of stress references on college freshmen Facebook profiles. Comput Inform Nurs CIN. 2011;29(10):586–92.
39. Cash SJ, Thelwall M, Peck SN, Ferrell JZ, Bridge JA. Adolescent suicide statements on MySpace. Cyberpsychology Behav Soc Netw. 2013;16(3):166–74.
40. Mitchell KJ, Ybarra ML. Online behavior of youth who engage in self-harm provides clues for preventive intervention. Prev Med. 2007;45(5):392–6.
41. Ybarra ML, Alexander C, Mitchell KJ. Depressive symptomatology, youth internet use, and online interactions: a national survey. J Adolesc Health. 2005;36(1):9–18.
42. Twitter Inc. 2014.
43. Cellan-Jones LK Dave Lee, Rory. Facebook artificial intelligence spots suicidal users. BBC News [Internet]. 2017 Mar 1 [cited 2017 Mar 20]; http://www.bbc.com/news/technology-39126027.
44. Kodratoff Y, Michalski RS. Machine learning: an artificial intelligence approach [Internet]. Vol. 3. Morgan Kaufmann; 2014 [cited 2016 Oct 31]. https://books.google.com/books?hl=en&lr=&id=vHyjBQAAQBAJ&oi=fnd&pg=PP1&dq=Kodratoff,+Y.,+%26+Michalski,+R.+S.+(2014).+Machine+learning:+an+artificial+intelligence+approach+(Vol.+3).+Morgan+Kaufmann.&ots=R3Y2U0zz7R&sig=Iyyr10ttpmZ2Ghr19Ufikkuvi08.
45. Jashinsky J, Burton SH, Hanson CL, West J, Giraud-Carrier C, Barnes MD, et al. Tracking suicide risk factors through twitter in the US. Crisis. 2014;35(1):51–9.
46. O'Dea B, Wan S, Batterham PJ, Calear AL, Paris C, Christensen H. Detecting suicidality on twitter. Internet Interv. 2015;2(2):183–8.
47. Braithwaite SR, Giraud-Carrier C, West J, Barnes MD, Hanson CL. Validating machine learning algorithms for twitter data against established measures of suicidality. JMIR Ment Health. 2016;3(2):e21.
48. De Choudhury M, Kiciman E, Dredze M, Coppersmith G, Kumar M. Discovering shifts to suicidal ideation from mental health content in social media. In: Proceedings of the 2016 CHI Conference on Human Factors in Computing Systems [Internet]. New York, NY: ACM; 2016 [cited 2017 Jan 13]. p. 2098–2110. (CHI '16). http://doi.acm.org/10.1145/2858036.2858207.
49. Coopersmith G. Emotion states based on social media data and activity states based on fitbit data. 2016.
50. Klein DF. Studying the clinician: judgment research and psychological assessment. Am J Psychiatry. 1999;156(7):1108.
51. The Durkheim Project Application [Internet]. http://www.durkheimproject.org/.
52. Thompson P, Poulin C, Bryan CJ. Predicting military and veteran suicide risk: cultural aspects. In: Proceedings of ACL [Internet]. 2014 [cited 2016 Oct 31]. p. 1–6. http://www.anthology.aclweb.org/W/W14/W14-32.pdf#page=13.
53. Laranjo L, Arguel A, Neves AL, Gallagher AM, Kaplan R, Mortimer N, et al. The influence of social networking sites on health behavior change: a systematic review and meta-analysis. J Am Med Inform Assoc. 2015;22(1):243–56.
54. Poulin C, Shiner B, Thompson P, Vepstas L, Young-Xu Y, Goertzel B, et al. Predicting the risk of suicide by analyzing the text of clinical notes. PLoS One. 2014;9(1):e85733.
55. Gilbody S, Littlewood E, Hewitt C, Brierley G, Tharmanathan P, Araya R, et al. Computerised cognitive behaviour therapy (cCBT) as treatment for depression in primary care (REEACT trial): large scale pragmatic randomised controlled trial. BMJ. 2015;351:h5627.
56. Chartier M, Stoep AV, McCauley E, Herting JR, Tracy M, Lymp J. Passive versus active parental permission: implications for the ability of school-based depression screening to reach youth at risk. J Sch Health. 2008;78(3):157–64.
57. Mohr D, Cuijpers P, Lehman K. Supportive accountability: a model for providing human support to enhance adherence to eHealth interventions. J Med Internet Res. 2011;13(1):e30.
58. Schueller SM, Tomasino KN, Mohr DC. Integrating human support into behavioral intervention technologies: the efficiency model of support. Clin Psychol Sci Pract. 2016;24(1):27–45.
59. Whitehill JM, Brockman LN, Moreno MA. "Just talk to me": communicating with college students about depression disclosures on Facebook. J Adolesc Health Off Publ Soc Adolesc Med. 2013;52(1):122–7.

60. Littlejohns P, Wyatt JC, Garvican L. Evaluating computerised health information systems: hard lessons still to be learnt. BMJ. 2003;326(7394):860–3.
61. Karsh B-T. Beyond usability: designing effective technology implementation systems to promote patient safety. Qual Saf Health Care. 2004;13(5):388–94.
62. ISO. Ergonomics of human-system interaction: part 210: human-centred design for interactive systems. Geneva: ISO; 2010.
63. Courage C, Baxter K. Understanding your users: a practical guide to user requirements: methods, tools, and techniques [Internet]. Gulf Professional Publishing; 2005 [cited 2016 Sep 8]. https://books.google.com/books?hl=en&lr=&id=bZ__HjU20hEC&oi=fnd&pg=PT24&dq=Understanding+your+users:+a+practical+guide+to+user+requirements+methods,+tools,+and+techniques&ots=Xhc5eL0Yc7&sig=ie0c5Rswr2FvJu0h0TFnvfFFNPo.
64. Pea RD. User centered system design: new perspectives on human-computer interaction. J Educ Comput Res. 1987;3(1):129–34.
65. Rubin J, Chisnell D. Handbook of usability testing: how to plan, design and conduct effective tests. Indianapolis, IN: Wiley; 2008.
66. Zhou R. How to quantify user experience: fuzzy comprehensive evaluation model based on summative usability testing. In: Aykin N, editor. Usability and internationalization global and local user interfaces [Internet]. Springer, Berlin; 2007 [cited 2016 Nov 1]. p. 564–73. (Lecture Notes in Computer Science). http://link.springer.com/chapter/10.1007/978-3-540-73289-1_65.
67. Lyon AR, Wasse JK, Ludwig K, Zachry M, Bruns EJ, Unützer J, et al. The contextualized technology adaptation process (CTAP): optimizing health information technology to improve mental health systems. Adm Policy Ment Health Ment Health Serv Res. 2015;13:1–16.
68. Eccles MP, Mittman BS. Welcome to implementation science. Implement Sci. 2006;1:1.
69. Proctor EK, Landsverk J, Aarons G, Chambers D, Glisson C, Mittman B. Implementation research in mental health services: an emerging science with conceptual, methodological, and training challenges. Adm Policy Ment Health Ment Health Serv Res. 2009;36(1):24–34.
70. Proctor E, Silmere H, Raghavan R, Hovmand P, Aarons G, Bunger A, et al. Outcomes for implementation research: conceptual distinctions, measurement challenges, and research agenda. Adm Policy Ment Health Ment Health Serv Res. 2010;38(2):65–76.
71. Curran GM, Bauer M, Mittman B, Pyne JM, Stetler C. Effectiveness-implementation hybrid designs. Med Care. 2012;50(3):217–26.
72. Obermeyer Z, Emanuel EJ. Predicting the future—big data, machine learning, and clinical medicine. N Engl J Med. 2016;375(13):1216–9.
73. Nock MK. Utilizing machine learning techniques to improve prediction and prevention of suicide and self-injury. New York: Association for Behavioral and Cognitive Therapies;2016.
74. Bickman LA. Measurement feedback system (MFS) is necessary to improve mental health outcomes. J Am Acad Child Adolesc Psychiatry. 2008;47(10):1114–9.
75. Lyon AR, Lewis CC. Designing health information technologies for uptake: development and implementation of measurement feedback systems in mental health service delivery. Adm Policy Ment Health Ment Health Serv Res. 2015;43(3):344–9.
76. Lyon AR, Lewis CC, Boyd MR, Hendrix E, Liu F. Capabilities and characteristics of digital measurement feedback systems: results from a comprehensive review. Adm Policy Ment Health Ment Health Serv Res. 2016;43(3):441–66.
77. Lyon AR, Lewis CC, Melvin A, Boyd M, Nicodimos S, Liu FF, et al. Health Information Technologies—Academic and Commercial Evaluation (HIT-ACE) methodology: description and application to clinical feedback systems. Implement Sci. 2016;11:128.
78. Yardi S, Bruckman A. Social and Technical Challenges in Parenting Teens' Social Media Use. In: Proceedings of the SIGCHI Conference on Human Factors in Computing Systems [Internet]. New York, NY, USA: ACM; 2011 [cited 2017 Mar 20]. p. 3237–3246. (CHI '11). http://doi.acm.org/10.1145/1978942.1979422.
79. Farmer EMZ, Burns BJ, Phillips SD, Angold A, Costello EJ. Pathways into and through mental health services for children and adolescents. Psychiatr Serv. 2003;54(1):60–6.
80. Bradshaw CP, Buckley JA, Ialongo NS. School-based service utilization among urban children with early onset educational and mental health problems: the squeaky wheel phenomenon. Sch Psychol Q. 2008;23(2):169–86.
81. De Leo D, Heller TS. Who are the kids who self-harm? An Australian self-report school survey. Med J Aust. 2004;181(3):140–4.
82. Scott MA, Wilcox HC, Schonfeld IS, Davies M, Hicks RC, Turner JB, et al. School-based screening to identify at-risk students not already known to school professionals: the columbia suicide screen. Am J Public Health. 2009;99(2):334–9.
83. Scott M, Wilcox H, Huo Y, Turner JB, Fisher P, Shaffer D. School-based screening for suicide risk: balancing costs and benefits. Am J Public Health. 2010;100(9):1648–52.
84. Walker B, Cheney D, Stage S, Blum C, Horner RH. Schoolwide screening and positive behavior supports identifying and supporting students at risk for school failure. J Posit Behav Interv. 2005;7(4):194–204.
85. Hayden DC, Lauer P. Prevalence of suicide programs in schools and roadblocks to implementation. Suicide Life Threat Behav. 2000;30(3):239–51.
86. Dever BV, Raines TC, Barclay CM. Chasing the unicorn: practical implementation of universal screening for behavioral and emotional risk. In: School Psychology Forum [Internet]. 2012 [cited 2016 Oct 31]. http://search.ebscohost.com/login.aspx?direct=true&profile=ehost&scope=site&authtype=crawler&jrnl=19382243&AN=95604496&h=aY%2FRkHcPCt8rVi3BL0CiPWb%2B%2FuivpJ6Ou1Qi7Ofrnpce%2FCkLiv5p8fRkxi0HLd7IddMyzwTLAxhS8VGHKmarlA%3D%3D&crl=c.

87. Fox JK, Halpern LF, Forsyth JP. Mental health check-ups for children and adolescents: a means to identify, prevent, and minimize suffering associated with anxiety and mood disorders. Clin Psychol Sci Pract. 2008;15(3):182–211.
88. Foster S, Rollefson M, Doksum T, Noonan D, Robinson G, Teich J. School mental health services in the United States, 2002–2003 [Internet]. SAMHSA's National Clearinghouse for Alcohol and Drug Information (NCADI); 2005 [cited 2016 Apr 7]. http://eric.ed.gov/?id=ED499056.
89. Romer D, McIntosh K. The roles and perspectives of school mental health professionals in promoting adolescent mental health. In: Evans DL, Foa EB, Gur RE, Hendin H, O'Brien CP, Seligman ME, et al., editors. Treating and preventing adolescent mental health disorders: what we know and what we don't know: a research agenda for improving the mental health of our youth. New York: Oxford University Press; 2005. p. 597–615.
90. Kalafat J, Brown CH. Suicide prevention and intervention: summary of a workshop. Natl Acad Sci. 2001, 2003;22
91. Prinstein MJ, Nock MK, Simon V, Aikins JW, Cheah CS, Spirito A. Longitudinal trajectories and predictors of adolescent suicidal ideation and attempts following inpatient hospitalization. J Consult Clin Psychol. 2008;76(1):92–103.
92. Adrian M, Miller AB, McCauley E, Vander Stoep A. Suicidal ideation in early to middle adolescence: sex-specific trajectories and predictors. J Child Psychol Psychiatry. 2016;57(5):645–53.
93. Lyon AR, Maras MA, Pate CM, Igusa T, VanderStoep A. Modeling the impact of school-based universal depression screening on additional service capacity needs: a system dynamics approach. Adm Policy Ment Health Ment Health Serv Res. 2015;43(2):168–88.

13 Telemental Health

Jennifer McWilliams and Kathleen Myers

Introduction

While one frequently thinks of numerous hazards and concerns when adolescents interact with technology, technology also offers tremendous potential to reach adolescents to improve their lives. One such example is the use of telemedicine to provide mental healthcare to teens who would otherwise not have access to care. According to the Substance Abuse and Mental Health Services Administration's report, "Behavioral Health Barometer [1]: United States (2014)," 10.7% of adolescents, ages 12–17 years old, reported having had a major depressive episode within the year prior to being surveyed. Of these teens, only 38.1% received treatment for their depression. Looking beyond depression, the National Institute of Mental Health estimates that over 20% of children and adolescents, either currently or at some point during their lives, have had a seriously debilitating mental disorder. These disorders often impair the adolescents' ability to function academically, socially, and within their families [2].

Despite this high need, access to care poses a significant barrier to meeting the need. Multiple factors have created a workforce shortage of qualified mental and behavioral health providers including a plateau in the percentage of medical students selecting a psychiatry residency and an economic and geographic maldistribution of providers [3, 4]. Further, over half of the practicing psychiatrists in the United States are over the age of 55 years old, and as these providers retire, the incoming rates of new graduates will not match the need [5]. The gap between the number of providers available and the number of adolescents in need of treatment for mental health disorders will grow. This gap is particularly notable in rural and poverty-stricken areas [6, 7]. According to their studies, less than 1% of rural counties have a child and adolescent psychiatrist, and no counties with greater than 50% of the population living below the poverty line have a child and adolescent psychiatrist practicing within their borders. A similar disparity has been noted for other mental health disciplines [8]. With adolescents' increasing need for mental healthcare, increasing eligibility with healthcare reform but shrinking resources that are not easily accessible, the

J. McWilliams, M.D., M.S.
Department of Behavioral Health, Children's Hospital & Medical Center, Omaha, NE, USA
e-mail: jmcwilliams@ChildrensOmaha.org

K. Myers, M.D., M.P.H., M.S., D.F.A.A.C.A.P., D.F.A.P.A., D.F.A.T.A. (✉)
Department of Psychiatry and Behavioral Sciences, University of Washington, Seattle, WA, USA

Department of Psychiatry and Behavioral Medicine, Seattle Children's Hospital, Seattle, WA, USA
e-mail: Kathleen.myers@seattlechildrens.org

M.A. Moreno, A. Radovic (eds.), *Technology and Adolescent Mental Health*,
https://doi.org/10.1007/978-3-319-69638-6_13

mental healthcare system will have to embrace different models of service delivery to meet the needs. Telemedicine offers one such solution.

There is no clear definition of telehealth-related activities, and some agencies do not distinguish between the terms telehealth and telemedicine. The Centers for Medicare and Medicaid Services (CMS) defines *telehealth* as the use of telecommunications and information technology to provide access to health assessment, diagnosis, intervention, consultation, supervision, and information across distance [9]. The CMS term *telehealth* designates a broad umbrella of services that involves telephones, facsimile machines, e-mail, radiographs, remote patient recording, patient portals, and other forms of electronic media. It does not necessarily meet the CMS definition of *telemedicine*.

CMS notes that "for purposes of Medicaid, *telemedicine* seeks to improve a patient's health by permitting two-way, real time interactive communication between the originating (i.e., patient) site and the distant (i.e., physician or provider) site. This electronic communication means the use of interactive telecommunications equipment that includes, at a minimum, audio and video equipment" [10, 11]. When telemedicine is used to provide psychiatric or more general mental health services, the terms "telepsychiatry" and "telemental health" (TMH), respectively, are generally used [12]. Telemental health is one of the most common telemedicine applications used in the United States.

Delivery Models

As discussed by Gloff and colleagues [13], numerous "studies show that services delivered through [telemental health] are feasible, acceptable, have been delivered across developmental status, and to young people with varied disorders." The evidence base supporting the efficacy of telemental health service delivery with youth is developing incrementally [14] and generally consistent with the larger adult evidence base that has shown that outcomes are equal to outcomes for comparable mental health services delivered in person.

Telemental health with youth has been utilized successfully in a number of settings including primary care clinics, schools, correctional facilities, and patients' homes. Additionally, different strategies, such as asynchronous delivery, are being explored to broaden access to care within these naturalistic settings. These variations in service delivery models highlight the potential for improving access to quality mental healthcare more equitably, more efficiently, and more effectively than usual community-based care.

Primary Care Clinics

Case: Mia is a 14-year-old girl who lives with her family in rural Hawaii. Her parents take her to the local medical clinic with concerns about her increasingly obsessive thoughts about her body image and refusal to eat. The medical provider is concerned about an eating disorder, but there are no resources specific to this disorder in the community. He recognizes the need for both acute consultation and ongoing care. He offers the family the options of traveling off island to a major medical center or obtaining a video consultation from a psychiatrist specializing in eating disorders at that medical center. The family agrees to start with video consultation. The telepsychiatrist met with Mia, her family, the medical provider, a nutritionist, and a community therapist. They constructed a multidisciplinary treatment plan that included each of these providers in Mia's care and monthly telepsychiatry consultation. The telepsychiatrist supervised the community therapist in the psychotherapy of youth with eating disorders and partnered with the medical provider in pharmacological interventions. The family continued this hybrid (i.e., combination of in-person and remote videoconferencing) model of care [15] without travel to a distant medical center until Mia's weight and nutritional intake normalized.

The use of telemental health technology in primary care settings is one of the most long-standing applications of telemental health. In this model, psychiatric providers at a distant location evaluate and treat patients and their families via videoconferencing technology at the patients' primary care providers' offices. Varying levels of care coordination exist. At the most basic level, there needs to be little coordination beyond the typical specialist-primary care relationship. The patient is referred to the specialist with a clinical question, and after evaluation and initiation of treatment by the specialist, the primary care provider receives feedback in the form of clinic notes or a letter and maintains care of the patient. Ideally the providers on both sides of the referral can use the technology to improve communication and coordination. With telemental health services available in the primary care office, essentially a virtual co-location model can be created, allowing the specialists and primary care providers to work side by side in treating teens with complex symptoms. Regardless of the level of coordination, the utilization of telemental health in primary care clinics improves youths' access to evidence-based mental healthcare and strengthens primary care providers' skills in caring for their young patients.

Emerging reimbursement models should encourage the use of telemental health in primary care. CMS provides a small care coordination fee paid to the patient site on a per patient, per month basis [11, 16] and recently announced plans to reimburse for care managers involved in collaborative care models [17].

Patient-Centered Medical Homes

James is a 17-year-old male who lives on a ranch in western Nebraska. He was recently diagnosed with bipolar disorder during psychiatric hospitalization in a bordering state. His discharge plan notes the need for psychiatric follow-up given severity of symptoms, partial remission with concerns for cycling into depression. His primary medical care is provided by a family physician in a patient-centered medical home in which primary providers collaborate with a general psychiatrist to deliver evidence-based care for their population of adults with mood and anxiety disorders. The psychiatrist collaborates through videoconferencing. As James is an older adolescent with psychiatric illness that usually onsets in adulthood, and the telepsychiatrist had the competencies to provide the needed care [14], James' family physician arranged his treatment in the patient-centered medical home in collaboration with the psychiatrist. Their shared electronic medical record (EMR) facilitated their collaboration.

In this model, telemental healthcare is used to support the development of the patient-centered medical home (PCMH) model. In addition to increasing access to mental healthcare, primary care providers are increasingly recognizing the complex interaction between physical and mental health [18]. Telemental health offers a tool to create a fully integrated team in which the psychiatrist and the primary care provider manage complex patients and/or to provide population-based care [19–21].

The "medical home" concept was introduced in 1967 by the American Academy of Pediatrics to centralize the care and medical records for children with special healthcare needs [22]. Since then, the concept of PCMH has expanded and evolved. Currently, there are several definitions of a PCMH, but the general principles consistently include a team-based approach toward improving the organization of healthcare delivery and developing a sustained partnership with patients. In order to qualify as a PCMH, primary care practices must provide comprehensive care and be responsible for the majority of patients' healthcare needs. Multidisciplinary teams are necessary to successfully establish this holistic focus [19, 20, 23].

With the workforce shortages within mental healthcare, this approach can be challenging. By using telemedicine technology, however, mental health providers can join as "remote" team members. In this model, the mental health provider treats the patient collaboratively with the primary care provider. The unique core feature of this model is the use of a care manager who liaises between the telepsychiatrist and the primary care provider who maintains responsibility for the patient, including pharmacotherapy. The telepsychiatrist supervises the care manager who administers screening tools, tracks treatment response through a patient registry, monitors patients to ensure adequate follow-up, and identify challenges to treatment adherence before they become problematic. The care manager also identifies patients who may need direct assessment with the consulting telepsychiatrist or other specialist.

Implementation of this model requires considerable effort to establish relationships, build clinical processes, alter clinic workflow, and, particularly, support the care manager's role [23]. Reimbursement remains a significant limitation to this model; however, the addition of the care coordination fee recently announced by CMS should make the model sustainable [17]. As the healthcare system in the United States evolves, the use of telemental health and the patient-centered medical home holds significant promise to redistribute the psychiatric workforce, supports primary care providers, and improves mental health outcomes. A new position of care manager is needed, and more work is needed to determine how these changes will affect costs and sustainability.

School-Based Telemental Healthcare

Case: At parent-teacher conferences, Thomas' guidance counselor at his urban high school expresses concern that he is struggling to pay attention, has been a distraction to his peers in classes, and has been getting in trouble in the lunch room. His mother notes longstanding academic difficulties and agrees that he is now having increasing behavioral difficulties and a "bad attitude" at home. She has been meaning to take him to see a therapist recommended by a friend, but she is working two jobs and cannot afford the long bus trip on the other side of the city. His school counselor suggests that he be evaluated by the psychologist who partners with the school guidance program via videoconferencing. His mother was pleased to be able to obtain services in the school with staff she trusted. The telepsychologist school staff met with Thomas and his mother who joined on her smartphone. The telepsychologist's evaluation indicated attention-deficit hyperactivity disorder (ADHD) and a reading disability that had not been noted earlier in his education. The telepsychologist made recommendations for special education assessment, undertook a brief therapy for adolescent ADHD, helped his mother with behavior management at home, and referred Thomas to his primary care provider for a medication evaluation [24]. The telepsychologist continued in this school-based brief intervention model of care for a total of five sessions at which time the community team continued with his new individualized education plan, and his primary care physician provided pharmacotherapy.

Some families lack ready access to primary care and a co-location model does not optimally meet their needs. As a result, there has been an increasing interest in providing primary care and, more recently, mental healthcare in school settings. While there is a growing body of literature regarding the benefits and shortcomings of school-based mental healthcare, there is a limited literature regarding the use of school-based telemental health programs, although such programs continue to be implemented. Cunningham and colleagues [25] have described the Prince George School Mental Health Initiative in Maryland that provides psychiatric consultation via videoconferencing to mental health providers practicing in the schools. Direct patient care is also provided by the consulting psychiatrists for the most challenging patients. Both the mental health providers and the psychiatrists have reported satisfaction with the model [25, 26]. The school clinicians reported that students appeared comfortable and possibly were more open regarding their concerns by using telemental health. Psychiatry fellows who provided the telemental healthcare were also satisfied, but noted that occasional on-site visits would help them to appreciate the students' milieu and the staff's resources, as well as the overall community.

Challenges to delivering telemental healthcare to schools are considerable and must be guided by the Family Educational Rights and Privacy Act [27] that specifies privacy rules for accessing student health information. The infrastructure needed for telemental health services may be difficult to establish in under-resourced, overcrowded schools, such as privacy and adequacy of the interview room.

Despite these challenges, the national trend to approve statewide Medicaid coverage of telemedicine, including the delivery of services to nontraditional sites such as schools [28], indicates further growth of school-based telemental healthcare. While more work is needed regarding the optimal delivery of telemental health services in schools and the outcomes of such care, school-based telemental health offers an opportunity to evaluate youth in naturalistic settings and collaborate with their educational staff.

Juvenile Justice System

Case: Bailey is a 16-year-old girl who has had longstanding struggles with ADHD, depression, and oppositional defiant disorder. She was recently sent to juvenile detention for multiple charges of shoplifting, vandalism, and disorderly conduct. In detention, she has become more depressed and anxious, is unable to sleep, and endorses suicidality to the detention center's healthcare provider. The provider arranges for her to be evaluated that afternoon by the telepsychiatrist who works part time for the facility. Initially, Bailey refused as she was concerned about privacy. The healthcare provider arranged for a nurse, rather than a detention staff, to accompany her to the session. Using tablets, the nurse scanned the examination room so that the telepsychiatrist could assess privacy and safety of the site. The telepsychiatrist's evaluation noted a major depressive disorder as well as exacerbating generalized anxiety disorder and suicide risk. The telepsychiatrist coordinated care with the healthcare provider who prescribed an antidepressant and placed Bailey on suicide observations. The telepsychiatrist implemented a brief course of mindfulness during and between the subsequent telepsychiatry sessions until she was adjudicated. In this model of care, the telepsychiatrist may have little control over the length or parameters of treatment and must adjust rapport building and treatment choice within the context of this uncertainty.

An unfortunate reality for many youth in the United States is involvement in the Juvenile Justice System (JJS). Oftentimes, these are the children and adolescents with undiagnosed mental health disorder, and most in need of mental healthcare, but with little access to care. Administrators within the corrections system have the daunting task of obtaining mental healthcare for their wards with limited resources. Telemental health provides a feasible and acceptable service model for this population across diagnoses and levels of care [29–31]. Clinicians in these settings must be aware of the risk of dual agency to their patients and the facilities by whom they are employed while balancing the needs of both. Privacy is a concern to youth, and the youth's healthcare team, rather than correctional staff, should be designated to participate in their telemental health sessions. A virtual tour of the clinical space and chart room will help to elucidate any concerns about security of the session and data storage. Often, juvenile corrections settings have on-site mental health staff who can implement a recommended course of therapy, or youth may prefer the relative anonymity of a teleprovider who is not on-site. Even with these challenges, telemental health can facilitate the provision of needed care to this underserved population and may help to alter their life course.

Home-Based Care

Case: Jamison is a 15-year-old young man with autism spectrum disorder and moderate intellectual disability who lives in a suburban community and is in treatment at an autism center. He has been increasingly aggressive and frequently tries to jump out of his parents' car when they take him to appointments. His family is very scared to transport him, but also knows that he needs to be reevaluated. His psychiatrist suggests that she evaluates him via videoconferencing in his home using the family's tablet. As Jamison is accustomed to using the tablet's communication board, he seems receptive to this approach. During the telesession, he was initially cooperative, but his frustration tolerance was limited. With the tablet, his parents were able to follow his movement around the house so that the autism team could appreciate his behaviors within the naturalistic setting of the home. They conducted a functional behavioral analysis [32] and implemented an interim treatment plan. Three months later, the family was able to transport him to the clinic for more routine care.

Within the last few years, attention has been given to delivering telemental healthcare to patients within their homes. Only a few studies have looked at delivering services to the home.

Early work has shown promise in this setting, however, as it allows the provider to observe and work with patients and their families in an ecologically environment. As described by Comer and colleagues [33, 34], this can be helpful especially when there are concerns about the impact of the home environment on the patient's mental health. Home-based care may also be helpful for teens who do not tolerate clinic settings, working parents, or for families that must move, for example, due to military assignments. The inability to control the multiple variables in this setting remains a significant limitation. Foremost, clinic staff are not available to assist with crises or urgent situations. Prior to commencing any services, a safety plan and protocol must be established [14]. Likewise, there are challenges to establishing privacy in the home. Teens may be more distractible when in their home environment, making it more difficult to engage them and for parents to redirect them [13]. Additionally, the home is not uniformly recognized as a site of care by many payers, although single case agreements can be made. Despite these concerns, telemental health to the patient's home is expected to increase over time as consumers request such services for youth who are not well served by traditional models of care.

Asynchronous Telemental Healthcare

Case: Caitlyn is a 14-year-old girl who lives with her family in a rural area of Alaska. She has been treated for attention-deficit hyperactivity disorder (ADHD) for several years by her family doctor. Recently, however, her grades have been slipping. At first, her parents and her doctor thought she was struggling to adjust to high school or that her recent growth spurt necessitated adjustment of her ADHD medication. After talking with Caitlyn, however, it becomes clear that she is struggling with symptoms of depression and anxiety and severe nightmares. She reveals that she recently began cutting herself. Her family doctor learned of the opportunity for asynchronous telepsychiatry consultation [35, 36] in Alaska. He records a standardized interview with Caitlyn that he then securely sends to the consulting child and adolescent psychiatrist for diagnostic and treatment recommendations. The psychiatrist determined a diagnosis of delayed post-traumatic stress disorder secondary to a trauma earlier in life prior to moving to Alaska. The psychiatrist made recommendations for medication that the family physician implemented and psychotherapy interventions with options to travel to a nearby center or to obtain through telemental health.

Regardless of the setting, most patients and providers think of telemental healthcare only as being provided in real time. In other fields of telemedicine, asynchronous, or "store and forward," care has become more commonplace. While it is easier to imagine how such a program would work for image-based fields such as radiology or remote monitoring such as cardiology, pioneering work has been done in telepsychiatry. In this model, a nonpsychiatric provider conducts and records a standardized interview with a patient, which is then later viewed by a psychiatric provider who provides diagnostic and treatment recommendations [35]. Alternatively, youth's behaviors in selected naturalistic settings, such as in school, may be recorded and uploaded onto a secure website for later observation and treatment planning [36]. This model can be particularly effective in healthcare systems that only employ part-time mental health providers, thus facilitating the timing of consultations, the efficiency of resource utilization, and possibly cost containment. It can also help child and adolescent providers to understand the variability of youths' behavior across settings. Currently, Alaska and Hawaii are conducting demonstration projects to test the feasibility, sustainability, and effectiveness of asynchronous telemental healthcare.

Logistics

While many aspects of telemental health are similar to in-person care, a number of logistical considerations must be addressed including technology options, space and staffing needs, and legal and regulatory obligations.

Technology

The various technology options available to providers interested in telemental health have evolved at a dizzying rate. While this can be overwhelming to providers, adolescent patients are accustomed to the rapid changes. Only a few years ago, the majority of practices utilized "standards-based" applications or platforms [37]. These platforms combine software with hardware specifically designed for telemedicine and use high bandwidth to transmit secure, high-quality synchronized audio and video signals through secure telephone-based systems. They provide excellent "telepresence." These systems are secure and offer the option of adding many peripheral features such as zoom and pan/tilt camera controls, dermatology-quality images, and stethoscopes. However, they require considerable initial financial investment, ongoing maintenance costs, and dedicated audiovisual technical staffing. Over the past decade, technological advances have converged with clinical need to provide "consumer-based" software platforms that transmit data via the Internet. These cloud-based platforms compress the bandwidth to approximate the high bandwidth offered by standards grade videoconferencing. They can be run on personal computers, tablets, or smartphones, making them more flexible and affordable to many practices. What they provide in flexibility, however, must be balanced by consideration of potential privacy and security compromise and limitations in adding peripheral features. Software vendors must sign a business agreement attesting compliance with the regulations established by the Health Information Portability and Accountability Act (HIPAA; [38]). Because the technology options change rapidly, providers are encouraged to review practice guidelines by organizations such as the American Telemedicine Association [14, 39] and to update and to reference resources such as the Telehealth Resource Centers (TRC; (40)).

Clinic Space

When developing a telemental health practice, providers need to consider space requirements, particularly at the patient, or originating, site, to develop a virtual therapeutic space. While there are no specific guidelines regarding the room in which the patients and their family members receive services, several recommendations have been proposed. In general, the room should be large enough to accommodate the teen and one or two adults, e.g., a parent and telepresenter. If the telemental health program plans on including more people, such as a multidisciplinary team at a school, a larger room is needed that can include all participants on-screen. Providers are cautioned from using a room that is too big as an oppositional teen could easily move outside of the scope of the camera. Likewise, medical examination rooms are often convenient locations, but create many distractions for patients. There is risk of damage to the medical equipment if the patients are not appropriately supervised.

Ideally, the patient room would be comfortably but sparsely decorated with a few age-appropriate implements to help the provider assess a patient's motor skills, attention span, relatedness, interests, and creativity. Of note, noisy items should be avoided as the sounds easily drown out voices on the sensitive microphone equipment [13]. Teens may simply prefer verbal interactions or want to share information on their smartphone or something they have written.

Lighting is crucial. Natural light from windows can fluctuate throughout the day and with weather changes. Bright overhead lights can cast distorting shadows. Lighting in back of participants will wash out that individual's image. Horizontal and indirect lighting are best. Prior to commencing services, the provider should work with a staff at the patient site to assess how the light affects the images on both the provider's and the patient's screens.

Finally, visual and auditory privacy of the rooms should be ensured so that patients and their family feel comfortable sharing sensitive information. The microphones are very sensitive. Thus, environmental noises, such as air conditioners or fans, rustling papers, and street sounds, should be minimized.

While there are no hard and fast rules regarding the location of the telemental health room, consideration of the physical space should be determined early in program development to ensure a therapeutic environment for the youth and family.

Staffing

The staff facilitating services at the patient/originating site, or "telepresenter" [41], can help to make a telemental health visit a safe and satisfying interaction. The Practice Guideline for Child and Adolescent Telemental Health defines a telepresenter as "An individual with a clinical background trained in the use of telehealth equipment who must be available at the originating site to "present" the patient, manage the cameras and perform any "hands-on" activities to complete the tele-exam successfully" [14]. Telepresenters may include licensed professionals or allied health professionals depending upon resources at the patient site. In some states, a telepresenter may be required, particularly for reimbursement from some payers. In addition to helping patients and their families navigate the telehealth session, the telepresenter can obtain vital signs, assist with completing rating scales, obtain laboratory testing results, liaise with the patients' primary care physicians or school, and provide collateral information regarding local concerns. They may share their observations of the patient outside of the telemental health session, e.g., while waiting in the lobby. They usually field calls from families between telemental health sessions and assist with medication refills, if needed. Telepresenters can also help patients and families identify local resources and, depending on their level of training, help provide psychoeducation for families. Most importantly, the telepresenter is a responsible staff member in whom the psychiatrist can rely for assistance between session and in urgent situation.

Legal and Regulatory Requirements

As telemental health continues to evolve, the legal and regulatory requirements are evolving as well. Currently, legislation and regulations regarding telemedicine practice are set at the state level. As a result, providers are strongly encouraged to determine the requirements governing their jurisdiction. If a provider chooses to treat a patient in another state, this can become even more complex, as the current recommendation is to adhere to the laws and regulations for the state in which the provider practices as well as the state in which the patient is receiving services.

Licensure is an important example of cross-state practice. In general, providers are expected to have a license in each state in which they practice. Of note, this does not represent the states in which patients *live*, but the states in which patients *receive care*. For example, if a patient who is receiving in-person services in one state moves to another state for college, and the psychiatrist wants to continue treatment through telemental health, he/she must be licensed in the patient's new state. Obtaining and maintaining multiple state licenses can be time-consuming and expensive. As a result, the Interstate Medical Licensure Compact [42] was introduced and has been adopted by several states. States participating in the Compact agree to standards of licensure and promise "increased efficiency in the licensing of physicians who practice in multiple states" [42]. Still, there is much variability in the requirements from state to state, and providers are encouraged to research the specifics for any state in which they wish to treat patients [43].

Beyond licensure, providers should also review other specific legislation for each state to which they plan to deliver services. Requirements for mandatory reporting of abuse and neglect can vary from state to state. Procedures and requirements for civil commitments differ by jurisdiction. Even the age of majority can differ. More specifically to telemedicine, some states have specific requirements regarding informed consent for telemedicine. The American Telemedicine Association has developed a State Telemedicine Legislation Tracker and a State Telemedicine Regulations Tracker to assist providers and organizations in identifying current requirements [44].

Credentialing and privileging pose local concerns. Providers are expected to have been credentialed and given privileges at each institution at which they practice. Like licensure, this can be a time-consuming and expensive undertaking. To facilitate this process, the Centers for Medicare & Medicaid Services [1] now allow "privileging by proxy" for telemedicine providers [45]. With this arrangement, one entity can accept the privileging decision of another entity. For example, rather than going through the time and expense of credentialing a telepsychiatrist, a rural hospital may accept the report of privileges from the urban hospital at which the telepsychiatrist is on staff. The Joint Commission has been supportive of this process as well.

Providing pharmacotherapy through telepsychiatry is a topic receiving national and state attention. Congress passed the Ryan Haight Online Pharmacy Consumer Protection Act of 2008 to prevent online pharmacies from illegitimately dispensing controlled substances without appropriate physician oversight [46]. This Act inadvertently caught legitimate medical and psychiatric practice in its broad net by placing restrictions around "the practice of prescribing by means of the Internet." While the Act specifically states that telemedicine is an exception to the Act, it technically requires that prescribers conduct at least one in-person evaluation of the patient prior to prescribing a controlled substance through telemedicine. Alternatively, patients being treated in and located in a hospital or clinic registered with the Drug Enforcement Administration (DEA) and in the presence of a DEA-registered practitioner may be prescribed a controlled substance during telemedicine. The letter of this legislation is difficult to follow and severely dilutes the value of telepsychiatry, or any telemedicine-related, practice. However, the DEA has noted that it does not intend to interfere with the legitimate prescribing of controlled substances during telemedicine practice [47]. While awaiting further clarification of rules around telemedicine prescribing several states have enacted legislation to allow the prescribing of controlled substances during telemedicine practice, particularly for telepsychiatry. Psychiatrists should carefully review federal and state guidelines in establishing their telepsychiatry practice regarding the prescription of controlled substances, as well as consider the best interests of their patients.

Risk Management

While the legal and regulatory requirements to practice telemental health can vary widely from state to state, there are some basic risk management strategies that can help alleviate risk. Specifically, providers should give close attention to informed consent, data security and privacy, and emergency procedures and protocols when developing a telemental health practice.

Just as with in-person care, informed consent is an important consideration for telemental health. As mentioned, several states have specific legislation regarding informed consent for telemedicine in particular, and providers are advised to research the local laws in their states. Key elements of informed consent include reviewing with patients and their families the requirements for confidentiality and the potential limits of that confidentiality when videoconferencing or other technology is utilized for the visit. Informed consent should also review how medical records will be maintained and stored and how those records will be shared between the patient site and the provider site. Informed consent should also outline the procedures for care in emergency situations and options for receiving care should the patient choose not to participate in telemental health. Finally, when developing informed consent policies, providers should be knowledgeable regarding the age of consent in each state in which they practice [39, 43].

Security and privacy are also issues that must be considered. At the most basic level, providers need to assess whether the technology they are utilizing is compliant with the HIPAA regulations [48]. As of April 2017, the Health and Human Services' website offers the following update regarding electronic personal health information privacy:

> The HIPAA Security Rule by 'the use of an algorithmic process to transform data into a form in which there is a low probability of assigning meaning without use of a confidential process or key' (45 CFR 164.304 definition of encryption) and such confidential process or key that might enable decryption has not been breached.

It is often quoted that the HIPAA standards require a minimum of 128-bit encryption for any electronic protected health information, but as technology evolves, this is expected to change and providers should clarify current requirements. Simply meeting the standard for HIPPA may not be sufficient, however, especially when mobile devices and wireless internet are employed, and additional encryption may be necessary.

As mentioned previously, choice of a patient room must consider privacy, including auditory privacy. Rooms should be sound-proofed. Telepsychiatry etiquette indicates that all participants should be visible on-screen. At the beginning of a patient encounter, providers are encouraged to introduce anyone else in the room with them and ask for the identity of anyone accompanying the teen. If perchance any participants are offscreen due to arrangements at the site, providers should clarify who else is attending the session and ask them to identify themselves if speaking.

Finally, prior to commencing any services, the provider and staff must develop a protocol regarding procedures and management for urgent situations. This includes identifying local resources, such as the nearest emergency room and law enforcement support. Additionally, the telepresenters and any other staff that have contact with patients should be trained regarding procedures for reporting suspected abuse to Child Protective Services, as well as for addressing situations in which other trauma is disclosed. The protocol should outline the roles of each individual on the telemental health team and responsibility for different aspects of the plan, such as who should contact local emergency support. Providers and staff should also consider how to maintain the appropriate level of privacy when initiating emergency protocols, especially for patients in small communities.

Overall, telemental health programs can increase access to and improve the quality of mental health services for youth. As with any mental healthcare practice, however, risks must be identified and actively managed to ensure safety and quality care. Teleproviders must establish competencies in delivering legal, safe, and team-based care that mitigates risk.

Evaluation and Treatment

The principles guiding the evaluation and treatment of adolescents' mental health concerns in person are the same for delivering these services through telemental health. Accommodations are made for service mode. Given the evolution of telemental health interventions, providers should maintain their competencies through familiarity with current guidelines provided by professional organizations, such as the American Telemedicine Association's Practice Guideline for Telemental Health with Children and Adolescents [14] and the American Academy of Child and Adolescent Psychiatry's Practice Parameter for Telepsychiatry with Children and Adolescents [49].

Evaluation

The first consideration in adapting evidence-based care to delivery through videoconferencing is determining if the adolescent is appropriate to receive care utilizing technology [14, 49]. While there are no absolute contraindications to telemental health, each provider must determine his/her competencies in treating the proposed population and selected disorders and whether the site's infrastructure is appropriate to the needed care. Cultural and language differences between the provider and patient can be challenging in telemental healthcare. Assessing important aspects of the mental status examination may require special approaches. For example, poor eye contact raises concerns about autism spectrum disorders, anxiety, depression, and psychosis. As the camera does not accurately convey eye contact, the provider needs to obtain input from the parent or telepresenter or clarification from the youth regarding the experience of eye contact. Concerns have been raised regarding the evaluation of psychosis via videoconferencing, although such concerns are unfounded. Nonetheless, providers must be sensitive to the possible need to adjust their communication style with patients experiencing paranoia or delusions. If standardized assessment tools are utilized, providers must account for any variations that may occur due to administration through videoconferencing [50]. Until more research is available, these concerns should not be considered contraindications to delivering evidence-based treatment through telemental health, but rather service delivery issues addressed by adjustment of style or use of collateral information.

Psychopharmacology

When developing a telepsychiatry program with the intention of prescribing medication, a number of factors must be considered. As noted previously, legal and regulatory issues must be addressed for each state to which services are delivered. The prescription of controlled substances has additional concerns [46, 47]. The technology chosen should be appropriate to the clinical service delivered as well as ensure visual and audio privacy. Bandwidth and screen resolution must be sufficient to assess medication side effects such as tics and more subtle effects such as affective blunting [14, 49]. Infrastructure and staffing at the patient site are needed to obtain vital signs, height, and weight, laboratory monitoring, and any needed information from the primary care provider, schools, or other referring sources. The Abnormal Involuntary Movement Scale can be administered through videoconferencing [51] although the telepresenter may be trained to assess cogwheel (www.rbha.net/presentations/AIMSDemo/player.html).

Overall, the principles of psychopharmacology treatment are the same as established for in-person care, but may require some creative logistical modifications.

Psychotherapy

As with initial evaluation and medication management, there are no absolute contraindications to providing psychotherapy to adolescents via telemental health [14]. Cognitive behavioral therapy for depression and anxiety is the most frequently reported therapy [52]. Other approaches have included behavioral interventions, such as for tics and obsessive-compulsive disorder, and parent management training for disruptive behaviors. Family and group therapy can be delivered using telemental health, but accommodations such as having a skilled facilitator at the patient site may be necessary. Although rarely used for adolescents, highly interactive therapies, such as parent-child interaction therapy [53], have been reported using telemental health technology.

As measurement-based care is becoming the standard for usual practice, providers should document the efficacy of psychotherapy using rating scales or other relevant approaches. Such assessments may be completed remotely and submitted to providers through patient portals, or deidentified email, or other secure methods.

Future Directions

Today's adolescents will help to guide the future of telemedicine, including telemental health. In 2001, Prensky coined the term "digital natives" to describe the generation born after 1980 [54]. As digital natives, current and future adolescents have always known the world of connectivity. They will increasingly demand that we meet them in their digital world. Healthcare systems are incorporating new telehealth technologies into usual healthcare. Their role in augmenting telemental healthcare remains to be determined. A role can readily be envisioned. For example, telemental health sessions in some underserved communities may be available to patients on a less than optimal schedule due to limited resources. Newer asynchronous telehealth technologies may provide interim information to guide decision-making during valuable, but limited, telemental health sessions.

Remote monitoring is commonplace in several medical specialties, such as cardiology. This type of remote monitoring can help improve compliance or adjust medications. For example, many teens with type I diabetes do not check their blood sugar as regularly. This could be mitigated by using monitors in insulin pumps that send reminders to the patients (or if necessary their parents) notifying them of abnormal values. Wearable technologies measure physical parameters from the number of steps a person takes, to their heart rate, to the number of hours that they sleep. Such remote monitoring can provide the consulting telepsychiatrist data to optimize subsequent sessions with youth who are resistant to managing their blood sugars, or youth whose increased physical activity suggests that medication effects have waned, or depressed youth whose sleep remains dysregulated.

Texting is becoming the preferred mode of communication for adolescents [55], and some psychotherapists have incorporated texting into their treatment to maintain engagement and safety with their patients. Texting may preclude the need for "phone tag" with youth or their families. With this asynchronous telehealth technology, however, comes the need to set boundaries with patients and families. For example, providers should discuss with patients and families when texting is appropriate and when it is not. In particular, providers should explicitly discuss whether it is acceptable for texting to be used for communication during crises. Unless providers are prepared to monitor text messages around the clock, texts cannot be used in emergencies, such as when a patient is experiencing suicidal ideation. Conversely, providers may use texting to reach out to teens and families, for example, to send automated reminders to take their medication or use their mood logs. Clinical infrastructure will have to be adapted to assist in monitoring and reviewing these interactions.

Adolescents report feeling more comfortable, honest, and engaged in therapeutic programs when there is anonymity [56–58]. Mobile applications (apps) may appeal to this preference. Many apps are available to help patients with anxiety to practice different coping skills such as breathing exercises. Other apps are designed to help patients to track and rate their mood, drug cravings, obsessive thoughts, or hallucinations. While many of these apps are available for free download or for a very limited cost, most have not been rigorously tested for their effectiveness, may not be based on evidence-based practice. Nonetheless, the use of asynchronous tools such as mobile apps offers the opportunity for youth to practice skills learned during telemental health sessions. They may be incorporated into integrated healthcare systems that "prescribe" an app prior to a higher level of care through telemental health or in-person care.

Finally, social media is a significant source of support for many adolescents. The benefits of social media are often cited as the ability to bring together people from social, economic, and geographic groups. Individuals isolated in their communities, due to a medical or psychiatric disorder, may find support through a social media site. While many concerns exist regarding safety, inappropriate communications, and difficulty in authenticating the identity of participants, many expectations are developing regarding therapeutic applications for social media. Telemental health providers in a contained healthcare system may find social media a mechanism to provide psychoeducation to their adolescent patients. Social media is a major presence in adolescents' lives. At a minimum, providers' familiarity with social media can help to channel their young patients toward safe and beneficial sites.

Going forward, many more psychiatrists and other medical and nonmedical providers are expected to incorporate telemental health into their practices, at healthcare organizations, in the public sector, and in private practice either through hybrid models of care [15] or as an alternative to traditional practice. While the process of establishing a telemental health service may seem daunting, there are multiple resources to assist the process. The first step is to determine the population to serve, followed by the model of care and partners. For example, school-based telemental health, community telemental health, or correctional settings will provide a defined population and support staff. The provider and partners must decide whether services will include consultation to primary care providers or direct service to youth or perhaps collaboration in co-managing care. Providers already practicing in these settings often substitute some videoconferencing hours for selected traditional in-person services. Others respond to advertisements for child and adolescent mental health specialists and offer telemental health approaches to service delivery. Providers seeking a patient population for typical psychotherapy and pharmacotherapy practice may seek to work with a commercial vendor or to "go it alone." The multitude of commercial vendors is readily appreciated by searching the Internet for "telepsychiatry jobs" or "telemental health jobs." These companies vary in their arrangements including time for patient sessions, support services, and reimbursement. Providers should interview these vendors just as they would for traditional employment. Providers seeking to establish their own private telepractice may consider joining national professional networking sites to share their interests in telemental health. Finally, several national organizations maintain website with timely, cutting-edge information on policy, resources, reimbursement, and other information needed to establish a sustainable telemental health practice [15, 28, 40, 59, 60].

Conclusion

As more adolescents struggle with mental health disorders, and become eligible for services with healthcare reform, but encounter dwindling resources for treatment, new approaches to mental healthcare are needed. Telemental health offers one approach. It helps to redistribute the existing mental healthcare workforce and to strengthen the skills of primary care physicians through collaborative models of care. Diverse populations and settings have profited from existing telemental health programs, and new programs are rapidly developing as technological and financial barriers to technology-driven care fall. Published guidelines of care can help prospective telemental health providers in establishing an evidence-based practice, but creativity may be needed to overcome any logistic hurdles to implementing services. Going forward, more research is needed to establish the effectiveness of telemental health services delivered to adolescents and to explore the role of asynchronous and other emerging telehealth technologies in augmenting telemental healthcare. Meanwhile, continued innovative program development indicates that telemental health appeals to adolescents' digital preferences to addressing their needs.

References

1. Substance Abuse and Mental Health Services Administration. Behavioral Health Barometer 2015. https://www.samhsa.gov. Accessed 1 Mar 2017.
2. Kieling C, Baker-Henningham H, Belfer M, Conti G, Ertem I, Omigbodun O, et al. Child and adolescent mental health worldwide: evidence for action. Lancet. 2011;378(9801):1515–25.
3. American Medical Association. AMA Physician Masterfile. http://www.ama-assn.org/ama/pub/about-ama/physician-data-resources/physician-masterfile.page. Accessed 14 Apr 2017.
4. Flaum M. Telemental health as a solution to the widening gap between supply and demand for mental health services. In: Myers K, Turvey C, editors. Telemental health: clinical, technical and administrative foundation for evidence-based practice. London: Elsvier Insights; 2013. p. 11–25.
5. Insel T. Where are we going? Director's Blog: Psychiatry: National Institute of Mental Health, 2011. http://www.nimh.nih.gov/about/director/2011/psychiatry-where-are-we-going.shtml. Accessed 14 Apr 2017.
6. Thomas C, Holzer C. The continuing shortage of child and adolescent psychiatrists. J Am Acad Child Adolesc Psychiatry. 2006;45(9):1023–31.
7. Thomas K, Ellis A, Konrad T, Holzer C, Morrissey J. County-level estimates of mental health professional shortage in the united states. Psychiatr Serv. 2009;60(10):1323–8.
8. Michalski DS, Kohout JL. The state of the psychology health service provider workforce. Am Psychol. 2011;66(9):825–34.
9. Center for Medicare and Medicaid. Telehealth. http://www.cms.gov/Medicare/Medicare-General-Information/Telehealth/index.html Accessed 14 Apr 2017.
10. Centers for Medicare & Medicaid Services. Telemedicine. 2014; https://www.medicaid.gov/medicaid-chip-program-information/by-topics/delivery-systems/telemedicine.html. Accessed 1 Mar 2017.
11. Centers for Medicare & Medicaid. Telemedicine. http://www.medicaid.gov/Medicaid-CHIP-Program-Information/By-Topics/Delivery-Systems/Telemedicine.html. Accessed 22 Apr 2017.
12. Yellowlees P, Shore J, Roberts L. Practice guidelines for videoconferencing-based telemental health—October 2009. Telemed J E Health. 2010;16(10):1074–89.
13. Gloff N, Lenoue S, Novins D, Myers K. Telemental health for children and adolescents. Int Rev Psychiatry. 2015;27(6):512–24.
14. Myers K, Nelson EL, Hilty DM, Rabinowitz T. Practice guidelines for child and adolescent telemental health. American Telemedicine Association, March 2017. http://www.americantelemed.org/. Accessed 22 Apr 2017.

15. Yellowlees P, Chan SR, Parish MB. The hybrid doctor-patient relationshp in the age of technology-Telepsychiatry consultations and the use of virtual space. Int Rev Psychiatry. 2015;27(6):476–89.
16. Center for Telehealth and e-Health Law. http://ctel.org/. Accessed 22 Apr 2017.
17. Unutzer J. Payment for important work gets approved. Psychiatric News, American Psychiatric Association, Published online August 26, 2016. http://psychnews.psychiatryonline.org/doi/full/10.1176/appi.pn.2016.9a11. Accessed 22 Apr 2017.
18. Blount F, Miller B. Addressing the workforce crisis in integrated primary care. J Clin Psychol Med Settings. 2009;16(3):113–9.
19. Fortney JC, Pyne JM, Mouden SB, Mittal D, Hudson TJ, Schroeder GW, et al. Practice-based versus telemedicine-based collaborative care for depression in rural federally qualified health centers: a pragmatic randomized comparative effectiveness trial. Am J Psychiatry. 2013;170(4):414–25.
20. Fortney JC, Pyne JM, Kimbrell TA, Hudson TJ, Robinson DE, Schneider R, Moore WM, Custer PJ, Grubbs KM, Schnurr PP. Telemedicine-based collaborative care for posttraumatic stress disorder: a randomized clinical trial. JAMA Psychiat. 2015;72(1):58–67.
21. Ratzliff A, Unutzer J, Katon W, Stephens KA. Integrated care: creating effective mental and primary health care teams. Malden: Wiley; 2016. 336 p.
22. Sia C, Tonniges TF, Osterhaus E, Taba S. History of the medical home concept. Pediatrics. 2004;113(5):1473–8.
23. McWilliams J. Integrating telemental healthcare with the patient-centered medical home model. J Child Adolesc Psychopharmacol. 2016;26(3):278–82.
24. Nelson E, Duncan AB, Peacock G, Bui T. Telemedicine and adherence to national guidelines for ADHD evaluation: a case study. Psychol Serv. 2012;9(3):293–7.
25. Cunningham D, Connors E, Lever N, Stephan S. Provider's perspectives: utilizing telepsychiatry in schools. Telemed e-Health. 2013;19(10):794–9.
26. Grady B, Lever N, Cunningham D, Stephan S. Telepsychiatry and school mental health. Child Adolesc Psychiatr Clin N Am. 2011;20(1):81–94.
27. U.S. Department of Education. 20 U.S.C. § 1232g; 34 CFR Part 99: Family Educational Rights and Privacy Act (FERPA). http://www2.ed.gov/policy/gen/guid/fpco/ferpa/index.html?src=rn. Accessed 14 Apr 2017.
28. Thomas L, Capistrant G. 50 State telemedicine gaps analysis: coverage & reimbursement. Washington, DC: American Telemedicine Association; 2016. https://higherlogicdownload.s3.amazonaws.com/AMERICANTELEMED/3c09839a-fffd-46f7-916c-692c11d78933/UploadedImages/Policy/State%20Policy%20Resource%20Center/Coverage%20-%202016_50-state-telehealth-gaps-analysis--coverage-and-reimbursement.pdf. Accessed 22 Apr 2017.
29. Myers K, Valentine J, Melzer S, Morganthaler R. Telepsychiatry with incarcerated youth. J Adol Health. 2006;38(6):643–8.
30. Fox K, Connor P, McCullers E, Walters T. Effect of a behavioral health and specialty care telemedicine programme on goal attainment for youths in juvenile detention. J Telemed Telecare. 2008;14:227–30.
31. Kaliebe K, Heneghan J, Kim T. Telepsychiatry in juvenile justice settings. Child Adol Psychiatr Clinics N Am. 2011;20(1):113–23.
32. Lee JF, Schieltz KM, Suess AN, Wacker DP, Romani PW, Lindgren SD, et al. Guidelines for developing telehealth services and troubleshooting problems with telehealth technology when coaching parents to conduct functional analyses and functional communication training in their homes. Behav Anal Practice. 2014;8(2):190–00.
33. Comer J, Elkins R, Chan P, Jones D. New methods of service delivery for children's mental health care. In: Alfano CA, Biedel D, editors. Comprehensive evidence-based interventions for school aged children and adolescents. New York: Wiley; 2014. p. 55–72.
34. Comer J, Furr J, Cooper-Vince C, Madigan R, Chow C, Chan P, et al. Rationale and considerations for the internet-based delivery of parent-child interaction therapy. Cogn Behavior Prac. 2015;22(3):302–16.
35. Yellowlees P, Odor A, Parish M, Iosif A, Haught K, Hilty D. A feasibility study of the use of asynchronous telepsychiatry for psychiatric consultations. Psychiatr Serv. 2010;61(8):838–40.
36. Nazneen N, Rozga A, Smith CJ, Oberleitner R, Abowd GD, Arriaga RI. A novel system for supporting autism diagnosis using home videos: iterative development and evaluation of system design. J Med Internet Res Mhealth Uhealth. 2015;3(2):e68. https://doi.org/10.2196/mhealth.4393.
37. Chou T, Comer JS, Turvey CL, Karr A, Spargo G. Technological considerations for the delivery of real-time child telemental health care. J Child Adolesc Psychopharmacol. 2016;26(3):192–7.
38. U.S. Department of Health and Human Services. Health Information Privacy: The Health Insurance Portability and Accountability Act (HIPAA) of 1996. 1996. http://www.hhs.gov/ocr/privacy/index.html. Accessed 22 Apr 2017.
39. Turvey C, Coleman M, Dennison O, Drude K, Goldenson M, Hirsch P, et al. ATA practice guidelines for video-based online mental health services. Telemed J E Health. 2013;19(9):722–30.
40. Office for the Advancement of Telehealth (OAT). Telehealth Resource Centers. 2015. http://www.telehealthresourcecenter.org/. Accessed 30 Apr 2017.
41. Leenknecht CK. The Telepresenting Standards and Guidelines Working Group. Expert consensus recommendations for videoconferencing-based telepresenting. 2011. http://dev.americantelemed.org/docs/default-source/standards/expert-consensus-recommendations-for-videoconferencing-based-telepresenting.pdf?sfvrsn=4. Accessed 22 Apr 2017.
42. Interstate Medical Licensure Compact. A faster pathway to medical licensure. https://imlcc.org/. Accessed 22 Apr 2017.
43. Kramer GM, Luxton DD. Telemental health for children and adolescents: an overview of legal, regulatory, and risk management issues. J Child Adolesc Psychopharmacol. 2016;26(3):198–203.

44. American Telemedicine Association's State Legislative & Regulatory Trackers. http://www.americantelemed.org/policy-page/state-policy-resource-center. Accessed 22 Apr 2017.
45. Centers for Medicare and Medicaid Services. 2011. http://www.jointcommission.org/assets/1/6/Revisions_telemedicine_standards.pdf. Accessed 22 Apr 2017.
46. Ryan Haight Online Pharmacy Consumer Protection Act. In: L P, ed. No. 110, H.R. 6353; 2008.
47. Arnold J, Chief of Policy Section, Drug Enforcement Administration, United States Department of Justice. Prescribing controlled substances via telemedicine. Presentation at the Short Course, 21st Annual Meeting of the American Telemedicine Association, Kaftarian E, Moderator; 2016 May 14–16; Minneapolis MN. http://hub.americantelemed.org/Go.aspx?MicrositeGroupTypeRouteDesignKey=cfbbf78e-e941-4c56-a54d-8d1903fa21b6&NavigationKey=c07d498f-c72b-42ab-8ecd-12367d8308f7.
48. U.S. Department of Health and Human Services. Guidance to render unsecured protective health information unusable, unreadable or undecipherable to unauthorized individuals. https://www.hhs.gov/hipaa/for-professionals/breach-notification/guidance/index.html. Accessed 15 Apr 2017.
49. American Academy of Child and Adolescent Psychiatry (AACAP) Committee on Telepsychiatry and AACAP Committee on Quality Isues. Clinical Update: Telepsychiatry with children and adolescents. J Am Acad Child Adol Psychiatry. 2017;56(10):875–93.
50. Cullum C, Grosh M. Special considerations in conducting neuropsychology assessment over videoteleconferencing. In: Myers K, Turvey C, editors. Telemental health: clinical, technical and administrative foundation for evidence-based practice. London: Elsvier Insights; 2013. p. 275–93.
51. Amarendran V, George A, Gersappe V, Krishnaswamy S, Warren C. The reliability of telepsychiatry for a neuropsychiatric assessment. Telemed J E Health. 2011;17(3):223–5.
52. Nelson E, Duncan A. Cognitive-behavioral therapy using televideo. Cogn Behav Pract. 2015;22(3):269–80.
53. Crum KI, Comer JS. Using synchronous videoconferencing to deliver family-based mental healthcare. J Child Adolesc Psychopharmacol. 2016;26(3):229–34.
54. Prensky M. Digital natives, digital immigrants, Part 1. On the Horizon. 2001;9(5):1–6. Emeraldinsight. http://www.pewinternet.org/2012/03/19/teens-smartphones-texting/.
55. Lenhart A. Teens, Smartphones and texting. Pew Internet and American Life Project, Washington, DC; 2012. http://www.pewinternet.org/2012/03/19/teens-smartphones-texting/. Accessed April 30, 2017.
56. Pretorius N, Rowlands L, Ringwood S, Schmidt U. Young people's perceptions of and reasons for accessing a web-based cognitive behavioural intervention for bulimia nervosa. Eur Eating Dis Rev. 2010 Apr;18(3):197–06.
57. Diamond JM, Block RM. Telepsychiatry assessments of child or adolescent behaviour disorders: a review of evidence and issues. Telemed e-Health. 2010;16(6):712–6.
58. Boydell KM, Hodgins M, Pignatiello A, Teshima J, Edwards H, Willis D. Using technology to deliver mental health services to children and youth: a scoping review. J Can Acad Child Adolesc Psychiatry. 2014;23(2):87–9.
59. Office for the Advancement of Telehealth, Health Resources and Services Administration, DHHS. Telehealth Resource Centers. http://www.telehealthresourcecenter.org/. Accessed May 24, 2017.
60. Center for Connected Health Policy. The National Telehealth Policy Resource Center. Office for the Advancement of Telehealth, Health Resources and Services Administration, DHHS. http://www.cchpca.org/. Accessed May 24, 2017.

14 Social Media Interventions for Adolescents and Young People with Depression and Psychosis

Olga Santesteban-Echarri, Mario Álvarez-Jiménez, John Gleeson, and Simon M. Rice

Social media refers to any web-based platform that allows social interaction. As a subset of social media, social networking sites (SNS) are web-based services that permit people to (1) create a public or semipublic profile within a bounded system, (2) easily organize a list of other users with whom they wish to connect, and (3) manage connections and contact with and between other users within the system [1, 2].

Below we differentiate and discuss outcomes associated with two broad types of websites. Firstly, we briefly summarize use of general social media sites with a non-specific purpose by adolescents experiencing mental illness. Secondly, we outline social media-based mental health interventions specifically developed for adolescents and young adults. These are social media sites designed with the specific purpose of providing mental health support and exchanging health-related knowledge, information, and personal experiences of users. We focus this section specifically on SNS, as they are the social media type most widely discussed in the mental health literature and the most frequently used by adolescents. We subsequently report findings for mood disorder (depression) and psychosis (schizophrenia or psychotic disorders).

O. Santesteban-Echarri (✉)
Orygen, The National Centre of Excellence in Youth Mental Health, Melbourne, VIC, Australia

Centre for Youth Mental Health, The University of Melbourne, Melbourne, VIC, Australia

Department of Psychology, Universitat Rovira i Virgili, Tarragona, Spain
e-mail: olga.santesteban@gmail.com

M. Álvarez-Jiménez • S.M. Rice
Orygen, The National Centre of Excellence in Youth Mental Health, Melbourne, VIC, Australia

Centre for Youth Mental Health, The University of Melbourne, Melbourne, VIC, Australia
e-mail: Mario.Alvarez@orygen.org.au; simon.rice@orygen.org.au

J. Gleeson
School of Psychology, Australian Catholic University, Melbourne, VIC, Australia
e-mail: John.Gleeson@acu.edu.au

Social Media Use by Adolescents

Use of the Internet is pervasive, with 92% of the adolescents connecting at least once a day [3]. Use of SNS has become ubiquitous, becoming the new context for social support and communications among young adults regardless of geographical location, background, and age [4]. The availability of mobile phones among adolescents is high. It has been estimated that 88% of adolescents own or have access to a mobile phone, with approximately 75% of adolescents owning a smartphone [5]. Among them, 91% use their mobile phone for social media at least occasionally, and 94% go online daily using their phone. Moreover, more than half of adolescents

M.A. Moreno, A. Radovic (eds.), *Technology and Adolescent Mental Health*,
https://doi.org/10.1007/978-3-319-69638-6_14

(58%) have a tablet computer, and nearly all adolescents (87%) have a computer or access to one. Therefore, technology is well integrated in the day-to-day life of adolescents, and the use of social media may increase adolescents' social and communication skills [6, 7]. For instance, adolescents and young adults can create, share, and follow events important to them (e.g., raising money for a cause, community events, etc.), share their creative projects (e.g., music and art), create videos or podcasts, and interact with peers (over shared interests and organize meet-ups).

In contrast to the potential education and social benefits, use of social media also carries potential risks for adolescents, such as cyberbullying, invasion of privacy, and problematic Internet use. Also, higher social media use, and nighttime-specific social media use, predicts poorer sleep quality, which may increase daytime tiredness and affect school performance and other daily activities of adolescents [8]. There are other risks such as the phenomena known as "parallel reality" and "presentation anxiety" [9] (i.e., need to look "cool" and desirable on Facebook), or the peer-based pressure to conform to unrealistic ideals in relation to glamor and wealth, which as a consequence may lead to poor self-esteem. Other issues include the perception that others are much happier, which may make the adolescent unhappier [10]. Finally, those adolescents who report greater discrepancies between their social network size and their desired number of social interactions tend to browse more and have less direct communications [11]. This may lead to a spiral of loneliness with diminishing opportunities for reparative face-to-face communication.

Social Media, Adolescence, and Mental Health

Adolescence is the most vulnerable developmental period for the onset of mental health problems. The incidence of mental disorders rises and peaks between adolescence and young adulthood [12]. Adolescents and young adults are usually reluctant to seek professional help, and the lack of help seeking among young males is especially concerning, with estimates indicating that only 13% of young males experiencing a need for mental health-care seek support [13]. Adolescents and young adults who finally seek help for mental health problems are usually encouraged to do so by their parents [14]. Nevertheless, online platforms appear to have impacted adolescents and young adults' help-seeking behaviors. For example, when there is an available online service, adolescents and young adults may be more likely to seek help independently via the Internet [15]. Given this, mental health services with integrated social media services may be especially relevant during adolescence. Improvements in other parameters related to engaging with health services have also been associated with the use of social media, including fewer missed appointments, increased medication adherence, improved health literacy [16], and enhanced communication with treating professionals [7]. In terms of mental health, the integration of online therapy and SNS may be a valid alternative or adjunct for some people who may prefer online support and peer-to-peer networking instead of face-to-face interventions [17]. However, researchers are still trying to disentangle whether using SNS as an alternative to therapy or as an adjunct would be more beneficial for some types of patient profiles, abilities, and preferences. Although "blended care" (i.e., combination of mobile or online components and face-to-face care) is gradually being used in mental health care, questions have arisen regarding the optimal combination; it is a complex question which needs further research [18].

Novel information and communication technologies may provide a good opportunity for improving and even transforming the delivery of intervention in psychiatric disorders [19]. Integrating SNS within online interventions may specifically bridge the gap between child and adolescent services, between community-based and primary care services, and between youth specialized services (such as headspace and the Early Psychosis Prevention and Intervention Centre in Australia and Australian national foundations that provide early intervention mental health services to support adolescents and young adults aged 12–25 [20, 21]) and usual care, serving to improve longer-term engagement with mental health services [22, 23]. The integration of SNS within mental health interventions is likely to be a cost-effective alternative to maintaining intervention gains from specialized early intervention services due to their potential to reach a substantial portion of people who need mental health assistance [24, 25]. Due to the general enthusiasm of adolescents and young adults for new technologies, social media-based interventions may be especially effective for, and attractive to, patients with mental health problems [26, 27]. Pioneering interventions using these technologies may play a pivotal role in the delivery of extended support to maintain the clinical gains of specialized face-to-face services. Moreover, new technologies may address substantial challenges in mental health such as the access to and engagement with services [22].

Despite their potential promise, the question remains as to whether social media-based interventions and increased online social interaction facilitate and improve long-term social functioning and quality of life. For example, although three out of four young patients diagnosed with first-episode psychosis (FEP) achieve symptom remission after treatment [28–30], many individuals with FEP experience poor functional recovery and remain socially isolated [29]. Also, 30% of adolescents and young adults with emerging mood disorders are functionally impaired [31]. Importantly, functional recovery (i.e., engagement with vocational and educational pathways) is the outcome most valued by patients [32]. Nevertheless, due to the early stage of the field of online mental health research, a major gap in the research literature relates to the lack of long-term studies on the impact of social media use and SNS interactions on general functioning. In the following sections, we outline social media-based mental health interventions specifically developed for adolescents and young adults.

Summing up, SNS studies are currently underway with adolescents and young adults with depression, and results are eagerly anticipated [33]. There are also significant opportunities to provide more timely and accessible support to young adults experiencing suicidal ideation and for those who are at risk of suicide. However, efforts in creating social networking interventions, which may bolster social connectedness and group affiliation (factors known to be protective for depression and suicide attempt), are still needed [34, 35]. We review some of these interventions in the following section.

Social Media-Based Interventions for Depression

The use of integrated, social media-based interventions for adolescent depression is a new phenomenon. In their early review of social networking interventions, Veretilo and Billick (2012, p. 386) reported: "…PubMed search revealed no articles addressing the use of Facebook or other social networking sites in child, adolescent or young adult psychiatric patient populations." A more recent systematic review of Internet-based interventions by Rice et al. for the treatment of depression for young people (age = 12–25) [36] identified 15 depression-specific online interventions, none of which were social media-based interventions. The same review identified 22 studies reporting on the association between SNS use and depression. These identified studies were divided in two main categories: (1) SNS (16 studies), defined as sites without a specific purpose, and (2) online support groups (OSG) (4 studies), defined as sites with a specific purpose (i.e., seeking health-related information and sharing associated personal experiences). Only one of these studies was intervention-based. Some were preventive studies to identify at-risk youth [37], others used pre-existing platforms to identify adolescents and young adults with depression [38–40], one sought to identify if social media use was associated with depression [41], and one reported a case study [42]. The only study with an intervention focus is described below.

Wright et al. (2012) employed a hybrid model of Facebook and a face-to-face support network to study communication, competence, social support, and depression among college students [43].

Based on a Relational Health Communication Competence Model (RHCCM) [44] (a process by which communication competence (i.e., empathic listening, nonverbal sensitivity) enhances information exchange and cooperation), Wright et al. (2012) reported that the increased face-to-face and computer-mediated competence were associated with higher social support network satisfaction and lower depression scores. However, the face-to-face network had larger effects than the Facebook support networking in the reduction of depression. Nevertheless, this study was undertaken with healthy students who may already have had more intact offline support networks. Applying the RHCCM model to SNS may have larger effects with adolescents and young adults experiencing clinically significant depression.

Since Rice's et al. (2014) review, a number of published studies specifically designed to target adolescents and young adults with depression have emerged. These interventions have typically sought to engage end users across all stages of development, based on participatory design principles. Mindful of the potential vulnerability of adolescents and young adolescents with depression, common characteristics of these sites include an emphasis on ensuring privacy and anonymity of participants, with a particular focus on disseminating positive (as opposed to negative) content within the social network. Moreover, these sites provide different levels of peer interaction and moderation by expert clinicians to maintain these foci. A common exclusion criterion in the studies published to date is active suicidality, or in some cases, a prior suicide attempt. Below we provide an overview of three innovative interventions for adolescents with depression—SOVA [45, 46], Project TECH [47], and Rebound [34]—each of which integrate peer-to-peer social networking.

The 6-week SOVA (Supporting Our Valued Adolescents, sova.pitt.edu) single-group pilot study tested the usability of a social media website for adolescents and young adults (age = 14–26, $N = 96$) experiencing depression or anxiety [45, 46]. The intervention was designed to change negative beliefs regarding depression and anxiety (i.e., stigma, negative attitudes toward therapy, or medication) and to improve mental health knowledge. SOVA included daily blog posts, peer support, and interaction with moderators through prompted discussion questions posted in response to blog post topics. Results showed that the SOVA site was feasible and acceptable, met usability criteria, and had no safety concerns. Although participants endorsed the content as easy to understand, and enjoyed the helpful and positive atmosphere, they nominated their preference for greater social interaction with peers. Future goals of SOVA include testing user engagement interventions and conducting a randomized controlled trial to establish whether it (along with a separate site for parents, wisesova.pitt.edu) is effective in increasing the frequency of mental health service use for adolescents referred for depression or anxiety treatment by their primary care provider.

The Project TECH (Teens Engaged in Collaborative Health) intervention, referred to as a behavioral intervention technology, was designed as a 10-week single-group CBT-based online intervention for youth depression (age = 14–19, $N = 13$) [47]. Project TECH followed a theory-driven model of online human support (i.e., supportive accountability [48]), which argues that adherence to e-Health interventions is increased through human support. The model underscores accountability (by setting clear and explicit process-oriented expectations at the induction process such as number of expected loggings and completion of modules) and reciprocity in the peer relations (capacity of network members to support and supervise the expected activities of others), which both interact with patient motivation (motivated patients need less support). Moderators only ensured safety without directly participating in the site. Project TECH relied on lay supporters (peer network) to promote accountability and adherence. Supportive accountability is incorporated in the Project TECH by different features: (1) the Activity Tracker: peer member tiles display different colors, which mirror logging expectations and adherence to the site (i.e., a brown color if the user has not logged in >4 days, a blue color if logging on is periodical) (peer users can click on an icon to send less active users a motivational email), and (2) Thought Journal: users are encouraged to post in other users' journals, which increases adherence and collaborative learning. Some visual examples of the site are shown in Ho et al. (2016). Results showed that adolescents were engaged with the site via the peer-to-peer networking feature. Usage rates of the intervention decreased over time, and system usage was found to be negatively associated with users' desire to log on or their desire to participate with group members. The Project TECH pilot study highlighted the potential effectiveness of the behavioral intervention technology and the supportive accountability model, especially when integrating the peer-networking component (i.e., capacity of network members to support and supervise the activities of others). However, the Project TECH intervention only included adolescents with high risk of suffering depression (individuals with severe depression were excluded).

The third published trial of a social networking-based study for depression—Rebound—is the first social networking-based intervention for depression relapse prevention in young adults [34]. Rebound is based on the moderated online social therapy (MOST) model, developed to integrate social networking technologies and delivery of therapeutic content [49, 50]. Rebound integrates (1) peer-to-peer social networking, (2) individually tailored interactive therapy content, and (3) professional and peer moderation. Similar to the Project TECH intervention, Rebound also follows a theory-driven model of online human support (i.e., supportive accountability [48]) and a positive psychotherapy model (i.e., strengths-based interventions [51]). Through a pilot study over 12 weeks (age = 15–25, N = 42), the Rebound intervention was shown to be acceptable, feasible, engaging, and safe in young adults with major depressive disorder (MDD). Exclusion criteria for this study included intellectual disability, non-English speakers, medical conditions requiring a high level of care, and diagnosis of conduct, antisocial, or borderline personality. Nearly 70% of users logged in more than ten times during the 12 weeks of the pilot study, and almost 80% of users remained logged in over at least 8 weeks of the trial. There was a significant improvement in depressive symptoms, and 85% of users reported that Rebound was helpful. Safety was denoted by (1) users stating that they felt adequately supported by moderators, (2) no unlawful entries into the system, and (3) all users recognized the system to be safe. Qualitative follow-up of user experience related to social networking, safety, and clinical benefit outcomes identified three overarching themes: (1) perception of helpfulness of the intervention, (2) protective environment, and (3) interest in social networking of the online platform [52]. Two clear groups emerged from the qualitative analysis regarding perceptions of the most helpful elements of the intervention: (1) young adults who preferred to engage in therapy following individualized content suggested by moderators and (2) young adults who perceived the SNS aspect as the most helpful component. Based on these findings, integration of SNS features appears to enhance intervention engagement for some young adults recovering from depression.

Social Media-Based Interventions for Suicide Behavior

Depression is the most common risk factor for suicide behavior, and among those adolescents who attempt suicide, between 60 and 80% had a diagnosis of depression [53]. Therefore, social media-based interventions specifically targeting suicide prevention among adolescents may be relevant. A recent review [34] examined two interventions: (1) Re-Frame IT [54, 55], a 12-week randomized controlled trial (RCT) school-based and CBT-based and moderated intervention (age = 14–18, N = 21), and (2) Safe Conversations [56], a 12-week single-group (pre-post comparisons) school-based suicide prevention intervention with an online SNS in the context of Facebook (age = 15–18, N = 11). These interventions included detailed protocols for the assessment of risk throughout the studies and utilized human support (i.e., moderation by expert clinicians) to ensure maintenance intervention adherence and safety. Findings showed that these interventions offered an opportunity to enhance feelings of connectedness in at-risk young adults. Re-Frame IT showed clinically meaningful changes with an overall decrease of depressive symptoms and suicidal ideation after the intervention [54, 55]. Safe Conversations showed that there are safe ways to talk about suicide with adolescents and young adults in schools, and none of the participants reported that the project made them feel suicidal [56].

Developing insights into the motivations underpinning adolescents and young adults' usage patterns of social networking interventions may assist to improve the effectiveness of social media-based interventions for adolescents and young adults with depression (i.e., the use and integration of SNS-based site within traditional psychoeducational sites have been informed by users who report that their main motivation to use the site is to share personal experiences and learn from other adolescents and young adults in similar circumstances). Online and social media-based interventions offer the possibility to improve feelings of connectedness through peer-networking components. Preliminary results for the growing body of literature show that they appear to be both feasible and safe (i.e., users' self-perception of safety and support by moderators, no unlawful entries to the sites, and improvement in depression scores and maintenance of remission rates for those asymptomatic at baseline) for adolescents and young adults with depression. Importantly, models of online human support can offer a structured and moderated environment to ensure safety to adolescents and young adults with depression. Nonetheless, evidence underscores the difficulties of maintaining engagement over time in online interventions; therefore, mechanisms to improve engagement and benefits of SNS need to be better understood, while flexible interventions that cater for the needs of different participants are necessary. Future generations of e-mental health interventions require controlled evaluation (i.e., larger effectiveness trials), where the participants have access to the intervention over a suitable duration of time (i.e., >12 months).

Social Media and Psychosis

The restructuring of psychiatric care accomplished in some countries (i.e., Australia) has led to major systems reforms including the emergence of early intervention programs and youth programs, which aim to offer support and timely entry into care for youth [57, 58]. Duration of care of specialist services (i.e., first-episode psychosis (FEP)) usually spans between 18 months and 2 years, and some studies have reported that benefits from early intervention may not persist at 5 years [59, 60]. Therefore, one of the major challenges is to ensure maintenance of treatment gains and improvement of patient functioning over the long term. Social isolation is a known risk factor for developing psychosis, worsening symptomatic presentation, and poorer functioning [61, 62]. Moreover, youth with psychosis have reduced social networks in relation to the general population [63]. In particular, positive symptoms of psychosis (i.e., delusions, hallucinations, thought disorder) may be related to active social avoidance, while negative symptoms (i.e., anhedonia, avolition, alogia, reduced affect) may be more related to passive/apathetic social withdrawal [64].

Given the potential benefits of online SNS for adolescents, the Internet may be the ideal environment for adolescents and young adults with psychosis to counteract isolation and improve their social network. However, psychotic disorders do not usually occur before age 14, with prevalence notably increasing between 15 and 17 years old [65, 66]. For example, the median age of presentation of first-episode psychosis at the Early Psychosis Prevention and Intervention Centre (EPPIC, Melbourne, Australia) is 22 years old (IQR 19–25). Because of the later onset of the illness (e.g., compared with depression) and the variability of age at onset, there has been a remarkable scarcity of research on social media and SNS use in adolescents with psychosis, and the majority of literature in the field also includes older cohorts. Therefore we cannot directly generalize results, and findings should be interpreted with caution.

Potential Benefits of Social Media Use for Young Adults with Psychosis

Due to the social difficulties experienced by adolescents and young adults with psychosis (i.e., social isolation, reduced social networks), online SNS use may be effective in facilitating social interactions. Some social media characteristics may benefit communication patterns among this population:

(a) Online conversations do not require an immediate response which can be difficult for individuals with psychosis who have impaired sustained attention and working memory [67].
(b) SNS do not require the use of nonverbal behaviors (i.e., gesture production and social perception), relevant as negative symptoms are associated with poorer interpersonal rapport [68] (i.e., more negative symptoms are associated with less nodding when listening and more gesture use when speaking [68]).
(c) social interactions may allow the user to contact people from an expanded network beyond and above their offline connections [69, 70].
(d) SNS are anonymous and due to the typical absence of hierarchy, they may enhance trust in collectively solving problems through social interactions [71].

Due to associated stigma, people with psychosis may also reduce their face-to-face interactions and instead gravitate to social contact via the Internet, where their mental illness may not be as apparent [72] and they can be anonymous. Furthermore, young adults with psychosis usually report high levels of social anxiety [73]. Because online social networking may be a less intimidating space for people with social anxiety [74], young adults with a comorbid diagnosis of psychosis and social anxiety may prefer to socially connect via SNS.

Social Media Use by Young Adults with Psychosis

Existing literature paints an interesting picture in relation to the use of SNS by young adults experiencing psychosis. A recent systematic review synthesized data from 11 studies examining the use of SNS by people with a diagnosis of psychosis [75]. The review found that most people with psychosis used SNS and engaged in online social interactions. Furthermore, rates of Internet usage and SNS participation varied greatly among studies. Findings suggested that people with psychosis spent more time using SNS in chat rooms, and playing online games, although they had fewer face-to-face contacts compared with control users. It has been suggested that young adults with psychosis may prefer particular SNS (i.e., smaller SNS, chat rooms, and Internet gaming) rather than sites with larger networks, such as Facebook [76]. This suggests that adolescents with psychosis are motivated to engage in social interaction online. Smaller SNS may provide the social environment that otherwise may be difficult to achieve because of the interpersonal difficulties they have. Spinzy et al. (2012) reported that psychotic symptom severity of people with psychosis was associated with reduced use of the Internet, although the mean time spent using SNS was still higher than nonpsychotic participants with affective disorders and the control group (healthy volunteers) regardless of the reduced Internet access [77]. Although this group reported having fewer friends than the comparison groups, of note, nearly 80% (total $N = 143$) of the people with psychosis expressed the desire to establish new online social connections in order to create a real-life connection through the Internet.

Online Peer Support and Help-Seeking Behaviors of People with Psychosis

It seems that social media platforms such as Facebook and Twitter are integrated in the daily lives of young adults with early psychosis [78] who are motivated to engage in social interaction. Therefore, HJ Chang [79] employed a network approach by examining posts from PTT (a popular bulletin board system in Taiwan) which contained supportive interactions by peers in an online unmoderated psychosis discussion group over 2.5 years. They identified five types of useful support received by peers:

1. *Informational support* for posts regarding health institutions, doctors, symptoms, and medication (one of the most searched issues [71])
2. *Esteem support* for posts related to positive comments about lessening guilty feelings and acknowledging patients' capabilities
3. *Network support* for posts showing empathy, companionship, and sharing similar personal situations
4. *Emotional support* for posts offering confidence and providing hope
5. *Thankfulness* for those posts expressing appreciation and gratefulness

Moreover, supportive interactions were centralized (i.e., users either gave support or received support but not usually both). The majority of the exchanged supportive interactions (76%) occurred between two and three people, users showing a preference for small groups. In Taiwan, the divulging of sensitive personal information such as a diagnosis of psychosis is not the norm. However, users engaged positively in the online setting with the majority (71.5%) writing at least one post. It seemed that the anonymity of the site and the gratefulness showed by members (at least 50% of the posts) facilitated their engagement, as these values are highly valued within this culture. Therefore, online settings could be a good environment to discuss stigmatizing issues, especially among collectivistic cultures.

Analysis of other self-help forums has identified similar self-help mechanisms (communicative skills to facilitate the increase of supportive relationships) [80]. Also, it seems that young adults with psychosis contribute in online self-help forums using the same self-help mechanisms and converse about similar themes [80] relative to people with other psychiatric disorders [81] and caregivers [82]. Nearly 50% of users disclosed personal experiences and provided information about their illness, followed by requests for information and expression of empathy (nearly 30%). However, percentages of self-help mechanisms (i.e., skills of communication that ease the development of supportive relationships) for gratitude or friendship were scarce (less than 10% of the interactions) [80], contrasting with previously discussed results from HJ Chang [79]. Some problems specifically related to psychosis that were frequently discussed in forums were difficulties with excessive amount of information, problems with concentration, risk factors, illness causes, paranoid ideas, and lack of energy [71]. These results show that the Internet is a significant source of information for patients with psychosis.

In order to disentangle patterns of social media use before, during, and after symptom onset, a recent study explored help-seeking behaviors and pathways to care in adolescents and youth with a psychotic spectrum disorder (PSD) over a 2-year period [78]. This study compared youth with nonpsychotic mood disorders with those with PSD. Results indicated that young adults with PSD used Facebook and Twitter when experiencing symptoms to gather information from these sources, which had a subsequent role in decision making related to help-seeking initiation. The Internet was the primary source used to find mental health-related information in the early stages of the illness. This is consistent with young adults' help-seeking preferences in the general population [83]. It may be the case that the potential stigma associated with mental health problems make young adults more reluctant to discuss symptoms with family, friends, and professionals [84]. Therefore, it seems that young adults choose one type of social media depending on their search purpose and personal preferences (i.e., Facebook and Twitter for seeking illness information, chatrooms for social networking).

Positive Outcomes of Social Media on Psychosis

Apart from the characteristics of social media use from people with psychosis, some beneficial outcomes have been described. It seems that receiving information and the discussion of illness-related problems with peers increase self-esteem and self-validation by helping others, reassurance through self-disclosing one's experiences [71]. Interacting in online forums or online chat services could decrease the risk of isolation and maintain or improve social networks for young adults experiencing symptoms of psychosis. The main reasons provided for using social networks identified in a systematic review of online social networking in people with psychosis [75] were to make new friends, reconnect with people they had lost contact with, and exchange peer support. Moreover, heterogeneity of methods and designs (i.e., inclusion of case studies) limits conclusions that can be drawn, with no formal diagnosis provided for five of the studies (i.e., only self-report measures used from people who had already being diagnosed with psychosis) [75].

Barriers, Risks, and Negative Outcomes of Social Media Use on Psychosis

Despite the positive outcomes and potential benefits of social media for young adults with psychosis, Kalk and Pothier [85] identified common barriers in this group, including access to a computer, technology, and connectivity problems, fear of computer viruses, or an inclination to use other sources of information and social connections. Also, young adults with psychosis usually perceive themselves as having lower social rank compared to others [86] which may increase their difficulties interacting with others if they do not perceive user similarity [52]. However, Schrank et al. (2010) reported on a study on how patients with schizophrenia used the Internet (adult sample) [71]. Among this sample, more significant barriers were noted regarding issues of suspicion and trusting unknown people and the desire of not being exposed to other people's psychosis stories. Some psychosis-related symptomatology (i.e., delusional interpretations or attention problems) may also interfere with Internet use, as websites providing information regarding psychosis can be difficult to understand. Moreover, they reported negative effects about the use of SNS among patients with psychosis, such as worsening of symptoms and negative coping responses when exposed to intense and difficult illness stories shared by peers. After being exposed to information online regarding medication, there was potential to cause changes in attitudes toward medication, prompting a more critical view regarding one's own medication. Furthermore, available information online can be misleading, maintaining stigma and sustaining wrong information related to mental health and psychosis in particular. This online environment may lead to treatment avoidance [78, 87]. Therefore, for this population, it may be especially important to have moderated forums by experts who can preserve the accuracy of the information and maintain safety when difficult stories were shared (i.e., creation of a wellness plan for relapse or worsening of symptoms, mechanisms to flag sensitive content so users can decide whether to read it or not, emergency contact telephones, etc.).

Social Media-Based Interventions for Psychosis

The development of interventions for psychosis involving online support, and in particular integrating peer support, comes from the idea that people who have faced difficulties can provide relevant and important assistance, advice, and hope to those overcoming similar adversities [88]. Although there are many online peer-support groups focusing particularly on mental health themes [89], very little is known yet about the effectiveness or adverse outcomes derived from well-designed social media-based interventions for people with psychosis. A study that involved patients with psychotic disorders and depression reported that taking part in an unstructured (i.e., no specific discussion format) and unmoderated peer-support group was not associated with clinical or psychological benefits [90]. This contradicts previous studies analyzing structured or moderated support groups in other populations [17, 91].

A recent systematic review on novel user-led interventions for psychosis identified that mobile-based and Internet interventions seem to be acceptable and feasible and may enhance clinical and social outcomes for psychosis [92]. However, the current research is heterogeneous and quality standards are poor. Out of the four RCTs included in the review, there was only one well-designed RCT; and out of the six uncontrolled studies, only three measured acceptability of the intervention and none included blinded assessors to study goals or methods. Out of the 12 studies included in the review, the majority were web-based psychoeducation sites, some were mobile-based interventions, and one included personalized advice-based monitoring. However, none of these interventions enabled peer-to-peer social interaction with other users. Only three interventions were social media-based interventions: a SNS and peer expert moderation site [93] and two web-based psychoeducation and moderated forums [94, 95], one of which was for family members and relatives of people with schizophrenia [94]. A more recent review and meta-analysis of the effectiveness of social media-based interventions for people with schizophrenia (age > 30) [96] identified only two randomized studies [90, 95]. The review focused on those interventions that entailed interactivity (user-to-user contact: patients, peers, and clinical staff) and social media (user-generated content) and social networking (websites that aimed to prevent, treat, or offer relapse prevention for depression) or interventions including Facebook, Twitter, YouTube, Instagram, blogs, and chats. Both studies showed an active role and a strong engagement in social media forums. Nevertheless, results showed that social media-based interventions were less effective than treatment as usual for social support and self-management [96]. Moreover, participants in the "high participation group" compared with their counterparts in the "low participation group" showed higher distress levels at follow-up [85]. Although positive symptoms were improved in the social media-based condition in Kaplan et al.'s study [85], Rotondi et al.'s study [90, 95] did not provide this information, and this variable was not included in the meta-analysis. It may be the case that forums and online chats unmoderated by professionals may increase anxiety among people with psychosis.

Three Examples of Social Media-Based Interventions for Psychosis

Although there is a scarcity of well-designed social media-based interventions, a number of published studies specifically designed to target people with psychosis have emerged. However, youth-specific interventions are still scant. Below we provide an overview of three innovative interventions—a Listservs Intervention or Bulletin Board Intervention support group (adult population) [90], SOAR (heterogeneous population of adolescents and adults) [95], and Horyzons (youth-specific intervention) [93, 97]—that integrate peer-to-peer social networking with therapy and moderation.

An RCT which allocated participants on the Listservs Intervention, Bulletin Board Intervention support group, or a waitlist control group, investigated the impact of an unmoderated, unstructured Internet peer-support site on the well-being of individuals diagnosed with schizophrenia spectrum or an affective disorder over 12 months [90]. Participants (age $\geq$ 18, N = 200) of the Peer Support Listserv (N = 101) (i.e., support through a group distribution email list) and Bulletin Board (N = 99) only accessible to them received instructions on safety, security, how to give and receive advice, and how to present themselves on the Internet. All the content was peer-directed, and research staff members were only available for technical help. There were no group differences in recovery, quality of life, empowerment, social support, and distress measures. The experimental sample was divided into high/low users. Participants who participated more, and those who reported a more positive experience, showed higher levels of psychological distress. Findings of this study showed that individuals with psychiatric disorders did not benefit by the use of an online support group to enhance their well-being although there was not increased psychological distress.

The Schizophrenia Online Access to Resources (SOAR), a 3-month intervention [95], was created to provide psychoeducation mainly (age $\geq$ 14, N = 30). The website offered three therapy forums (for patients with schizophrenia, for support people, and one combining both groups). Therapeutic tools emphasized problem-solving discussions and encouraged creation of a supportive peer network. The investigators adapted written materials to compensate for cognitive limitations of people with psychosis (i.e., use of two-tiered appearance of text, where a summary is presented before the text, and use of nontechnical language, easy-level reading, up-to-date medical information, relevant day-to-day information, etc.). Results showed that users with schizophrenia had logged in more than expected and endorsed lower perceived stress and higher levels of perceived social support at 3 months compared to a control group (i.e., treatment as usual). Finally, after the trial, some of the participants reported that the site was an important resource for their well-being, where they could always refer to if needed.

As opposed to the previous interventions more centered on schizophrenia, the Horyzons study [93, 97] is a moderated online social therapy (MOST) [49, 50] designed to improve long-term outcomes in young adults with first-episode psychosis (FEP). Horyzons was developed iteratively following participatory design principles [98] through a process of testing and systematic feedback with focus groups of stakeholders (clinicians and FEP patients). Horyzons predates the Rebound intervention for depression relapse prevention (discussed above; both developed by our group (Melbourne, Australia)) and similarly integrates (a) peer-to-peer social networking, (b) individually tailored interactive therapy content, and (c) professional and peer moderation using supportive accountability [48] and positive psychotherapy models [51]. Over a 1-month pilot study (age = 15–25, N = 20), the Horyzons intervention was found to be acceptable, feasible, safe, and engaging among young adults with FEP. Seventy percent of users utilized the system for at least 3 weeks, and 95% used the SNS features and reported feeling more socially connected. Further, the study revealed a significant reduction in depression symptoms at 1-month follow-up, specifically in those with more frequent use of the website [93]. Importantly, despite the personality traits of young adults with FEP, symptoms such as suspiciousness (which may be intensified in an online environment [99]), and the importance of safety due to the vulnerability of FEP patients, young adults recovering from psychosis reported feeling safe, and there were no incidents (i.e., inappropriate usage or adverse events) during the study. First, the online SNS was password protected and only available for consumers from the Early Psychosis Prevention and Intervention Centre (EPPIC) in Melbourne, Australia. Second, young adults reported feeling safe within the Horyzons platform due to the moderation by expert clinicians, who offered a close monitoring and intervention for any signs of deterioration.

Following the example described in D'Alfonso et al. (2017), each user's main page is a newsfeed Café page, a Facebook-style newsfeed where users can add posts and comments, react to posts from other users' share experiences, give and obtain support, and gain perspectives and validation (see Fig. 14.1). Additionally, each user also has access to therapy content, where moderator suggestions appear to the left, posts advertising content just taken by other users appear in the newsfeed, and therapy recommendations relative to a user's posts are made upon their submission. Therapy content is organized in Steps (interactive therapy modules with increased difficulty designed to exercise and develop a range of psychological skills alphabetically—ordered in a

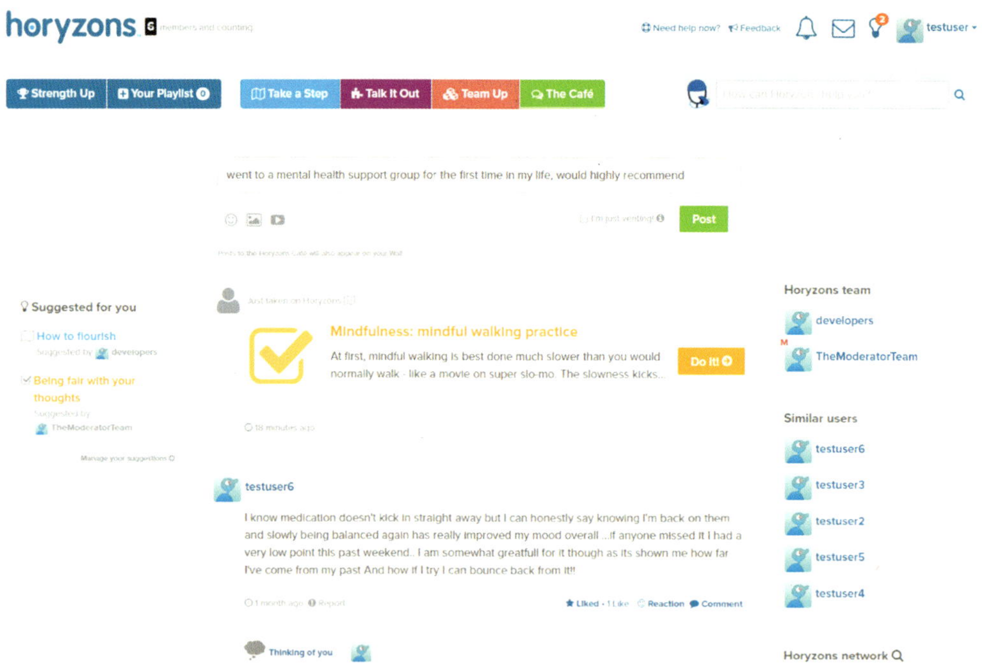

Fig. 14.1 The Café newsfeed (Horyzons)

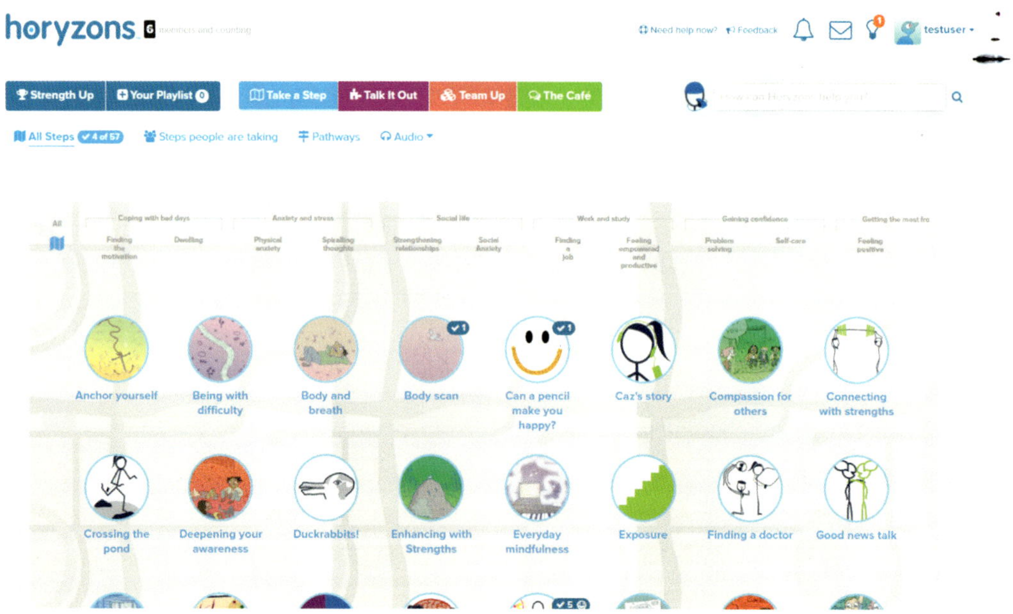

Fig. 14.2 Part of the Steps grid page (Horyzons)

grid with respective icons, as shown in Fig. 14.2). An example of one Step—"How to Flourish"—is illustrated in Fig. 14.3. Users can interact with the Step and contribute to a "mini-newsfeed" by commenting on a Talking Point (Fig. 14.4). Upon completing the Step, they can feed back into The

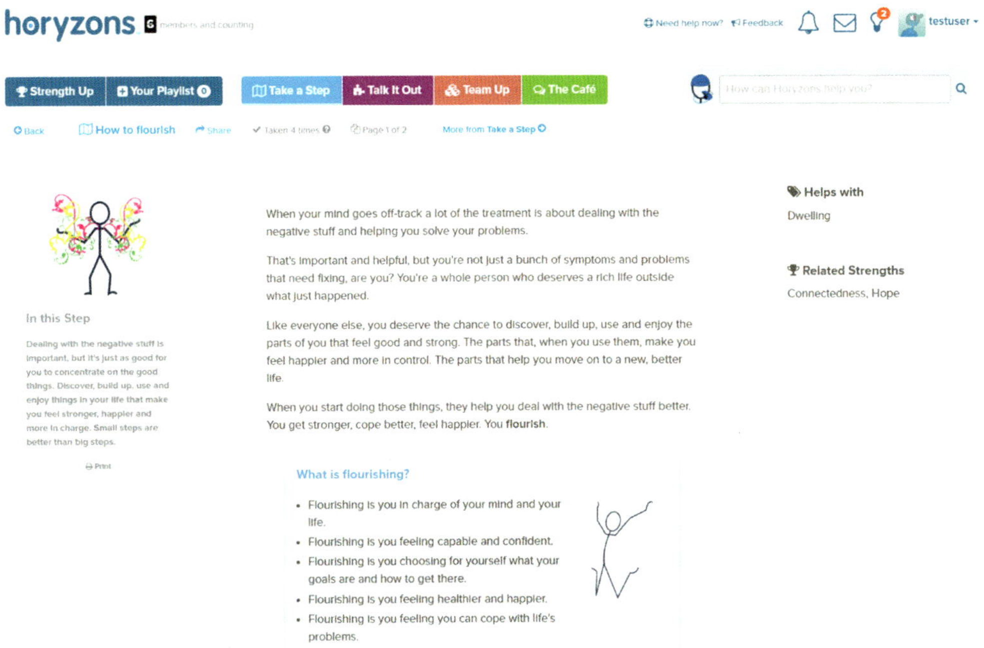

Fig. 14.3 Part of a Step, "How to Flourish" (Horyzons)

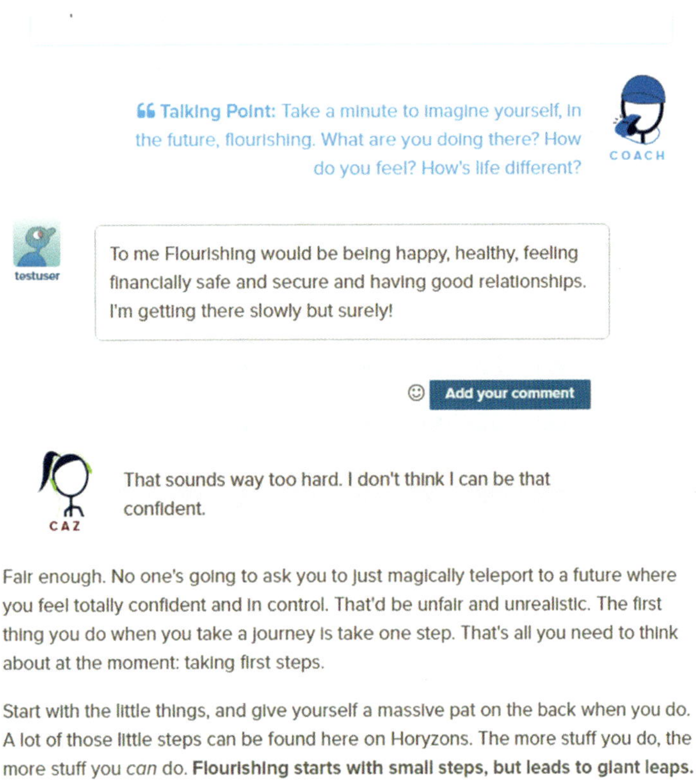

Fig. 14.4 Talking Point from one Step "How to Flourish" (Horyzons)

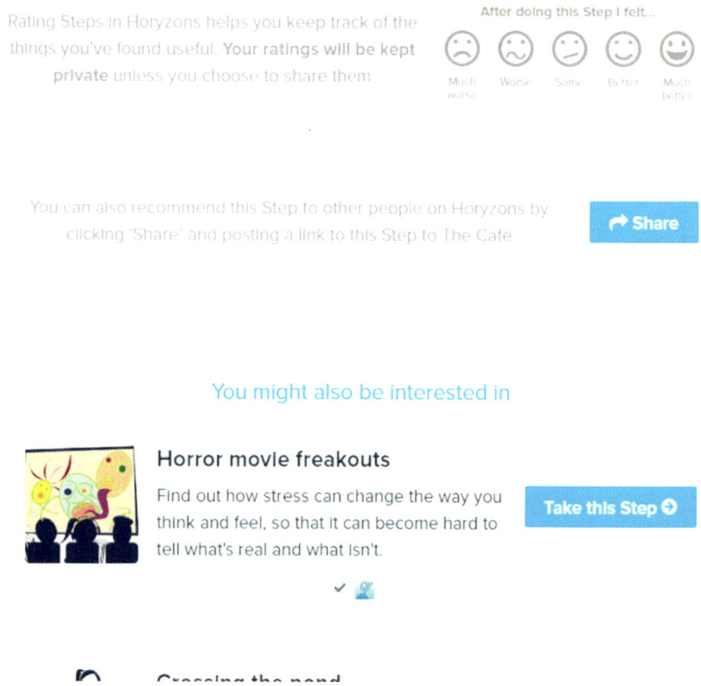

Fig. 14.5 Finishing a Step "How to Flourish" (Horyzons)

Café by sharing a link to the Step or rating the Step and sharing this rating with a message. Finally, the system suggests other relevant Steps the user might like to try (Fig. 14.5) [100].

Therefore, the use of an integrated SNS with therapy content, peer support, and expert moderation may enhance social connectedness and empowerment in FEP. The question remains however as to whether increased online social interaction may facilitate social functioning in other domains. While promising, these findings need to be validated. A major 5-year RCT of the Horyzons platform is currently in progress at Orygen, The National Centre of Excellence in Youth Mental Health, Australia.

The point of distinction of the Horyzons intervention compared with the SOAR trial and the Listservs Intervention or Bulletin Board Intervention support group related to the structured and moderated environment. In line with the supportive accountability model, these factors may be crucial to ensure safety and provide longer-term intervention to young adults with psychosis, who may especially benefit from a structured and moderated online setting due to the nature of their mental health illness. This type of intervention may especially benefit adolescents and young adults with first-episode psychosis compared to adults with schizophrenia (i.e., associated with the high burden of disease, chronicity, and disability [101]). SNS usage and the feasibility of technology-based interventions may be more limited among people diagnosed with schizophrenia due to the nature of the illness with symptoms such as disorganization, paranoia, and a progressive cognitive impairment [102]. Therefore, their capacity to engage or their attitudes toward online tools (i.e., reluctance to use SNS) may be diminished compared with those in the early stage of illness [102]. Moreover, the benefits of specialist FEP services are likely to persist when patients continue to receive specialized treatment [103]. Therefore, these technologies can be particularly useful in early stages of illness for maintaining treatment gains and engagement over time when transitioning from specialized to usual care services.

Implications and Future Directions

We expect that integration of social media and social networking-based interventions with youth-focused treatment services will proliferate exponentially over the next decade. Although we have only focused on the use of social media in adolescent depression and psychosis, there are wide-ranging applications for other disorders. In particular, social networking interventions ideally lend themselves to help-seeking populations who may be in the early/prodromal illness phase. Providing accessible and timely online support to families and caregivers of adolescents who are experiencing mental illness is also much needed. SNS studies are currently underway with such populations, and results are eagerly anticipated [33]. There are also significant opportunities to provide more timely and accessible support to young adults experiencing suicidal ideation or at risk of suicide. In this way, social networking interventions may bolster social connectedness and group affiliation, factors known to be protective for suicide attempts [34, 35, 54].

The grand challenges of online mental health interventions, yet to be solved, relate to longer-term engagement and attrition [104] and whether online engagement will translate into long-term improved social functioning and quality of life. The integration of social media and social networking within online interventions is likely to be an effective mechanism for maintaining and even enhancing user engagement and creating supportive therapeutic communities. To do this well, interventions require thoughtful integration of human support [48]. The development of effective models of online clinical moderation is central to this, and we call on clinicians and researchers in the field of youth mental health to further develop, manualize, and test over time theory-driven models currently in use [34, 45, 46, 93]. As reported in the review, online intervention research is heterogeneous (mixed age ranges, diagnosis, objectives of the interventions, lack of structured moderation which may impact safety, etc.), making it difficult to create individualized treatment plans and provide sufficient support for more vulnerable adolescents. The next generation of social media-based interventions ideally should be adjunctive, that is, integrated with face-to-face therapy rather than being implemented independently from usual care, allowing clinicians' involvement in the development of the online tools [25]. Future analyses of these systems need to target and report engagement and clinical results (i.e., whether the intervention reduced symptoms). We need a much deeper understanding of how these sites may respond to the needs of adolescents and what the processes are to foster meaningful and empowering social connections via these interventions.

Finally, there is room for significant SNS advances on intervention delivery since development of cost-effectiveness interventions and improvement of accessibility is still a challenge. Expansion of online SNS may offer exciting new prospects beyond user content analysis [100]. Some possibilities include development of automated content by the implementation of therapy chatbots [105, 106] (i.e., computer program that simulates interaction with users via a chat interface), making therapeutic suggestions based on geolocation data [107] (i.e., determining the location of a user with their mobile phone in order to translate therapy into day-to-day situations), and self-monitoring/self-sensing data [108] (i.e., detecting physiological measures, which correlate with the physiological characteristics of the onset of a panic attack to deliver suitable therapy content).

Conclusion

Social media and social networking-based interventions for adolescents are increasing exponentially and appear to be an effective mechanism for maintaining user engagement and creating supportive therapeutic communities. Nevertheless, due to the vulnerability of adolescents with mental health difficulties (i.e., depression and psychosis), implementation of these studies should include protocols mindful of risk, ethical issues, and utilizing human support (i.e., moderation by expert clinicians) to maintain longer-term intervention adherence and ensure safety. Further, well-designed studies (i.e., randomized control trials with long-term follow-up periods) are required to demonstrate intervention efficacy and whether increased online social interaction may facilitate offline social functioning.

References

1. Boyd DM, Ellison NB. Social network sites: definition, history, and scholarship. J Comput-Mediat Commun. 2008;13:210–30.
2. Ellison NB, Boyd DM. Sociality through social network sites. In: Dutton WH, editor. The Oxford handbook of Internet studies. Oxford: Oxford University Press; 2013. p. 151–72.
3. Pew Research Center. Pew Internet & American Life Project. Washington, DC: Pew Research Center; 2014.
4. ACMA. The ACMA communications report 2014–15. In:Australian Communications and Media Authority. 2015. p. 146.
5. Lenehart A, Duggan M, Perrin A, et al. Teens, social media & technology overview 2015. Washington, DC: Pew Research Center; 2015.
6. Hauk L. Clinical report—the impact of social media on children, adolescents, and families. Pediatrics. 2011;127:800–4.
7. O'keeffe GS, Clarke-Pearson K. The impact of social media on children, adolescents, and families. Pediatrics. 2011;127:800–4.
8. Woods HC, Scott H. #Sleepyteens: social media use in adolescence is associated with poor sleep quality, anxiety, depression and low self-esteem. J Adolesc. 2016;51:41–9.
9. Turkle S. Alone together: why we expect more from technology and less from each other, Social Studies of Science. New York: Basic Books; 2011. p. 1–5.
10. Jordan AH, Monin B, Dweck CS, et al. Misery has more company than people think: underestimating the prevalence of others' negative emotions. Personal Soc Psychol Bull. 2011;37:120–35.
11. Burke M, Marlow C, Lento T. Social network activity and social well-being. In: Proceedings of the 28th International Conference on Human Factors in Computing Systems (CHI 2010). 2010. p. 1909.
12. Polanczyk GV, Salum GA, Sugaya LS, et al. Annual research review: a meta-analysis of the worldwide prevalence of mental disorders in children and adolescents. J Child Psychol Psychiatry. 2015;56:345–65.
13. Slade T, Johnston A, Teesson M et al. The mental health of Australians 2. Report on the 2007 National Survey of mental health and wellbeing. Department of Health and Ageing, Canberra. 2009.
14. Rickwood D, Deane F, Wilson CJ, et al. Young people's help-seeking for mental health problems. Advancement of Mental Health. 2005;4:1–34.
15. Rickwood D, Mazzer KR, Telford NR. Social influences on seeking help from mental health services, in-person and online, during adolescence and young adulthood. BMC Psychiatry. 2015;15:40.
16. Krishna S, Austin-Boren S, Balas EA. Healthcare via cell phones: a systematic review. Telemedicine e-Health. 2009;15:2–4.
17. Houston TK, Houston TK, Cooper LA, et al. Internet support groups for depression: a 1-year prospective cohort study. Am J Psychiatr. 2002;159:2062–8.
18. Wentzel J, Van Der Vaart R, Bohlmeijer ET, et al. Mixing online and face-to-face therapy: how to benefit from blended care in mental health care. JMIR Mental Health. 2016;3:e9.
19. Ben-Zeev D. Mobile technologies in the study, assessment, and treatment of schizophrenia. Schizophr Bull. 2012;38:384–5.
20. Rickwood D, Telford N, Mazzer K, et al. The services provided to young people by headspace centres in Australia. Med J Aust. 2015;202:533–7.
21. Rickwood DJ, Telford NR, Parker AG, et al. Headspace—Australia's innovation in youth mental health: who are the clients and why are they presenting? Med J Aust. 2014;200:108–11.
22. Álvarez-Jiménez M, Gleeson JF, Bendall S, et al. Internet-based interventions for psychosis: a sneak-peek into the future. Psychiatr Clin N Am. 2012; 35:735–47.
23. Andersson G, Titov N. Advantages and limitations of Internet-based interventions for common mental disorders. World Psychiatry. 2014;13:4–11.
24. Álvarez-Jiménez M, Gleeson JF, Rice S, et al. Online peer-to-peer support in youth mental health: seizing the opportunity. Epidemiol Psychiatr Sci. 2016;25(2):123–6.
25. Fraser S, Randell A, Desilva S, et al. E-mental health: the future of youth mental health? In: Research Bulletin. Melbourne, Victoria. 2016.
26. Burns J, Morey C. Technology and young people's mental health and wellbeing. In: Bennet DL, Towns SJ, Elliot EJ, Merrick J, editors. Challenges in adolescent health: an Australian perspective. Melbourne: International Academic Press; 2008.
27. Park J, Lee DS, Shablack H, et al. When perceptions defy reality: the relationships between depression and actual and perceived Facebook social support. J Affect Disord. 2016;200:37–44.
28. Cassidy CM, Norman R, Manchanda R, et al. Testing definitions of symptom remission in first-episode psychosis for prediction of functional outcome at 2 years. Schizophr Bull. 2010;36:1001–8.
29. Lieberman J, Jody D, Geisler S, et al. Time course and biologic correlates of treatment response in first-episode schizophrenia. Arch Gen Psychiatry. 1993;50:369–76.
30. Tohen M, Strakowski SM, Zarate C, et al. The McLean-Harvard first-episode project: 6-month symptomatic and functional outcome in affective and nonaffective psychosis. Biol Psychiatry. 2000; 48:467–76.

31. Scott J, Scott EM, Hermens DF, et al. Functional impairment in adolescents and young adults with emerging mood disorders. Br J Psychiatry. 2014;205:362–8.
32. Iyer SN, Mangala R, Thara R, et al. Preliminary findings from a study of first-episode psychosis in Montreal, Canada and Chennai, India: comparison of outcomes. Schizophr Res. 2010;121:227–33.
33. Gleeson J, Lederman R, Herrman H, et al. Moderated online social therapy for carers of young people recovering from first-episode psychosis: study protocol for a randomised controlled trial. Trials. 2017;18:27.
34. Rice S, Robinson J, Bendall S, et al. Online and social media suicide prevention interventions for young people: a focus on implementation and moderation. J Can Acad Child Adolesc Psychiatry. 2016;25:80–6.
35. Robinson J, Cox G, Bailey E, et al. Social media and suicide prevention: a systematic review. Early Interv Psychiatry. 2016;10:103–21.
36. Rice SM, Goodall J, Hetrick SE, et al. Online and social networking interventions for the treatment of depression in young people: a systematic review. J Med Internet Res. 2014;16:1–16.
37. Silenzio VMB, Duberstein PR, Tang W, et al. Connecting the invisible dots: reaching lesbian, gay, and bisexual adolescents and young adults at risk for suicide through online social networks. Soc Sci Med. 2009;69:469–74.
38. Holleran SE. The early detection of depression from social networking sites. Tucson: The University of Arizona; 2010. p. 86.
39. Moreno MA, Christakis DA, Egan KG, et al. A pilot evaluation of associations between displayed depression references on Facebook and self-reported depression using a clinical scale. J Behav Health Serv Res. 2012;39:295–304.
40. Moreno MA, Jelenchick LA, Egan KG, et al. Feeling bad on Facebook: depression disclosures by college students on a social networking site. Depress Anxiety. 2011;28:447–55.
41. Jelenchick LA, Eickhoff JC, Moreno MA. Facebook depression? Social networking site use and depression in older adolescents. J Adolesc Health. 2013; 52:128–30.
42. Veretilo P, Billick SB. Psychiatric illness and Facebook: a case report. Psychiatry Q. 2012;83: 385–9.
43. Wright KB, Rosenberg J, Egbert N, et al. Communication competence, social support, and depression among college students: a model of Facebook and face-to-face support network influence. J Health Commun. 2012;0730:1–17.
44. Kreps GL. Relational communication in health care. Southern Speech Commun J. 1988;53:344–59.
45. Radovic A, Demand A, Gmelin T, et al. SOVA: design of a stakeholder informed social media website for depressed adolescents and their parents. J Adolesc Health. 2016;58:S58–9.
46. Radovic A, Gmelin TA, Venkatakrishnan K, et al. SOVA: acceptability and usability of a social media website for adolescents with depression or anxiety. J Adolesc Health. 2017;60:S93.
47. Ho J, Corden ME, Caccamo L, et al. Design and evaluation of a peer network to support adherence to a web-based intervention for adolescents. Internet Interventions. 2016;6:50–6.
48. Mohr DC, Cuijpers P, Lehman K. Supportive accountability: a model for providing human support to enhance adherence to eHealth interventions. J Med Internet Res. 2011;13:1–11.
49. Lederman R, Wadley G, Gleeson JF, et al. Moderated online social therapy: designing and evaluating technology for mental health. ACM Trans Computer-Human Interaction. 2014;2:1–27.
50. Wadley G, Lederman R, Gleeson J, et al. Participatory design of an online therapy for youth mental health. In: OZCHI'13. 2013.
51. Seligman MEP, Rashid T, Parks AC. Positive psychotherapy. Am Psychol. 2006;61:774–88.
52. Santesteban-Echarri O, Rice S, Wadley G, et al. A next-generation social media-based relapse prevention intervention for youth depression: qualitative data on user experience outcomes for social networking, safety and clinical benefit. Internet Interventions. 2017;9(C):65–73.
53. Cash SJ, Thelwall M, Peck SN, et al. Adolescent suicide statements on MySpace. Cyberpsychol Behav Soc Netw. 2013;16:1–9.
54. Robinson J, Hetrick S, Cox G, et al. Can an Internet-based intervention reduce suicidal ideation, depression and hopelessness among secondary school students: results from a pilot study. Early Interv Psychiatry. 2016;10:28–35.
55. Robinson J, Hetrick S, Cox G, et al. The safety and acceptability of delivering an online intervention to secondary students at risk of suicide: findings from a pilot study. Early Interv Psychiatry. 2015;9: 498–506.
56. Robinson J, Bailey E, Hetrick S, et al. Suicide and social media: the bayside Safe Conversations project. New York, NY: International Association for Suicide Prevention;2015.
57. Mcgorry PD, Edwards J, Mihalopoulos C, et al. EPPIC: an evolving system of early detection and optimal management. Schizophr Bull. 1996; 22:305–26.
58. Mcgorry PD, Yung AR. Early intervention in psychosis. Aust N Z J Psychiatry. 2003;37:393–8.
59. Bertelsen M, Jeppesen P, Petersen L, et al. Five-year follow-up of a randomized multicenter trial of intensive early intervention vs standard treatment for patients with a first episode of psychotic illness: the OPUS trial. Arch Gen Psychiaty. 2008;65:| 762–71.
60. Gafoor R, Nitsch D, Mccrone P, et al. Effect of early intervention on 5-year outcome in non-affective psychosis. Br J Psychiatry. 2010;196:372–6.

61. Norman RMG, Malla AK, Manchanda R, et al. Social support and three-year symptom and admission outcomes for first episode psychosis. Schizophr Res. 2005;80:227–34.
62. Norman RMG, Windell D, Manchanda R, et al. Social support and functional outcomes in an early intervention program. Schizophr Res. 2012;140:37–40.
63. Goldberg RW, Rollins A, Lehman A. Social network correlates among people with psychiatric disabilities. Psychiatr Rehabil J. 2003;26:393–402.
64. Hansen CF, Torgalsbøen A-K, Melle I, et al. Passive/apathetic social withdrawal and active social avoidance in schizophrenia difference in underlying psychological processes. J Nerv Ment Dis. 2009;197:274–7.
65. Kessler RC, Amminger GP, Aguilar-Gaxiola S, et al. Age of onset of mental disorders: a review of recent literature. Curr Opin Psychiatry. 2007;20:359–64.
66. Thomsen PH. Schizophrenia with childhood and adolescent onset. A nationwide register-based study. Acta psychiatrica Scandinavica. 1996;94:187–93.
67. Docherty NM, Hawkins KA, Hoffman RE, et al. Working memory, attention, and communication disturbances in schizophrenia. J Abnorm Psychol. 1996;105:212–9.
68. Lavelle M, Healey PGT, Mccabe R. Is nonverbal communication disrupted in interactions involving patients with schizophrenia? Schizophr Bull. 2013;39:1150–8.
69. Indian M, Grieve R. When Facebook is easier than face-to-face: social support derived from Facebook in socially anxious individuals. Personal Individ Differ. 2014;59:102–6.
70. Kiesler S, Siegel J, Mcguire TW. Social psychological aspects of computer-mediated communication. Am Psychol. 1984;39:1123–34.
71. Schrank B, Sibitz I, Unger A, et al. How patients with schizophrenia use the Internet: qualitative study. J Med Internet Res. 2010;12:e70.
72. Ellison N, Mason O, Scior K. Bipolar disorder and stigma: a systematic review of the literature. J Affect Disord. 2013;151:805–20.
73. Michail M, Birchwood M. Social anxiety disorder in first-episode psychosis: incidence, phenomenology and relationship with paranoia. Br J Psychiatry. 2009;195:234–41.
74. Cechnicki A, Angermeyer MC, Bielańska A. Anticipated and experienced stigma among people with schizophrenia: its nature and correlates. Soc Psychiatry Psychiatr Epidemiol. 2011;46:643–50.
75. Highton-Williamson E, Priebe S, Giacco D. Online social networking in people with psychosis: a systematic review. Int J Soc Psychiatry. 2015;61:92–101.
76. Mittal VA, Tessner KD, Walker EF. Elevated social Internet use and schizotypal personality disorder in adolescents. Schizophr Res. 2007;94:5–57.
77. Spinzy Y, Nitzan U, Becker G, et al. Does the Internet offer social opportunities for individuals with schizophrenia? A cross-sectional pilot study. Psychiatry Res. 2012;198:319–20.
78. Birnbaum ML, Rizvi AF, Correll CU, et al. Role of social media and the Internet in pathways to care for adolescents and young adults with psychotic disorders and non-psychotic mood disorders. Early Interv Psychiatry. 2017;11(4):290–5.
79. Chang HJ. Online supportive interactions: using a network approach to examine communication patterns within a psychosis social support group in Taiwan. J Am Soc Inform Sci Technol. 2009; 60:1504–18.
80. Haker H, Lauber C, Rössler W. Internet forums: a self-help approach for individuals with schizophrenia? Acta Psychiatr Scand. 2005;112:474–7.
81. Finn J. An exploration of helping processes in an online self-help group focusing on issues of disability. National Assoc Soc Workers. 1999;24:220–31.
82. Perron B. Online support for caregivers of people with a mental illness. Psychiatr Rehabil J. 2002;26:70–7.
83. Cave L, Fildes J, Luckett G, et al. Mission Australia. Youth survey report. 2015.
84. Gerlinger G, Hauser M, De Hert M, et al. Personal stigma in schizophrenia spectrum disorders: a systematic review of prevalence rates, correlates, impact and interventions. World Psychiatry. 2013;12:155–64.
85. Kalk NJ, Pothier DD. Patient information on schizophrenia on the Internet. Psychiatric Bulletin. 2008;32:409–11.
86. Gilbert P. The relationship of shame, social anxiety and depression: the role of the evaluation of social rank. Clin Psychol Psychother. 2000;7:174–89.
87. Birnbaum ML, Candan K, Libby I, et al. Impact of online resources and social media on help-seeking behaviour in youth with psychotic symptoms. Early Interv Psychiatry. 2016;10:397–403.
88. Davidson L, Chinman M, Sells D, et al. Peer support among adults with serious mental illness: a report from the field. Schizophr Bull. 2006;32:443–50.
89. Ali K, Farrer L, Gulliver A, et al. Online peer-to-peer support for young people with mental health problems: a systematic review. JMIR Mental Health. 2015;2:e19.
90. Kaplan K, Salzer MS, Solomon P, et al. Internet peer support for individuals with psychiatric disabilities: a randomized controlled trial. Soc Sci Med. 2011;72:54–62.
91. Lieberman MA, Goldstein BA. Not all negative emotions are equal: the role of emotional expression in online support groups for women with breast cancer. Psycho-Oncology. 2006;15:160–8.
92. Alvarez-Jimenez M, Alcazar-Corcoles MA, González-Blanch C, et al. Online, social media and mobile technologies for psychosis treatment: a systematic review on novel user-led interventions. Schizophr Res. 2014;156:96–106.

93. Alvarez-Jimenez M, Bendall S, Lederman R, et al. On the HORYZON: Moderated online social therapy for long-term recovery in first episode psychosis. Schizophr Res. 2013;143:143–9.
94. Glynn SM, Randolph ET, Garrick T, et al. A proof of concept trial of an online psychoeducational program for relatives of both veterans and civilians living with schizophrenia. Psychiatr Rehabil J. 2010;33:278–87.
95. Rotondi AJ, Haas GL, Anderson CM, et al. A clinical trial to test the feasibility of a telehealth psychoeducational intervention for persons with schizophrenia and their families: intervention and 3-month findings. Rehabil Psychol. 2005;50:325–36.
96. Välimäki M, Athanasopoulou C, Lahti M, et al. Effectiveness of social media interventions for people with schizophrenia: a systematic review and meta-analysis. J Med Internet Res. 2016;18(4):e92.
97. Gleeson JF, Lederman R, Wadley G, et al. Safety and privacy outcomes from a people with first-episode psychosis safety and privacy outcomes from a moderated online social therapy for young people with first-episode psychosis. Psychiatr Serv. 2014;65:546–50.
98. Schuler D, Namioka A. Participatory design: principles and practices. Hillsdale: Lawrence Erlbaum Associates; 1993.
99. Nitzan U, Shoshan E, Lev-Ran S, et al. Internet-related psychosis—a sign of the times? Isr J Psychiatry Relat Sci. 2011;48:207–11.
100. D'alfonso S, Santesteban-Echarri O, Rice S, et al. Artificial intelligence-assisted online social therapy for youth mental health. Front Psychol. 2017;8:1–13.
101. World Health Organization. Burden of disease: DALYs. Geneva: World Health Organization; 2015.
102. Ennis L, Rose D, Denis M, et al. Can't surf, won't surf: the digital divide in mental health. J Ment Health. 2012;21:395–403.
103. Norman RM, Manchanda R, Malla AK, et al. Symptom and functional outcomes for a 5 year early intervention program for psychoses. Schizophr Res. 2011;129:111–5.
104. Eysenbach G. The law of attrition. J Med Internet Res. 2005;7:1–9.
105. Abdul-Kader SA, Woods J. Survey on chatbot design techniques in speech conversation systems. Int J Adv Comput Sci Appl. 2015;6:72–80.
106. Pinto MD, Hickman RL Jr, Clochesy J, et al. Avatar-based depression self-management technology: promising approach to improve depressive symptoms among young adults. Appl Nurs Res. 2013;26:45–8.
107. Dredze M, Paul M, Bergsma S, et al. Carmen: a twitter geolocation system with applications to public health. In: Proc. AAAI. 2013.
108. Matthews M, Abdullah S, Gay G, et al. Tracking mental well-being: balancing rich sensing and patient needs. Comput Hum Behav. 2014;47:36–43.

15 The Role of Texting in Addressing Mental Health

Megan L. Ranney, Anthony R. Pisani, and Lauren S. Chernick

Case Introduction

You are working in a busy emergency department. Your next patient is Jayson, a 14-year-old boy with a chief complaint of "twisted ankle." Jayson reports that he twisted his ankle playing basketball with friends. His x-ray shows no fracture, and you note only mild swelling inferior to the lateral malleolus. While explaining the diagnosis and treatment for ankle sprain to Jayson and his family, you are struck by Jayson's flat affect.

You ask how he's feeling. Jayson says that he's feeling very down, because "basketball was the one thing that made me happy." On further questioning, Jayson tells you that "life sucks" since his girlfriend broke up with him 6 months ago. He endorses symptoms consistent with mild depression—apathy, insomnia, irritability with increased aggressiveness (a fistfight after school a month ago), and decreased appetite. Jayson denies suicidal ideation and is still getting good grades in school. With his mother out of the room, he confides that he drinks alcohol and smokes marijuana "to make myself feel better." He says that he has been feeling worse lately, because his ex-girlfriend started dating someone new.

Jayson says that his primary care doctor wanted him to see a therapist a couple years ago, after a prior stressor, but he does not think it would help. He says he would not be able to go to an appointment anyhow; his mom works two jobs, he cannot drive, and he has heard "bad stories" about the local counseling center. Now that this ankle sprain will take him out of basketball, he's concerned that he might start feeling even worse. Jayson's mother reports that Jayson's father is an alcoholic and left the family years ago. The father's side of the family may also have a history of suicide, although she is not sure "because they all live in my old country." She confirms that she has neither time nor resources to take her son to counseling but says "I wish there were some way to help him. I don't want him to go downhill."

Unfortunately, that's all you have time for—there are 15 patients in the waiting room and 2 consultants on hold. While writing up the chart, you rack your brain for solutions; a referral to

M.L. Ranney, M.D., M.P.H., F.A.C.E.P. (✉)
Emergency Digital Health Innovation program, Department of Emergency Medicine, Alpert Medical School, Brown University, Providence, RI, USA
e-mail: megan_ranney@brown.edu

A.R. Pisani, Ph.D.
Department of Psychiatry (Psychology) and Pediatrics, University of Rochester Medical Center, Rochester, NY, USA

L.S. Chernick, M.D., M.Sc.
Pediatric Emergency Department, New York-Presbyterian Children's Hospital, Columbia University Medical Center, New York, NY, USA

M.A. Moreno, A. Radovic (eds.), *Technology and Adolescent Mental Health*,
https://doi.org/10.1007/978-3-319-69638-6_15

one of the local counseling services is unlikely to be accepted. You remember a text-message program that one of your colleagues is conducting research on and wonder whether this teen would be appropriate for her study.

Why Use Text Messaging?

Advantages Over Other Forms of Technology

Text messaging is ubiquitous, easy to use, and inexpensive. Over 90% of adolescents—in essence, all adolescents with access to a mobile phone—communicate via text messages [1, 2]. Girls text slightly more often than boys, but, in contrast to other forms of technology, there are limited differences in rates of texting by socioeconomic status, race, or ethnicity [1–3]. Partly due to its high availability and use, texting is highly engaging for adolescents, with some studies suggesting that it is more engaging than other forms of technology-based interventions, because it "feels comfortable" to teens [4–8]. From a user experience perspective, the use of text messaging is standard; therefore, there is a limited need for explanation about the features of a text-message program. Finally, phone apps can easily be erased from a phone, while the ability to send or receive text messages is inherent to a phone [9].

Text-message interventions are also relatively inexpensive to develop and maintain. No formal design experience is needed to create an engaging text-message intervention, as there is no graphical user interface to design (although, as will be discussed below, it is still important to conduct high-quality formative development work). Texts cost a fraction of a penny to send, and most users have unlimited texting plans, so there is rarely an added cost to patients to receive the messages. Text messaging is platform-agnostic, so no programming is required for different phone operating systems, nor does it need to be updated when operating systems change.

Most importantly, as will be discussed below, there is extensive evidence that text messaging is effective in changing health behaviors, including behaviors associated with serious mental illness, when well-designed and well-implemented [7, 10–14].

A Growing Body of Evidence for Text-message interventions for Adolescent Mental Health

Self-Monitoring

One of the oldest, and easiest, ways to use text messaging for mental healthcare is as an assessment tool. Dating back to the mid-2000s, researchers and clinicians have used regular (twice-daily, daily, weekly) text-message assessments to track patient symptoms and predict worsening symptoms. These assessments range from complex surveys (such as the "mobiletype" research program), which texted teens daily with questions about a mood, stress, alcohol use, and other daily activities and then synthesized the information for their primary care provider [15] to simpler single-question daily assessments and appointment reminders [16]. These text-message-based momentary assessments are highly feasible and have high rates of completion. They have high correlation with traditional measurements of mental illness (particularly for depressive symptoms) [16, 17]. Some studies suggest that by simply conducting daily text assessments, adolescents may experience improved emotional self-awareness, reduced depressive symptoms, and reduced anxiety symptoms [17, 18]. Daily self-assessments may also increase adolescent primary care practitioners' likelihood of engaging patients in appropriate outpatient mental health services [18]. Commercial web-based services, such as Mood 24/7 (https://www.mood247.com/), also exist to facilitate such assessments and integrate them into health records.

Depression

Multiple studies have been shown that text messaging can improve patient engagement in and coordination with depression care and compliance with appointments and medications [13, 19, 20]. Only a few studies of text messaging as an adjunct to mental healthcare have been completed with adolescents. One study showed that text messaging facilitates coordination with mental health outreach workers, although this study did not have a comparison group [21]. Another small study showed that regular texting with a therapist (in conjunction with other technology-augmented cognitive behavioral therapy trainings) significantly improved adolescents' therapeutic alliance and comprehension of CBT concepts [22]. In this case, texting did not significantly improve depressive symptoms compared to usual care, although changes might have been difficult to detect due to the small sample size (total $n = 72$).

Two interventions (MEMO and iDOVE) have examined the use of text messaging for primary or secondary depression prevention. MEMO was studied in New Zealand as a school-based universal prevention technique [23]. It consisted of 9 weeks of twice-daily automated text messages (including pure text, links to videos and cartoons, and access to a mobile website). Preliminary results from a randomized trial of 855 students (aged 13–17) showed high acceptability and engagement, with over 75% of intervention participants viewing at least one text message. Although preliminary results suggested higher subjective positivity among intervention participants than control participants, to our knowledge, formal outcomes have not been published.

iDOVE (intervention for DepressiOn and Violence prevention in the Emergency department) targets high-risk adolescents with mild-to-moderate depressive symptoms and a history of peer physical violence who visit the emergency department. The iDOVE intervention consists of a brief in-person motivational interviewing session, followed by 8 weeks of automated daily mood assessments and automated, tailored CBT-based text curriculum. A pilot study showed high engagement (with 80% of daily texts receiving a response) and a significant decrease in depressive symptoms among intervention participants, although there was no comparison group [24]. A pilot randomized controlled trial showed a trend toward improved depressive symptoms in youth who were more symptomatic at baseline, compared to enhanced usual care [25]. A fully powered randomized controlled trial is in planning stages.

Suicide

The potential for text messaging in suicide prevention falls into three categories along the prevention continuum: extension of preventive interventions, crisis text intervention, and post-crisis text support.

School-based universal prevention programs show promise for reducing youth suicide [26, 27]. Help-seeking norms and behaviors, youth–adult connectedness, and strategies for emotion regulation are promising targets [26, 28, 29]. However, reaching a diverse array of young students with intervention content is a challenge. One program currently being piloted seeks to overcome this challenge by using text messaging to reinforce and extend school-based suicide prevention. Text4Strength [30, 31] is being tested as an extension of Sources of Strength [26], evidence-based peer network intervention for schools. Text4Strength uses text- and video-based testimonials from school peer leaders to encourage help-seeking, youth–adult connectedness, and strategies for emotion self-regulation. In a small pilot [Pisani, personal communication], the intervention was found to be feasible and appealing. The authors found two surprising results that inform adolescent future school or other universal texting interventions. First, students found texts useful regardless of whether they replied often; this finding suggests that students perceived the texts as invitations to interact when an interest or need arose. Understanding this attitude can help set realistic expectations about participation. Second, few students watched the videos. Students reported being limited by time, location, and bandwidth/capability. It is possible that texting and video are not a natural fit for interventions; text messaging is an on-the-go medium but videos require you to stop and watch. At the time of this publication, a randomized trial is under way to test the efficacy of a revised version of Text4Strength that does not rely on videos.

Crisis counseling via text is a second promising new avenue for addressing youth suicidal behavior. Young people at risk for suicide have historically been reluctant to seek help from crisis services. Shame and over reliance on self have been primary barriers to adolescents seeking help from crisis services [32]. Text messaging may overcome these barriers by offering added protection from emotional exposure and vulnerability. Crisis Text Line (http://www.crisistextline.org/) is by far the nation's largest provider of crisis services via text with more than 450,000 young people projected to reach out for help in 2017—many at high risk for suicide (Personal communication, Pisani). Research is under way to understand the population of texters, their reasons for texting an anonymous crisis line, and how they view their access to support from adults in their lives. This information is critical for improving and evaluating crisis text services and ultimately for developing text counseling approaches that not only relieve suicidal crises but put youth on a path toward greater support in their natural environments. The raw number of youth who reach out to the service speaks to the unmet need among young people for an anonymous source of help and empathy and the desire to interact using their predominant and most comfortable communication medium.

Finally, automated text messages may be a powerful way to extend caring contacts and safety information to individuals who have experienced a suicidal crisis or attempt. Post-acute crisis interventions have been piloted and are currently being tested [33]. These interventions generally deliver "caring contacts" [34, 35] and information related to help-seeking, distress tolerance, and safety planning. For example, the "suicide intervention assisted by messages" (SIAM) sends text messages to patients starting 2 days after discharge from an inpatient service. Approximately ten different messages are sent at increasing time intervals (1 week, 1 month) for 6 months; these messages communicate care for the patient's experience and suffering, remind them of their discharge plans, and provide contact numbers for help-seeking [33]. A randomized trial of the intervention is currently under way.

Alcohol, Smoking, and Substance Abuse

Use of alcohol, cigarettes, and substances often coexists with mental illness. As such, texting interventions that show promise in reducing adolescent and young adult alcohol abuse, smoking cessation, and substance abuse may be useful to patients with mental illness.

In a smoking cessation intervention using text messaging, investigators designed messages to be nonjudgmental, build rapport, and encourage participants to stop smoking based on the principles of motivational interviewing [36]. Those in the texting intervention experienced a reduction in smoking days. To address alcohol abuse, the Texting to Reduce Alcohol Consumption trial randomized a subset of young adults who received texting assessments and feedback when asked to respond to drinking-related queries and received real-time texting feedback both before and after the weekend [37]. The intervention group reduced self-reported binge drinking and drinks consumed by day as compared to controls. Similarly showing promising results, in Project ESQYIR (Educating and Supporting Inquisitive Youth in Recovery), a mobile-based aftercare intervention for youth transitioning out of a substance abuse treatment program, participants were sent three types of text messages for 12 weeks: daily self-monitoring texts, a daily wellness recovery tip, and substance abuse education and social support resource information on weekends [38]. Automated texts were sent to youth based on predetermined rules linking to patient characteristics and resulted in sustained recovery over time compared to the aftercare-as-usual group.

How to Design and Select a Text-Message Intervention

Understanding how to evaluate mental health text-message programs requires knowledge of what makes a texting platform both effective and engaging [7, 37–39]. In this section, we will discuss the essential features to examine when choosing a texting platform that converses with, educates, and counsels adolescent patients.

Engagement

To catch the attention of a technologically savvy adolescent, the program must be engaging. Three strategies to increase patient engagement are personalization or tailoring, interactivity, and recognition of adolescents' preferences for a positive, relatable voice [8, 40].

Personalized communication engages teens to read, think, and act [41, 42]. Personalized text messaging can incorporate anything from the user's name and area of residence to prewritten statements written by respondents to be incorporated into their text messages. Texts can be tailored, meaning that information about that individual is used to determine which context he or she will receive. Adolescent opinions vary on preferred timing of messages, ranging from random to regular, and on tone, with preference ranging from professional without abbreviations to conversational without slang [43, 44]. Texts can also be personalized based on preferred time of day, frequency, or tone. For example, in iDOVE (described above) [24], three streams of messages were created based on violence levels and gender. The streams were alike in content but differed in types of behavioral activity, and adolescent participants received the stream that matched their baseline characteristics.

Interactivity is key to engaging youth with texting [37, 40, 45, 46]. Two-way texting mimics a digital conversation between the clinician and participant, creating the feeling of a "pocket counselor" [6, 39]. This can be in the form of a live-clinician texting back in real time or can be achieved by automated texting algorithms [47].

Finally, given the 160-character limit that most carriers still impose, every word of a text message is important. There is a robust body of evidence that messages that are positive, or gain-framing, are the most likely to promote prevention behaviors. Such messages highlight the benefits of engaging in a particular behavior rather than stressing the consequences of failing to engage in the behavior (loss-frame) [48]. Several qualitative studies have also highlighted adolescent preferences for messages that were positive, relevant, funny, short, and non-accusatory [43, 49].

Rigorous Design

It is important for clinicians and researchers alike to consider "good design" when developing or choosing a text-message program for patients. Below, we describe the characteristics of a rigorously designed text-message mental health intervention. If a clinician is evaluating potential programs for their patients, this description may serve to guide their questions for the intervention developer.

An effective text-message intervention is more likely to be based on strong theory and extensive formative research, conducted prior to and after the design of a text-message intervention [23, 50, 51]. Text-message interventions based on theory and behavioral change methods lead to greater intervention effect [52]. Popular theories or models such as the health belief model, theory of planned behavior, social cognitive theory, and transtheoretical stages of change have been used as a foundation for successful text-message interventions [53]. The psychology of cognitive behavioral therapy and motivational interviewing (MI) has also been translated into text messages [24, 36]. Often, each text corresponds to a theory, model, or psychology and, in essence, has a reason for being there.

Also important to the design of an effective texting intervention is the collaboration of a multidisciplinary team of researchers and patient stakeholders, including adolescents, to define the curriculum that the text messages intend to teach. For instance, in designing Text4Strength, a school-based universal texting intervention described above, suicide prevention researchers and human–computer interaction specialists built the intervention based on a prior theory-based, efficacious program (Sources of Strength [26]) and adapted the evidence-based content with extensive involvement of high school peer "opinion leaders" [30].

After the texting curriculum is built, participatory design is critical to build an intervention that matches adolescent perspectives. This can take the form of semi-structured interviews, focus groups, or quantitative assessments. For example, to design a pregnancy prevention texting intervention, researchers conducted semi-structured interviews with adolescent females focusing on the barriers and enablers to initiating contraception; such information was then reformatted into text messages [54]. Focus groups were conducted by investigators in Australia to examine behavior change after implementing a texting intervention to promote safer sex behaviors [55]. Lastly, to quantitatively assess messages, researchers are turning to the Internet and crowd surfing to gather large samples [56, 57]. One popular mechanism is through Amazon Mechanical Turk (mTurk), an online communication platform where participants can perform human intelligence tasks (HITs). By gathering such feedback, texts can be edited iteratively, both increasing user acceptability and making the mental health intervention patient-centered.

Potential Challenges for Text-Message Mental Health Interventions

Privacy and Security

The United States' Health Insurance Portability and Accountability Act (HIPAA) and Health Information Technology for Economic and Clinical Health (HITECH) Act establish standards for privacy, security, and confidentiality of healthcare data. Recent clarifications of HIPAA and HITECH from the US government state that unencrypted text messaging is *not* permissible between providers. The extent to which healthcare providers can engage in unencrypted text messaging with patients (with explicit patient permission) is under debate [58, 59]. Some healthcare organizations have concerns that text messaging may violate their obligation to protect patients' health information. Others use unencrypted text messaging (with proper legal releases from the patient), arguing that not doing so violates patients' rights to accessing medical care when and how it is desired. This debate suggests that, prior to engaging in text-message interventions with patients, providers should consult with their hospital or practice risk management and legal team.

Additionally, clinicians should consider issues of ambient privacy (in which another person sees a text message, just by being next to the recipient) and issues with parental monitoring of text messages. These potential violations of patient privacy should be discussed at the time of patient enrollment in a text-message interventions.

Not a Substitute for In-Person Care

It is critically important to emphasize that text messaging is not a substitute for in-person care, particularly for serious mental illness. As texting may not be able to replace the personal one-on-one clinical patient connection, many interventions use texting as an addendum to a clinician's practice [47]. As described above, many studies suggest that such a multimodal approach may improve compliance and increase efficacy.

Many text-message interventions also include stringent ethical safeguards, to ensure that patients with acute mental health crises are adequately cared for. These safeguards range from automated "crisis" responses (responses sent to the texting server that are received outside of the expected time range or responses containing information that does not meet the system's expected criteria) to immediate notification of licensed independent mental health providers on receipt of an unexpected message from a patient and to direction to real-time, nonaffiliated crisis services (such as Crisis Text Line, Samaritans, or local mental health crisis counselors). To our knowledge, no formal evaluation of adverse effects of text-message-based mental health interventions has been conducted, although evaluations of nonmental-health text-message interventions suggest limited risk [60].

Lack of Commercially Available Programs

Finally, as is true for all mental health interventions, it is essential for providers to demand evidence of efficacy prior to deployment of an intervention. Unfortunately, to our knowledge, no commercially based mental health text-message interventions have efficacy data from rigorous, randomized controlled trials. In general, few well-developed, efficacious text-message interventions are commercially available. To overcome this barrier, we suggest that interested health systems contact the designers of potentially interested text-message interventions.

Future Directions for Text-Message Mental Health Interventions

The long-term potential for text-based mental health interventions extends beyond current technologies for exchanging text. The platforms and protocols for exchanging text messages continually advance. Older technologies such as short messaging systems (the classic form of "text messaging") are rapidly being replaced worldwide by Internet-enabled applications such as WhatsApp, Twitter direct messaging, and Facebook Messenger. Emojis, images, and other media commonly accompany text. Nevertheless, the lessons learned from research on classical "text-message" interventions will likely translate well to the broader category of interactive text interventions that will emerge in the future.

Additionally, computers' advancing ability to understand and interact intelligently with human texters will have a profound impact. As artificial intelligence (AI) improves, text-message interventions will get better and smarter. Rhee and colleagues [61] demonstrated feasibility of using AI in a text-messaging youth asthma intervention in which adolescents received open-ended prompts each morning inquiring about their symptoms. Based on the texter's response, the computer delivered management advice. To address cases where AI was not sufficient to understand and respond, the developers made creative use of a human "wizard," a staff person who could be alerted if the computer could not decipher the message and temporarily take over the interaction. While this achievement is impressive, an even greater degree of AI technology is likely to be needed in the complex context of mental health interventions, where symptoms are often harder to pinpoint or even recognize. Going forward, improved AI in interactions in mental health texting interventions would improve the conformability (the degree to which a technology fits into one's life) of current text-message interventions.

Finally, the field awaits true "dissemination and implementation" studies—in which text-message mental health interventions are put into place in real-world settings.

Case Resolution

After quickly reviewing the literature and talking to your colleague, you realize that Jayson would be eligible for the text-message intervention. He enthusiastically consents to the study. You also call Jayson's pediatrician to let her know about your findings and to encourage follow-up.

A couple of months later, you get an email from the pediatrician, thanking you for your care. She tells you that Jayson has "improved a lot," particularly by developing improved emotional awareness and decreasing his involvement in physical fights. He also reached out to a school-based therapist based on his increased awareness of his mood variability from participating in the program. She wants to know if the program is available to her other patients. You tell her that you'll get back to her!

References

1. Lenhart A. Teens, Social Media & Technology Overview 2015. April 2015, Pew Research Center.
2. Ranney ML, et al. Adolescents' preference for technology-based emergency department behavioral interventions: does it depend on risky behaviors? Pediatr Emerg Care. 2013;29(4):475–81.
3. Vyas AN, et al. Public health interventions: reaching Latino adolescents via Short Message Service and social media. J Med Internet Res. 2012;14(4):e99.
4. Gibson K, Cartwright C. Young people's experiences of mobile phone text counselling: balancing connection and control. Child Youth Serv Rev. 2014;43:96–104.
5. Underwood MK, et al. The BlackBerry project: capturing the content of adolescents' text messaging. Dev Psychol. 2012;48(2):295–302.
6. Ranney ML, et al. 'You need to get them where they feel it': conflicting perspectives on how to maximize the structure of text-message psychological interventions for adolescents. In: Proceedings of the 48th Annual Hawaii International Conference on System Sciences. 2015. IEEE & Computer Society Press. p. 3247–3255.
7. Mason M, et al. Text messaging interventions for adolescent and young adult substance use: a meta-analysis. Prev Sci. 2015;16(2):181–8.
8. Head KJ, et al. Efficacy of text messaging-based interventions for health promotion: a meta-analysis. Soc Sci Med. 2013;97:41–8.
9. IMS Institute for Healthcare Informatics. Patient apps for improved healthcare: from novelty to mainstream. Parsipanny, NJ: IMS Institute; 2013.
10. Armanasco AA, et al. Preventive health behavior change text message interventions: a meta-analysis. Am J Prev Med. 2017;52(3):391–402.
11. Alvarez-Jimenez M, et al. Online, social media and mobile technologies for psychosis treatment: a systematic review on novel user-led interventions. Schizophr Res. 2014;156(1):96–106.
12. Menon V, Rajan TM, Sarkar S. Psychotherapeutic applications of mobile phone-based technologies: a systematic review of current research and trends. Indian J Psychol Med. 2017;39(1):4–11.
13. Agyapong VI, et al. Cross-sectional survey evaluating Text4Mood: mobile health program to reduce psychological treatment gap in mental healthcare in Alberta through daily supportive text messages. BMC Psychiatry. 2016;16(1):378.
14. McKay FH, et al. Evaluating mobile phone applications for health behaviour change: a systematic review. J Telemed Telecare. 2016.
15. Kauer SD, et al. Investigating the utility of mobile phones for collecting data about adolescent alcohol use and related mood, stress and coping behaviours: lessons and recommendations. Drug Alcohol Rev. 2009;28(1):25–30.
16. Aguilera A, Schueller SM, Leykin Y. Daily mood ratings via text message as a proxy for clinic based depression assessment. J Affect Disord. 2015;175:471–4.
17. Kauer SD, et al. Self-monitoring using mobile phones in the early stages of adolescent depression: randomized controlled trial. J Med Internet Res. 2012;14(3):e67.
18. Reid SC, et al. A mobile phone application for the assessment and management of youth mental health problems in primary care: a randomised controlled trial. BMC Fam Pract. 2011;12:131.
19. Aguilera A, Munoz RF. Text messaging as an adjunct to CBT in low-income populations: a usability and feasibility pilot study. Prof Psychol Res Pr. 2011;42(6):472–8.
20. Agyapong VI, et al. Supportive text messaging for depression and comorbid alcohol use disorder: single-blind randomised trial. J Affect Disord. 2012;141(2–3):168–76.
21. Furber GV, et al. How adolescents use SMS (short message service) to micro-coordinate contact with youth mental health outreach services. J Adolesc Health. 2011;48(1):113–5.
22. Kobak KA, Mundt JC, Kennard B. Integrating technology into cognitive behavior therapy for adolescent depression: a pilot study. Ann General Psychiatry. 2015;14:37.
23. Whittaker R, et al. MEMO—a mobile phone depression prevention intervention for adolescents: development process and postprogram findings on acceptability from a randomized controlled trial. J Med Internet Res. 2012;14(1):e13.
24. Ranney ML, et al. A depression prevention intervention for adolescents in the emergency department. J Adolesc Health. 2016;59(4):401–10.
25. Ranney M, et al. An emergency department text message program to reduce peer violence and depressive symptoms among at-risk youth: evidence for future adaptive interventions. Psychol Serv. Under review.
26. Wyman PA, et al. An outcome evaluation of the Sources of Strength suicide prevention program delivered by adolescent peer leaders in high schools. Am J Public Health. 2010;100(9):1653–61.
27. Schilling EA, Aseltine RH Jr, James A. The SOS suicide prevention program: further evidence of efficacy and effectiveness. Prev Sci. 2016;17(2):157–66.
28. Pisani AR, et al. Associations between suicidal high school students' help-seeking and their attitudes and perceptions of social environment. J Youth Adolesc. 2012;41(10):1312–24.
29. Pisani AR, et al. Emotion regulation difficulties, youth–adult relationships, and suicide attempts among

high school students in underserved communities. J Youth Adolesc. 2013;42(6):807–20.
30. Thiha P, et al. Efficacy of web-based collection of strength-based testimonials for text message extension of youth suicide prevention program: randomized controlled experiment. JMIR Public Health Surveill. 2016;2(2):e164.
31. Pisani AR, et al. Diverse uses for text messaging in suicide prevention: three New York State projects and interactive discussion of implications. In: Firstst Annual Conference of the Suicide Prevention Center of New York. 2016. Albany, NY.
32. Gould MS, et al. Teenagers' attitudes about seeking help from telephone crisis services (hotlines). Suicide Life Threat Behav. 2006;36(6):601–13.
33. Berrouiguet S, et al. SIAM (suicide intervention assisted by messages): the development of a post-acute crisis text messaging outreach for suicide prevention. BMC Psychiatry. 2014;14:294.
34. Luxton DD, June JD, Comtois KA. Can postdischarge follow-up contacts prevent suicide and suicidal behavior? Crisis. 2013;34(1):32–41.
35. Motto JA, Bostrom AG. A randomized controlled trial of postcrisis suicide prevention. Psychiatr Serv. 2001;52(6):828–33.
36. Mason M, et al. Text message delivered peer network counseling for adolescent smokers: a randomized controlled trial. J Prim Prev. 2016;37(5):403–20.
37. Suffoletto B, et al. A text message alcohol intervention for young adult emergency department patients: a randomized clinical trial. Ann Emerg Med. 2014;64(6):664–72. e4
38. Gonzales R, et al. Substance use recovery outcomes among a cohort of youth participating in a mobile-based texting aftercare pilot program. J Subst Abus Treat. 2014;47(1):20–6.
39. Gonzales R, et al. Youth recovery outcomes at 6 and 9 months following participation in a mobile texting recovery support aftercare pilot study. Am J Addict. 2016;25(1):62–8.
40. Fjeldsoe BS, Marshall AL, Miller YD. Behavior change interventions delivered by mobile telephone short-message service. Am J Prev Med. 2009;36(2):165–73.
41. Hawkins RP, et al. Understanding tailoring in communicating about health. Health Educ Res. 2008; 23(3):454–66.
42. Noar SM, Benac CN, Harris MS. Does tailoring matter? Meta-analytic review of tailored print health behavior change interventions. Psychol Bull. 2007;133(4):673–93.
43. Chernick LS, et al. Adolescent female text messaging preferences to prevent pregnancy after an emergency department visit: a qualitative analysis. J Med Internet Res. 2016;18(9):e261.
44. Ranney ML, et al. "You need to get them where they feel it": conflicting perspectives on how to maximize the structure of text-message psychological interventions for adolescents. Proc Annu Hawaii Int Conf Syst Sci. 2015;2015:3247–55.
45. Devine S, et al. Enhancing a teen pregnancy prevention program with text messaging: engaging minority youth to develop TOP (R) plus text. J Adolesc Health. 2014;54(3 Suppl):S78–83.
46. Suffoletto B, et al. A sex risk reduction text-message program for young adult females discharged from the emergency department. J Adolesc Health. 2013; 53(3):387–93.
47. Seko Y, et al. Youth mental health interventions via mobile phones: a scoping review. Cyberpsychol Behav Soc Netw. 2014;17(9):591–602.
48. Gallagher K, Updegraff J. Health message framing effects on attitudes, intentions, and behavior: a meta-analytic review. Ann Behav Med. 2012;43(1):101–16.
49. Ranney ML, et al. Acceptability, language, and structure of text message-based behavioral interventions for high-risk adolescent females: a qualitative study. J Adolesc Health. 2014;55(1):33–40.
50. Pisani AR, et al. Human subjects protection and technology in prevention science: selected opportunities and challenges. Prev Sci. 2016;17(6):765–78.
51. Abroms LC, et al. Developing and pretesting a text messaging program for health behavior change: recommended steps. JMIR Mhealth Uhealth. 2015; 3(4):e107.
52. Glanz K. The role of behavioral science theory in development and implementation of public health interventions. Annu Rev Public Health. 2010;31:399–418.
53. Lopez LM, et al. Theory-based interventions for contraception. Cochrane Database Syst Rev. 2016; 11:CD007249.
54. Chernick LS, et al. Barriers to and enablers of contraceptive use among adolescent females and their interest in an emergency department based intervention. Contraception. 2015;91(3):217–25.
55. Gold J, et al. What's in a message? Delivering sexual health promotion to young people in Australia via text messaging. BMC Public Health. 2010;10:792.
56. Kristan J, Suffoletto B. Using online crowdsourcing to understand young adult attitudes toward expert-authored messages aimed at reducing hazardous alcohol consumption and to collect peer-authored messages. Transl Behav Med. 2015;5(1):45–52.
57. Muench F, et al. Understanding messaging preferences to inform development of mobile goal-directed behavioral interventions. J Med Internet Res. 2014;16(2):e14.
58. Text messaging and HIPAA. [April 26, 2017]. https://hipaaqsportal.hhs.gov/a/dtd/Text-messaging-and-HIPAA/135929-36899.
59. Drolet BC. Text messaging and protected health information: what is permitted? JAMA. 2017;317 (23):2369–70.
60. Christofferson DE, Hamlett-Berry K, Augustson E. Suicide prevention referrals in a mobile health smoking cessation intervention. Am J Public Health. 2015;105(8):e7–9.
61. Rhee H, et al. Mobile phone-based asthma self-management aid for adolescents (mASMAA): a feasibility study. Patient Prefer Adherence. 2014;8:63–72.

Check for updates

16 Online Therapy for Adolescent Mental Health

Huma Ali Khan, Karen Bernstein, and Benjamin Van Voorhees

Patient Case

Angela is a 17-year-old female who presents to her outpatient family practice clinic in rural Idaho with her mother and has complaints of difficulty sleeping, decreased energy, loss of appetite, and "feeling down." She also notes that she frequently worries about her school, work, health, and well-being of her family. Angela's family recently moved to Idaho from Connecticut, which was also stressful for Angela. Her mother has a history of depression and has been treated with SSRIs and psychotherapy in the past. Angela and her mother are both interested in Angela starting therapy for her anxiety and depressed mood. Unfortunately, there are no certified mental health professionals in the area. Angela asks about other options for therapy; she has heard about a clinic in a nearby city that offers computerized cognitive behavioral therapy.

Angela and mom ask about the effectiveness of computerized therapy and its utility in treating anxiety and depression in adolescents.

Since the early 2000s, there have been increasing interest and efforts in improving the efficiency and availability of mental health services. E-mental health, defined as "mental health services and information delivered or enhanced through the Internet and related technologies" [1], is a growing field of research that has aided in the development of Internet-/technology-based health applications and programs [2]. Benefits of e-mental health programs and interventions include improved accessibility for hard-to-reach populations, convenience, and self-paced services [3], anonymity for those who feel stigma from traditional services, and cost-efficiency [2]. Additionally, studies have shown that young adults use e-mental health care as a means of self-help which can enhance conventional care [4, 5]; one review reported a mean of 38.4% (range 18–53%) of young people who use e-mental health care for self-help [6]. Although

H.A. Khan, M.D., F.A.A.P. (✉)
University of Illinois Hospital, Chicago;
John H. Stroger, Jr. Hospital of Cook County, Chicago, IL, USA
e-mail: hakhan@UIC.EDU

K. Bernstein, M.D., M.P.H.
Division of Adolescent Medicine, University of Illinois Hospital, Chicago, Chicago, IL, USA

B. Van Voorhees, M.D., M.P.H.
Department of Pediatrics, University of Illinois Hospital, Chicago, Chicago, IL, USA

M.A. Moreno, A. Radovic (eds.), *Technology and Adolescent Mental Health*,
https://doi.org/10.1007/978-3-319-69638-6_16

there has been concern that e-mental health applications would hinder the outreach to mental professionals, there has been no evidence of reduction of mental health-seeking behavior [4]. The efficacy of online mental health therapy can be dependent on the design of the intervention. A meta-analysis of Internet-based cognitive behavioral therapy (iCBT) studies showed that high effect size for reduction of mood symptoms was related to the presence of therapist support (monitoring and feedback) vs. iCBT with no therapist support [7]. Another review suggested that accurate diagnoses and targeted iCBT can help create a better patient to treatment match [8]. Internet-based cognitive behavioral therapy has been studied in both adults and adolescents and offers a unique, effective, and cost-efficient strategy in treatment of depression, anxiety, and other mental health disorders (Table 16.1). Other online-therapy modalities, such as e-counseling, have been used for both early intervention and treatment [9]. As Internet-based therapy continues to develop, medical and mental health-care systems and providers will need to adapt to integrate this new technology into standard care [9]. The following is a review of the most recent and more widely studied adult Internet-based and computerized therapies as well as the developing literature on the efficacy of e-mental health services for adolescents. Research on implementation of e-mental health programs in clinic and school settings as well as in worldwide adaptations has demonstrated the benefits, challenges, and potential solutions for effective dissemination of online and computerized therapy.

Internet-Based Cognitive Behavioral Therapy (iCBT) in Adults

A cross-sectional survey of a sample of US-accredited training programs in psychiatry, psychology, and social work showed a gap between scientific evidence for psychotherapy and clinical training, resulting in a lack of mental health providers with adequate evidence-based training [10]. This is one of the reasons why Internet-based cognitive behavioral therapy (iCBT) and computerized CBT (cCBT, CBT over a computer in clinic) for adults are the attractive treatment options. In the past decade, several meta-analyses of adult e-mental health therapy studies have demonstrated the efficacy of computerized therapy for treatment of depression and anxiety. One meta-analysis of 23 adult randomized controlled trials (RCT) comparing effects of computerized psychotherapy (CBT or exposure therapy) vs. a control or face-to-face therapy for anxiety disorders reported a large effect size over control conditions (Cohen's $d = 1.1$); computerized psychotherapy as a whole was as effective as face-to-face psychotherapy [11]. Another meta-analysis of 12 randomized controlled trials (RCT) on adult computerized therapy for depression showed a moderate effect size (0.42), with greater effect size for therapist-supported therapy [12]. In 2010, a meta-analysis by Andrews et al. [3] evaluated 22 randomized controlled trials of computerized or Internet-based CBT for adults with major depression, social phobia, panic disorder, or generalized anxiety disorder and showed superiority of computerized therapy (cCBT and iCBT) over the control group (mean effect size 0.88); five studies compared computerized CBT with face-to-face CBT and both modes were equally effective [3]. A more recent meta-analysis [13] of 16 randomized controlled trials on adults with depressive symptoms receiving self-guided iCBT compared with controls (usual care, waiting list, attention control) showed that participants with iCBT had lower depression symptom severity and a greater treatment response compared to participants in the control group; also, there were no significant differences in iCBT treatment outcomes associated with sociodemographic characteristics [13].

The need for evidence-based and accessible mental health care, specifically iCBT, has led to the development of a free online service for adults, the MindSpot Clinic [14]. Australia's government-funded e-mental health strategy, the MindSpot Clinic, was designed to provide therapist-guided e-mental health services for more than 10,000 adults with anxiety and depression per year [15]. Through the MindSpot Clinic, four iCBT treatment courses are offered over 4–6

Table 16.1 Adolescent studies on cCBT and iCBT for depression and anxiety

	Condition	Sample	Intervention	Design	Attrition	Findings	Country	Availability
Abeles et al. (2009) [39]	Depression	$N = 23$ Age 12–16	*Stressbusters* Unmonitored Eight sessions 30–45 min	No control Pre-/post-intervention comparison	70% completed all sessions	78% of completers diagnosis free post-intervention 93% diagnosis free at 3 months	England	
Calear et al. (2009) [50]	Depression and anxiety	$N = 1477$ Age 12–17 years	*MoodGym* 5 iCBT modules over 5 weeks administered by school teachers	RCT 1. *MoodGym* 2. Control group	32.7% completed all modules	Significant reduction in anxiety for *MoodGym* compared to control (Cohen's *d*: 0.15–0.25) Significant reduction in depression among males (Cohen's 0.27–0.43)	Australia	Available online to the public for a small annual fee
Khanna and Kendall (2010) [36]	Anxiety	$N = 49$ Age 7–13 years	*Camp-Cope-A-Lot (CCAL)* 12 therapist-monitored CBT sessions	RCT 1. CCAL 2. Individual CBT (ICBT) 3. Computer-assisted education, support, and attention (CESA)	92% completed all sessions	Significant reduction in anxiety for CCAL and ICBT compared to control Posttreatment, 81% of CCAL participants, 70 % of ICBT participants, and 19% of CESA participants no longer met criteria for primary anxiety diagnosis Parents and children rated CCAL acceptable	Australia	Software available for purchase online for individuals and institutions
March et al. (2008) [33]	Anxiety	$N = 73$ Age 7–12 years	*BRAVE* Ten weekly 60-min child CBT sessions Six weekly 60-min parent CBT sessions Booster sessions at 1 and 3 months Therapist guided	RCT 1. Internet-based CBT (NET) 2. Wait-list control	Posttreatment: 33% children, 60% adults completed all sessions 6-month follow-up: 62% children, 72% adults completed all sessions	Posttreatment, NET participants had small but significant reduction in anxiety and functioning compared to control 6-month follow-up: 75% of NET children free of primary anxiety diagnosis	Australia	Available online to the public (in and out of Australia) for a fee

(continued)

Table 16.1 (continued)

	Condition	Sample	Intervention	Design	Attrition	Findings	Country	Availability
Robinson et al. (2016) [48]	Depression with suicidal ideation	*N* = 32 Age 14–18 years	*Reframe-IT* 8-week intervention School based Therapist-monitored cCBT modules focused on suicide ideation management	Pilot study Pre-/posttest intervention comparison	65% completed all eight sessions	Significant reduction in depressive symptoms (moderate effect size 0.6), suicidal ideation (moderate effect size, 0.66), and hopelessness (small effect size, 0.46) after intervention	Australia	
Santucci et al. (2013) [56]	Depression and anxiety	*N* = 44 Age 18–32 years (mean age 23)	*Beating the Blues* Eight weekly 50-min sessions University based	Pilot study 1. cCBT with email reminder 2. cCBT with no reminder	1. cCBT with reminder: 14% completed eight sessions 2. cCBT with no reminder: 13% completed eight sessions	1. Significant reductions in anxiety, depressive symptoms, and functional impairment after treatment completion 2. High attrition rate 3. No difference in session completion between email reminder and no reminder groups	United States	Available online to the public for a fee
Spence et al. (2011) [35]	Anxiety	*N* = 115 Age 12–18 years	*BRAVE* Ten weekly 60-min child iCBT sessions Six weekly 60-min parent iCBT sessions Therapist guided booster sessions at 1 and 3 months	RCT 1. Internet-based treatment (NET) 2. Clinic-based treatment (CLIN) 3. Wait-list control (WLC)	12-month follow-up: NET: 57 % adolescents, 79% parents completed all sessions CLIN: 79% adolescents, 79% parents completed all sessions	Significantly greater reductions in anxiety symptoms for NET and CLIN participants compared to WLC at 12 weeks 12-month follow-up: 78.4% in NET and 80.6% in CLIN conditions free of primary anxiety diagnosis Adolescent satisfaction ratings equal for NET and CLIN conditions Parent satisfaction slightly higher for CLIN condition	Australia	Available online for a fee for children, teens, and parents

Spence et al. (2006) [32]	Anxiety	$N = 72$ Age 7–14 years	Combined clinic and Internet-delivered CBT (CLIN-NET) 10 weeks total, 5/10 were 60-min iCBT sessions	RCT 1. CLIN-NET 2. Clinic- based group CBT (CLINIC) 3. Wait-list control	90% completed all sessions	1. Significant reduction in anxiety posttreatment and at 12-month follow-up for CLIN-NET and CLINIC compared to control 2. CLIN-NET: high levels of acceptability, compliance, and retention for children and parents	Australia	(See above for *BRAVE*)
Tillfors et al. (2011) [38]	Anxiety	$N = 19$ Age 15–21 years	iCBT 9-week course Minimal therapist support	RCT 1. iCBT 2. Wait-list control	On average, 32% completed all iCBT modules No iCBT participants completed iCBT on time	iCBT group had significant improvements in social anxiety, general anxiety, and depression Improvements maintained at 1-year follow-up Average within and between group effect sizes (Cohen's d) for anxiety scales posttreatment 0.98 and 1.38, respectively	Sweden	
van der Zanden et al. (2012) [43]	Subthreshold or mild depression	$N = 244$ Age 16–25	*Master Your Mood* Monitored by mental health professional Six sessions 90 min each	Wait-list control	194/244, 80% completed all sessions	Significant improvement in depressive symptoms for intervention group vs. control Large effect size ($d = 0.94$) Improvement maintained at 6 months	Netherlands	Free online access with registration at info@gripopjedip.nl (Dutch version)

(continued)

Table 16.1 (continued)

	Condition	Sample	Intervention	Design	Attrition	Findings	Country	Availability
Van Voorhees et al. (2009) [46]	Subthreshold depression	*N* = 84 Age 14–21 years	*CATCH-IT* iCBT 14 modules Interpersonal therapy and behavioral activation Physician interviews pre-/post-intervention MI group: three motivational phone calls from social workers	RCT Two groups: 1. Brief advice (BA) + cCBT 2. Motivational interviewing (MI) + cCBT	MI: 61% completed all modules BA: 67% completed all modules Overall 7/84 dropped out	Significant reduction in depressive symptoms for both groups post-intervention MI: Significant reduction in thoughts of self-harm and hopelessness	United States	A culturally adapted version of *CATCH-IT*, called CURB (Chicago Urban Resiliency Building) [94], is available for free online at www.mycheck.uic.edu
Wuthrich et al. (2012) [37]	Anxiety	*N* = 43 Age 14–17 years	*Cool Teens* 12-week therapist-supported cCBT	RCT 1. *Cool Teens* 2. Wait-list control	86% completed all sessions	Significant reduction in anxiety symptoms and severity in *Cool Teens* group vs. control	Australia	

weeks: a Wellbeing course for anxiety and depression for adults 18–60 years, a Wellbeing Plus course for adults over 60 years, an OCD course, and a PTSD course [15]. A prospective noncontrolled cohort study of the MindSpot Clinic reported results of iCBT given as routine clinical care. The course completion rate was 71.8%, and there were moderate to large effect sizes (Cohen's d = 0.67–1.66, 95% confidence interval = 0.08–2.07) from assessment to 3-month follow-up; with the exception of the OCD course, the treatment courses had effect sizes >1.3 on anxiety and depression measures [15].

E-Mental Health in Usual Care Settings

Primary Care

Primary care implementation of Internet-based cognitive behavioral therapy for adults has also been studied in recent years showing promising results for incorporation of computerized therapy in clinic settings. A randomized controlled trial evaluating 16 primary care centers providing iCBT in Sweden showed that there were no significant differences in depression symptoms found among adults receiving iCBT with minimal therapist support and those receiving treatment as usual over a 12-month period; these findings provided evidence of equal effectiveness of iCBT and face-to-face therapy in primary care [16]. In 2011, Hoifodt et al. [17] reviewed eight randomized controlled trials of provider-assisted cCBT or iCBT in primary care clinics and showed that these modes of therapy were effective in treatment of mild to moderate depression as well as anxiety in adolescents and adults [17]. *Beating the Blues* [18], an evidence-based computerized cognitive behavioral therapy program for adults with depression and/or anxiety, has been disseminated for routine practice in the UK [11]. *Beating the Blues* uses an interactive, multimedia format to deliver an introductory 15-min video, followed by weekly 50-min therapy sessions with customized homework projects at on-site clinic settings. This cCBT program has significantly reduced depression and anxiety symptoms among adult primary care patients and also improved work and social adjustment [18]. Furthermore, *Beating the Blues* has demonstrated efficacy for mild to severe depression in primary care settings [18]. A Dutch study evaluating performance of iCBT in routine clinical practice showed that a clinic-based therapist-assisted CBT for depression, panic disorder, posttraumatic stress, and burnout had reductions in symptomology for adult patents for up to 1 year; 79% of patients completed posttreatment measurements, and 71% completed every step of the treatment [19]. In the Randomized Evaluation of the Effectiveness and Acceptability of Computerized Therapy (REEACT) trial, primary care-based cCBT interventions, a free-to-use cCBT program *MoodGym*, and a commercial pay-to-use cCBT program *Beating the Blues* were compared in addition to usual general practitioner care [20]. *MoodGym,* in a community-based setting, has been found to reduce dysfunctional thinking and depressive symptoms when used with a weekly contact [21]. *MoodGym*, a widely available Internet-based program in Australia, has been recommended as a population-level intervention for depression and anxiety [22]. It has shown effectiveness in improving symptoms of depression, general psychological distress, and anxiety for adults, but adherence rates have been problematic, sometimes falling below 10% [22]. The REEACT trial, a multicenter randomized controlled trial, showed no difference in outcome between either cCBT intervention and usual general practitioner care [20]. There was low uptake of all cCBT programs, despite regular phone support [23], and neither *Beating the Blues* nor *MoodGym* showed evidence of cost-effectiveness, compared to treatment as usual with a general practitioner [20]. Qualitative evidence from the REEACT trial showed that some participants lacked motivation to access the computer-based programs due to their depressed mood [20]. Also, some participants stated they would prefer more therapeutic input [20]. Participants in the trial received weekly telephone calls designed to provide technical support, but no psychotherapy [20]. Follow-up was also offered over the phone or face to face, but not for therapeutic purposes [20]. Overall, the REEACT trial demonstrated that computerized CBT in primary care led to no difference in clinical outcomes than usual care, and commercially developed cCBT products had little to no benefit over free, open-access sites [23].

Specialty Care

One study at specialty mental health clinics (Kaiser Permanente, northern California) assessed the effectiveness of an Internet-delivered care management and patient self-management program, *eCare for Moods*, for adults with recurrent or chronic depression (N = 103) [24]. *ECare* offered patients personalized self-monitoring, confidential messaging with a psychiatric nurse care manager, and depression education based on CBT interventions [24]. Those participants randomly assigned to *eCare* had significant improvements in depression symptoms over 2 years, compared to those who had usual mental health care [24]. This study showed that even in specialty settings, Internet-delivered mental health services can provide continuous access to care and better outcomes than treatment as usual [24].

Despite promising results for iCBT use in primary and specialty care, and some studies citing good patient adherence and acceptability [3], various shortcomings exist regarding patient participation and completion. Limitations that have been noted in studies of iCBT include poor adherence rate and high dropout rates [25], especially for open-access websites [19, 26], and unguided iCBT [13]. Factors associated with poor adherence include disease severity, treatment length, and chronicity [26].

E-Mental Health and Youth

There is significant value in the use of Internet-based mental health care for adolescents. An Australian study of *eheadspace,* a web-based counseling site, compared demographics of adolescents who sought care through *eheadspace* vs. those who received similar in-person counseling [27]. Those who preferred the online mental health care were mainly female (80%), highly distressed, earlier in the development of a mental illness, and interested in help with depression, anxiety, and relationship problems [27]. These findings support the need for Internet-based services in reaching a unique population who may not otherwise seek help [27]. Internet-based interventions can be used as preventative tools and also serve as effective gateways and complimentary adjuncts to face-to-face therapy, rather than replacements for traditional therapy [28].

There is a growing body of literature on school- and clinic-based e-mental health interventions, mainly iCBT, geared toward adolescents, aged 12–18 years, who are in need of therapy for anxiety and depression [29]. A recent meta-analysis of 13 randomized controlled trials on Internet- and computer-based cognitive behavioral therapy for youth with depression and anxiety demonstrated significant moderate to large treatment effects on symptoms of anxiety and depression, similar to effect sizes for traditional face-to-face CBT (NNT 2.56) [30]. Although both adolescent anxiety and depression have been evaluated for response to iCBT, there has been more evidence of equal effectiveness of online CBT with remote therapist support compared to face-to-face CBT for anxiety disorders [29]. Further evidence of effectiveness in different populations and settings is needed prior to full integration of e-mental health services into standard mental health care for US adolescents [29].

Studies on iCBT and cCBT in Adolescents with Anxiety

The feasibility of Internet-based CBT used with clinic-based CBT was studied by Spence and colleagues [31]. In this randomized controlled trial, 72 clinically anxious children age 7–14 years were randomly assigned to clinic-based group CBT (CLINIC), clinic- and Internet-based CBT (CLIN-NET), or a wait-list control [31]. In the CLIN-NET program, five of the ten sessions were delivered via Internet as well as a 3-month booster session [31]. Additionally, three of six supportive parent sessions and 3-month booster session were delivered via the Internet [31]. Program content consisted of interactive, animated sessions covering CBT topics like physiologic symptoms of anxiety, relaxation skills, problem solving, self-reinforcement, and using anxiety-management skills [31]. The CLIN-NET treatment was associated with high levels of compliance with Internet sessions and high retention over the 10-week period, as well as high levels of acceptability and child/parent satisfaction [31]. There was minimal difference in outcomes between the CLINIC and CLIN-NET interventions, and children in both treatment groups showed significantly greater reductions in anxiety symptoms posttreatment and at 12-month follow-up than those in the wait-list group [31].

BRAVE-online (**B**ody signs, **R**elaxation, **A**ctive helpful thoughts, **V**ictory over your fears, **E**njoy! Reward yourself) is an Australian-based Internet CBT tool, developed by researchers at the University of Queensland [32], available to the public, and targeting children age 7–13 years with separation anxiety disorder, social phobia, generalized anxiety disorder, and specific phobia [33]. For instance, a recent study in New Zealand demonstrated the feasibility and utility of BRAVE online for reduction of child and adolescent anxiety related to a recent natural disaster (Canterbury earthquakes) [34]. Parent involvement and minimal therapist support (phone or email) are components of the online therapy that uses an engaging, interactive, and animated interface to educate users on physiologic symptoms of anxiety, relaxation techniques, self-talk coping strategies, problem solving, gradual exposure, and cognitive restructuring [33]. A study comparing BRAVE-online to equivalent clinic-based (face-to-face) CBT and a wait-list control showed that 78% of adolescents in the BRAVE-online group and 80.6% in the face-to-face clinic group were free of their primary anxiety diagnosis at the 12-month follow-up; adolescents in both groups had significant reductions in anxiety symptoms at 12 weeks, compared to those in the control group [35]. Furthermore, adolescent satisfaction was equivalent in both the BRAVE-online and clinic-based group [35]. Effect sizes were not significantly different between the online and face-to-face groups [29], indicating equal efficacy of the online BRAVE treatment and treatment as usual [32, 35]. However, completion of Internet sessions has been an issue in studies of this intervention; March et al. (2009) [33] found that 33% of children and 60% of parents completed all sessions post-intervention, and 62% of children and 72.3% of parents completed all sessions at the 6-month follow-up.

Another computer-based CBT model, Camp-Cope-A-Lot (CCAL), is designed to address anxiety in youth in a nonthreatening way [36]. Camp-Cope-A-Lot is a 12-session computerized program for anxious children, age 7–13 years [36]. Sessions include flash animation, cartoons, and a reward system to create an interactive and fun setting for children. The first six levels are designed for independent work and skill-building, and the remaining six levels involve exposure and rehearsal and are completed with a coach (therapist) [36]. In a study of CCAL, participants were randomly assigned to CCAL, individual CBT, or computer-assisted education, support, and attention (CESA) [36]. After completion of treatment, the individual CBT and CCAL participants had significant improvements in symptomology compared to the CESA children; 70% of individual CBT participants, 81% of CCAL participants, and 19% of CESA participants no longer met criteria for primary anxiety diagnosis posttreatment [36]. Also, parents and children rated CCAL acceptable and gave it higher scores for satisfaction than CESA. Overall, CCAL was found to be feasible, acceptable to teens, and beneficial [36].

Another computerized CBT-based intervention, *Cool Teens*, is geared toward anxious adolescents age 14–17 years and, in contrast to *BRAVE*, is inclusive of all types of anxiety disorders [37]. *Cool Teens* is CD-ROM based and composed of eight 30-min modules using live video, cartoons, illustrations, and text teaching CBT skills [37]. Minimal therapist involvement via brief conversations with adolescents and parents occurs throughout the 12-week intervention [37]. A randomized controlled trial of 43 adolescents randomly assigned to complete *Cool Teens* program or wait-list found that those who completed the program had significant reductions in number of anxiety disorders and severity of anxiety symptoms [37].

Adolescent social anxiety was the focus of an Internet-based CBT study in Sweden [38]. Nineteen high-school students were randomized to either a 9-week Internet-based CBT group or a wait-list control [38]. Participants in the treatment group received nine weekly CBT modules, accessible via the Internet, that provided information on social anxiety disorder, cognitive restructuring, exposure, social skills, and relapse prevention [38]. Internet therapists monitored weekly homework assignments and provided feedback [38]. Adolescents in the iCBT group had significant improvements in social anxiety, general anxiety, and depression, compared to the control group, that were maintained at a 1-year follow-up [38]. Also, average within and between group effect sizes (Cohen's *d*) for anxiety scales posttreatment was 0.98 and 1.38, respectively [38]. However, timely completion of modules was a noted problem in the study (0 participants completed modules on time) and only an average of 2.9/9 modules over the 9-week treatment period [38]. These findings again demonstrated the efficacy of iCBT for adolescent anxiety as well as the pervasive problem with participant adherence.

Studies on iCBT and cCBT for Depressed Adolescents

In recent years, cCBT interventions specifically created for depressed adolescents have been tested and become available for certain populations. *Stressbusters* [39] is a multimedia and interactive cCBT program developed in England that uses graphics, narration, video case vignettes, and animation to deliver information on psychoeducation about depression, behavioral activation, identifying and changing negative automatic thoughts, problem solving, social skills, and relapse prevention [39, 40]. Adolescents who completed eight sessions of *Stressbusters* were found to be depression-free at post-intervention and at 3-month follow-up (78% and 93%, respectively) [39, 40]. There were also improvements in global functioning and automatic thoughts and cognitions, post-intervention [39, 40]. In a RCT [41] evaluating effectiveness of *Stressbusters* for managing depressed adolescents in a school setting, the cCBT program was associated with significant and clinically meaningful reductions in depression symptomatology, post-intervention and at 3 and 6 months [41].

A publicly available group chat format, *Master Your Mood*, has also been studied in the Netherlands and found to be efficacious for adolescent depression [42]. The group chat intervention, available at www.gripopjedip.nl (Dutch website), was adapted from a face-to-face CBT course Grip op je dip and designed with a chat box allowing group conversations with a mental health professional. The eight sessions focused on detection of negative thoughts patterns, medication of negative thought patterns, and creation of positive thought processes and activities [42]. This online intervention was monitored by a mental health professional and included review of course material and homework. In an initial study of 189 adolescents with subthreshold depression who enrolled in the course, only 35.7% completed it [40, 42]. Important findings were that the target group of adolescents at risk for major depression was reached and anonymity was valued by participants and mental health professionals. Dropout rate due to technical difficulties, duration of the course, and participants' difficulties facing their depressive symptoms was problematic [40, 42]. A randomized controlled trial comparing the *Master Your Mood* program to a wait-listed control group found that adolescents who completed the online group chat course showed significantly greater improvements in depressive symptoms than the control group, with a large between group effect size ($d = 0.94$) [43].

A US multi-site primary care-based intervention, *Competent Adulthood Transition with Cognitive Behavioral Humanistic and Interpersonal Training* (*CATCH-IT*), used a self-guided, online strategy to prevent depression in adolescents [44, 45]. This public health-focused Internet-based initiative taught resiliency skills through teen-friendly modules to at-risk adolescents with subthreshold depression symptoms. The *CATCH-IT* intervention included Internet modules (14 teen and 4 parent modules) as well as motivational interviewing by a primary care provider (at months 0, 2, and 12) and 1–3 staff coaching phone calls [45]. It also incorporated primary care provider motivational support and parental courses on behavioral change [45]. An initial study on engaging adolescents with an Internet-based preventive strategy, *CATCH-IT*, found that adolescents were engaged with the Internet site and had significant reduction in depressive symptoms post-intervention up to 2.5 years after enrollment. Those who received motivational interviewing by a primary care provider, instead of brief advice, in addition to the *CATCH-IT* Internet program were significantly less likely to experience a depressive episode or hopelessness [46]. A randomized controlled trial of a Chinese language version of CATCH-IT, "Grasp the Opportunity," demonstrated reductions in depressed mood in adolescents at 12 months compared to an attention-control group [47]. The longitudinal 5-year randomized controlled trial (outcomes pending) comparing *CATCH-IT* to a health education, attentional control group will provide a systematic and cost-efficient approach to how primary care settings can mass screen adolescents at risk for depression and implement iCBT programs that are supported by trained providers [45].

One study targeting suicidal youth piloted an Internet program for adolescents at risk for suicide called Reframe-IT [48]. In the pilot, 21 students were enrolled from 9 schools in Melbourne, Australia [48]. The study demonstrated that participants found the program enjoyable and would recommend it to a friend. Also, the modules did not trigger any distress or suicidal thoughts. The program used a "host" character who delivered the CBT-based therapy that focused on suicidal thinking and behaviors [48]. In addition to using the site at school, participants also accessed the site at home. Student well-being staff checked responses to weekly suicide screens and responded appropriately; a research therapist also checked message boards and responded as needed [48]. This small and uncontrolled trial has been followed by a randomized controlled trial comparing outcomes for adolescents who completed a 10-week in-school intervention administered by a student well-being staff member vs. a treatment-as-usual group. Outcomes are still pending [49]. There is limited evidence of effectiveness of e-mental health interventions for adolescents at risk for suicide, and further studies may better demonstrate how Internet-based programs can reach this subgroup.

Adolescent School-Based Interventions

School-based e-mental health applications for adolescents have demonstrated similar efficacy. The YouthMood Project [50] sought to test the effectiveness of the *MoodGym* in a large and diverse group of adolescents attending 32 schools in Australia. The *MoodGym* is a cognitive behavioral program that is delivered online, fully automated, self-directed, and available outside the classroom free of charge [50]. Participants ($N = 1477$) were either randomly assigned to the wait-list-control group or the *MoodGym* intervention that was delivered in class weekly for 5 weeks and supervised by the classroom teacher [50]. Post-intervention and at 6-month follow-up, there were significant reductions in anxiety for *MoodGym* participants, compared to those in the control group (Cohen's *d*: 0.15–0.25) and significant reductions in depression among males (Cohen's 0.27–0.43) [50]. Although effect sizes were small to moderate, this program provided evidence of the effectiveness of school-based iCBT for adolescents [50]. Adolescent adherence to the *MoodGym* iCBT intervention has been found to be greater in monitored school settings vs. open-access community settings [51]. A follow-up study on YouthMood project adherence showed that both males and females who had high adherence in the *MoodGym* online intervention had stronger intervention effects for anxiety and depression than those with low adherence or those in the control group; the findings suggest that small nonsignificant effects for females in the original study were due to females' poor adherence with the *MoodGym* program [52]. The *YouthMood* Project showed promising results for school-based iCBT for adolescents, yet again confirmed the known limitation of iCBT, poor adherence.

Adolescents with social anxiety have been known to have biased information processing [53], attentional bias toward a threat [54], and negatively interpret ambiguous information [55]. One computerized intervention, focused on adolescents (N = 240) age 13–15 years with social anxiety, compared an Internet-based cognitive bias modification to a school-based cognitive behavioral therapy and a control group [53]. In this study conducted in the Netherlands, cognitive bias modification sessions targeted attentional bias, interpretive bias, dysfunctional associations, and self-esteem through social scenarios and visual probes [53]. The adolescents randomly assigned to the Internet-based cognitive bias modification program completed 20 sessions (40 min each) that were delivered biweekly on the Internet and received email reminders [53]. Compared to teens who received in-school group CBT, those who completed the online CBM sessions had a similar trend in reduction of social anxiety symptoms at 6-month follow-up, with small to moderate range effect sizes and a greater decrease of negative automatic associations than the CBT and control groups at 12-month follow-up [53]. However, a noted limitation of this study was lower training attendance in the CBM condition which may be improved with reduction of technical problems in the online CBM treatment, including browser-independent programs that do not require additional installation of plug-ins [53]. Overall, these findings suggest that online CBM training could be effective for adolescents with social anxiety. The *Beating the Blues* Internet-based cognitive behavioral program has also been piloted in a university setting as a potential intervention for young adults (18–32 years, mean age 23 years) [56]. Results of the study showed that participants (N = 43) reported significant improvement in symptoms of anxiety and depression as well as functional improvement [56]. However, a large number of participants (88%) did not complete all eight sessions, and weekly email reminders did not improve adherence [56]. Overall, this study provided initial evidence that cCBT could be implemented in a university health center with positive mental health outcomes; however, similar to other studies, strategies for improved adherence are needed.

ICBT for Other Mental Health Disorders

Internet-based CBT programs have also been designed to manage and treat other disorders including PTSD, OCD, body dysmorphia, and insomnia. A recent study of war-traumatized Arab adults (18–56 years, mean age 28.1 years, N = 159) with PTSD showed that those assigned to a 5-week Internet-based Arabic-translated CBT program had significant reductions in PTSD symptoms, compared to the control group [57]. The treatment included written assignments that were reviewed by therapists and covered self-confrontation with the trauma, cognitive restructuring, and social sharing. This study showed the feasibility and potential benefits of administering Internet-based CBT to people suffering from PTSD in war-torn and unstable environments [57]. An Australian RCT of adults with PTSD (N = 44) had similar results demonstrating that those who completed an 8-week therapist-supported iCBT course had significant reductions in PTSD symptoms, with large within-group effects, pre- to posttreatment (>0.8); participants also expressed satisfaction with the intervention [58].

There have been fewer definitive studies providing evidence of the efficacy of cCBT for OCD in youth [59]. A recent RCT of adults with OCD compared two low-intensity versions of CBT (guided self-help and supported cCBT) and showed neither low-intensity version of CBT led to clinically significant benefits in patient outcomes [59]. Access to "low-intensity" interventions led to significant reductions in uptake of CBT with a therapist over 12 months; however, there was no evidence that lower uptake of therapist-led CBT was associated with worse outcomes in 12 months [59]. Also, the widespread literature has shown contrary findings that those who used web-based interventions had greater participation in health care [59, 60]. Preliminary findings from a recent Australian study on OCD-focused iCBT demonstrated that adolescents (ages 12–18 years) who completed an eight-stage self-guided online program, "OCD? Not me!," [61] had significant reductions in OCD symptoms and severity posttreatment [62]. These preliminary results show the potential therapeutic use of self-guided iCBT for young people with OCD.

An Internet-based CBT intervention for adults with body dysmorphic disorder (BDD) was evaluated in a Swedish RCT ($N = 94$) [63]. Participants who completed a 12-week iCBT program had significant improvements in body dysmorphic disorder symptoms compared to those who only received supportive therapy and also reported satisfaction with the intervention [63]. Findings of this study showed the feasibility of use of a BDD-focused iCBT intervention by a general practitioner or other mental health professional treating patients with mild to moderate symptoms of BDD [63]. A randomized controlled trial on prevention of eating disorders among high-risk college students demonstrated effectiveness of an 8-week iCBT intervention in reducing weight and body image concerns (effect size, $d = 0.81$) and high adherence (79% of assignments completed) to the intervention [64]. The preventative eating disorder program included an online discussion group moderated by a clinical psychologist and completion of weekly online assignments and journal entries. Subjects also received weekly emails to enhance participation [64]. A more recent study evaluated the utility of the online-guided discussion group of the same iCBT intervention for college-age women at risk for eating disorder and showed that weight and body image concerns were reduced significantly more among those who received the online discussion group vs. those who had no discussion group (p .002; $d = 0.52$) [65].

There has been established evidence of the utility of iCBT for patients with insomnia improving sleep-related symptoms, as well as some evidence that individuals treated with iCBT for insomnia also experience a reduction in depressive symptoms [66]. A recent RCT in the Netherlands was the first to evaluate adolescents with insomnia ($N = 116$, mean age = 15.6 years) and showed that those who completed 6 weeks of insomnia-focused, therapist-monitored iCBT as well as those in group therapy improved significantly in sleep efficiency, sleep onset latency, and total sleep post-intervention (medium to large effect sizes), compared to a wait-list control [67]. These findings further demonstrated potential benefits of promoting Internet treatment for adolescent in mental health centers [67].

Other E-Mental Health Interventions

While the majority of the literature focuses on CBT, several other online mental health modalities have been studied and used for adolescents with depression, anxiety, and PTSD. Behavioral activation (BA) is a useful treatment for depression and focuses on the relationship between an individual and the environment, as well as triggers and maladaptive behaviors that may worsen depressive symptoms [68]. *Bounce Back Now* (*BBN*) is an online, evidence-based intervention, with a BA focus, for adolescents who have been victims of disasters [68]. The goal of the *BBN* intervention is to provide adolescents with specific guidance in returning to functional activities: helping others, learning, socializing, or applying for a job [68]. Qualitative data from preliminary studies showed that the BA intervention was well received by teens and that teens responded favorably to the program. Overall, this study demonstrated the willingness of teens to engage in an Internet BA intervention after a stressful life event [68].

An avatar-based depression self-management intervention for young adults, Electronic Self-Management Resource Training for Mental Health (eSMART-MH), has been evaluated in a longitudinal randomized controlled trial ($N = 28$) [69]. eSMART-MH is a novel avatar-based self-management tool for depressed adolescents that allows users to interact with virtual mental health-care providers and a virtual health coach in a virtual primary care environment [69]. Initial results of participants (age 18–25 years) in the eSMART-MH group had significant reductions in depressive symptoms over 4 months, compared to those assigned to the attention-control condition [69]. This study was the first to evaluate an avatar-based mental health intervention for young adults and demonstrated the feasibility of this mode of virtual depression self-management [69].

BiteBack is an Australian-based publicly available website geared to address positive psychology for adolescents [70]. A recent study of Australian youth sought to determine the feasibility of using an online positive psychology program to improve well-being and address mental health problems [70]. The *BiteBack* website uses interactive sessions that incorporate various positive psychology topics: flow, optimism, meaning, hope, mindfulness, character strengths, healthy lifestyle, and positive relationships. The website, targeting adolescents age 13–17 years, also provides skill-building strategies and includes online discussions [70]. The randomized controlled trial (N = 235) comparing *BiteBack* to control websites showed that 79% of *BiteBack* users had positive experiences with the website, and 89% stated they would use the intervention after 6-week study completion [70]. Those with high adherence (website use of 30+ min/week) had significant decreases in stress and depression and improvements in well-being [70]. Overall, the potential success of online positive psychology websites for use in improvement of well-being in adolescents was shown in the *BiteBack* study [70]. However, a school-based study, evaluating the efficacy of a 6-week *BiteBack* intervention in a monitored setting, showed no difference between the *BiteBack* condition and a control in reduction of depressive symptomology [71].

Studies on online exposure therapy have shown promising results for those with specific phobias, specifically spider phobia [72]. Mathews et al. (2015) [72] evaluated the use of online real and "hyper-real" (exaggerated features) images of spiders in a graded exposure therapy. The online exposure to the images resulted in significant improvements in spider phobia symptoms and behavioral avoidance among adults with spider phobia [72]. These findings provided interesting implications for future interventions using online image-based exposure therapy [72].

E-Mental Health Therapy: Barriers and Solutions for Care

Although the utility of e-mental health modalities for youth is promising, there are barriers to successful implementation of Internet and computerized therapy programs. Uptake of computer-based psychological treatment in the United States remains relatively low [73]. Certain factors, as noted in one Delphi study [74], increase the likelihood of adolescents' use of website interventions. Important motivators for adolescents, as far as first site visit, are a positive recommendation by word of mouth and an attractive website interface [74]. Adolescent adherence may be dependent on discreetness of website, time to complete intervention, and a built-in commitment to revisit the site [74]. Another recommendation for improved uptake of computerized mental health intervention is increasing awareness of computer-based psychological treatment programs by PCPs, HMOs, or insurance companies [73]. Adherence to e-health programs has been shown to be problematic [52], especially in open-access or community formats [4, 21, 51]. For adolescents, predictors of better adherence include female gender, living in a rural area, higher pretest depression scores [51], and higher levels of initial motivation [75]. Providers' thoughts and opinions on effectiveness and reliability of e-mental health therapy may also affect likelihood of recommendations to adolescent patients [4] and may also affect adolescent experience [76]. Disadvantaged or ethnic minority groups may require additional efforts to engage with the program and may have additional preferences including use of adjunct discussion groups, cultural adaptation, engagement in high trust settings (community centers rather than physician offices), and stigma and privacy concerns [77, 78].

Another concern with online therapy is how to deal with a mental health emergency or crisis [79]. Safety procedures undoubtedly need to be in place in order to continually monitor for suicidality and homicidality [75]. However, two studies of online approaches have demonstrated that self-harm thoughts do not appear to increase and may actually decline [45, 80, 81]. Also, participants must be accurately screened in order to engage in therapy; those who are in inpatient settings or with severe psychiatric conditions are not good candidates for e-mental health interventions [75].

Implementation of Computer- and Internet-Based Therapy: Efforts Around the World

Of the e-mental health programs developed around the globe, the majority originate from Australia, a leader in web interventions [82]. A focus for many of these interventions are generalized anxiety disorder and panic disorder, depression, and stress; fewer target bipolar disorder and social anxiety [82]. Comparatively, countries in Asia and the Middle East are lacking in the development and use of e-mental health technologies [78]. In Hyderabad, India, where there is a lack of accessible mental health services and a pervasive mental health stigma, a randomized controlled trial was recently initiated to be the first to evaluate the effectiveness of guided and unguided iCBT for Indian university students with generalized anxiety disorder (outcomes pending) [83]. If found to be effective and feasible, programs delivered to Hyderabadi university students could help close the substantial mental health treatment gap in India [83]. While Australia continues to be the international leader in Internet-based mental health interventions, the United States and Canada are now becoming leaders in mobile phone-based mental health technologies [82]. Furthermore, a Western-based depression prevention tool, *CATCH-IT*, has been adapted to be used cross-culturally, for Chinese adolescents [47] as well as for Arab youth [84]. A proposed model for the cultural adaptation of a preventative Internet-based mental health intervention (CATCH-IT) for Arab youth used a theoretical framework (PEN-3) to evaluate cultural identity, relationships and expectations, and cultural empowerment in Arab communities. An expert panel also provided feedback on proposed changes to the CATCH-IT website for Arab youth [84]. The Western-developed iCBT intervention CATCH-IT was also adapted and translated for Chinese youth (grasping the opportunity) and found to be effective in reducing symptoms of depression in Chinese adolescents [47]. This adaptation was based on a theoretical analysis using data from focus groups, an expert panel, public health campaign, and a primary care physician-social worker review group [85]. These international efforts provide the basis for future success in worldwide prevention and management of adolescent mental illness.

Future Directions: Implementation

The broad reach of e-mental health interventions for youth is encouraging [73]. The incorporation of online CBT in routine mental health care and primary care has shown promising results of improvements, comparable to face-to-face interventions, for symptoms of depression, panic disorder, posttraumatic stress, and burnout [19]. Furthermore, economic analysis has showed that cCBT is the most efficient mode of therapy compared to treatment as usual [86]. Successful widespread dissemination and implementation of e-mental health modalities for adolescents will require alignment of focus and objectives of all stakeholders including clinicians, researchers, health-care administration, and policymakers [87–89]. Areas of research focus should include not only patient satisfaction and acceptability of Internet-based mental health but also cost, penetration, and feasibility of interventions [87]. For e-mental health interventions to successfully achieve the promise of their public health reach, much greater attention must be devoted to implementation and motivation [90]. A range of motivational frameworks need to be considered including traditional marketing, motivational interviewing, and even short persuasive engagement materials [46, 91]. Attention must be devoted to creating a positive user experience including user narratives, videos, games, and social media like experiences [92] that will sustain adolescent interest and increase likelihood of an effective dose [93]. Implementation in medical and educational systems is very complex—despite the ease in which the intervention may be accessed. Not integrating these approaches into "bricks and mortar" systems is likely to result in only a small fraction of youth using these interventions in a sufficiently organized manner to achieve an effective dose [89].

From a global and public health perspective, adolescents have attributes that make them uniquely suited to receive and benefit from Internet-based preventative and intervention programs. In the near future, larger longitudinal trials evaluating at-risk cohorts, different geographic locations, and clinic sites will provide important information on how to implement effective e-mental health services. Considerable efficiencies can be gained by adapting existing interventions from other cultures given many underlying therapeutic principles may be somewhat universal. For example, a single intervention could be adapted and translated into Arabic, Chinese, Spanish, and French and cover a large portion of world youth [84, 85]. Although online therapy has become more evidence-based, program implementation and overcoming structural barriers will be a key area of research that may shed light on how to better reach and manage adolescents with or at risk for mental illness.

References

1. Christensen H, Griffiths KM, Evans K. e-Mental health in Australia: implications of the Internet and related technologies for policy. Commonwealth Department of Health and Ageing: Canberra; 2002.
2. Lal S, Adair CE. E-mental health: a rapid review of the literature. Psychiatr Serv. 2014;65(1):24–32.
3. Andrews G, Cuijpers P, Craske MG, McEvoy P, Titov N. Computer therapy for the anxiety and depressive disorders is effective, acceptable and practical health care: a meta-analysis. PLoS One. 2010;5(10):e13196.
4. Christensen H, Reynolds J, Griffiths KM. The use of e-health applications for anxiety and depression in young people: challenges and solutions. Early Interv Psychiatry. 2011;5(s1):58–62.
5. Younes N, Chollet A, Menard E, Melchior M. E-mental health care among young adults and help-seeking behaviors: a transversal study in a community sample. J Med Internet Res. 2015;17(5):e123.
6. Kauer SD, Mangan C, Sanci L. Do online mental health services improve help-seeking for young people? A systematic review. J Med Internet Res. 2014;16(3):e66.
7. Spek V, Cuijpers PI, Nyklíček I, Riper H, Keyzer J, Pop V. Internet-based cognitive behaviour therapy for symptoms of depression and anxiety: a meta-analysis. Psychol Med. 2007;37(3):319–28.
8. Andersson G, Carlbring P, Berger T, Almlöv J, Cuijpers P. What makes Internet therapy work? Cogn Behav Ther. 2009;38(S1):55–60.
9. Rickwood D. Entering the e-spectrum: an examination of new interventions for youth mental health. Youth Studies Australia. 2012;31(4):18.
10. Weissman MM, Verdeli H, Gameroff MJ, Bledsoe SE, Betts K, Mufson L, Fitterling H, Wickramaratne P. National survey of psychotherapy training in psychiatry, psychology, and social work. Arch Gen Psychiatry. 2006;63(8):925–34.
11. Cuijpers P, Marks IM, van Straten A, Cavanagh K, Gega L, Andersson G. Computer-aided psychotherapy for anxiety disorders: a meta-analytic review. Cogn Behav Ther. 2009;38(2):66–82.
12. Andersson G, Cuijpers P. Internet-based and other computerized psychological treatments for adult depression: a meta-analysis. Cogn Behav Ther. 2009;38(4):196–205.
13. Karyotaki E, Riper H, Twisk J, Hoogendoorn A, Kleiboer A, Mira A, Mackinnon A, Meyer B, Botella C, Littlewood E, Andersson G. Efficacy of self-guided Internet-based cognitive behavioral therapy in the treatment of depressive symptoms: a meta-analysis of individual participant data. JAMA Psychiat. 2017;74(4):351–9.
14. Mindspot. Online assessment and treatment for anxiety and depression. https://mindspot.org.au/. Accessed 2nd August 2017.
15. Titov N, Dear BF, Staples LG, Bennett-Levy J, Klein B, Rapee RM, Shann C, Richards D, Andersson G, Ritterband L, Purtell C. MindSpot clinic: an accessible, efficient, and effective online treatment service for anxiety and depression. Psychiatr Serv. 2015;66(10):1043–50.
16. Eriksson MC, Kivi M, Hange D, Petersson EL, Ariai N, Häggblad P, Ågren H, Spak F, Lindblad U, Johansson B, Björkelund C. Long-term effects of Internet-delivered cognitive behavioral therapy for depression in primary care—the PRIM-NET controlled trial. Scand J Prim Health Care. 2017:126–36.
17. Høifødt RS, Strøm C, Kolstrup N, Eisemann M, Waterloo K. Effectiveness of cognitive behavioural therapy in primary health care: a review. Fam Pract. 2011;28(5):489–504.

18. Proudfoot J, Ryden C, Everitt B, Shapiro DA, Goldberg D, Mann A, Tylee A, Marks I, Gray JA. Clinical efficacy of computerised cognitive–behavioural therapy for anxiety and depression in primary care: randomised controlled trial. Br J Psychiatry. 2004;185(1):46–54.
19. Ruwaard J, Lange A, Schrieken B, Dolan CV, Emmelkamp P. The effectiveness of online cognitive behavioral treatment in routine clinical practice. PLoS One. 2012;7(7):e40089.
20. Littlewood E, Duarte A, Hewitt C, Knowles S, Palmer S, Walker S, Andersen P, Araya R, Barkham M, Bower P, Brabyn SA. randomised controlled trial of computerised cognitive behaviour therapy for the treatment of depression in primary care: the Randomised Evaluation of the Effectiveness and Acceptability of Computerised Therapy (REEACT) trial. Health Technol Assess (Winch Eng). 2015;19(101):1.
21. Christensen H, Griffiths KM, Jorm AF. Delivering interventions for depression by using the Internet: randomised controlled trial. BMJ. 2004;328(7434):265.
22. Twomey C, O'Reilly G. Effectiveness of a freely available computerised cognitive behavioural therapy programme (MoodGYM) for depression: meta-analysis. Aust N Z J Psychiatry. 2017;51(3):260–9.
23. Gilbody S, Littlewood E, Hewitt C, Brierley G, Tharmanathan P, Araya R, Barkham M, Bower P, Cooper C, Gask L, Kessler D. Computerised cognitive behaviour therapy (cCBT) as treatment for depression in primary care (REEACT trial): large scale pragmatic randomised controlled trial. BMJ. 2015;351:h5627.
24. Hunkeler EM, Hargreaves WA, Fireman B, Terdiman J, Meresman JF, Porterfield Y, Lee J, Dea R, Simon GE, Bauer MS, Unützer J. A web-delivered care management and patient self-management program for recurrent depression: a randomized trial. Psychiatr Serv. 2012;63(11):1063–71.
25. de Graaf LE, Hollon SD, Huibers MJ. Predicting outcome in computerized cognitive behavioral therapy for depression in primary care: a randomized trial. J Consult Clin Psychol. 2010;78(2):184.
26. Christensen H, Griffiths KM, Farrer L. Adherence in Internet interventions for anxiety and depression: systematic review. J Med Internet Res. 2009;11(2):e13.
27. Rickwood D, Webb M, Kennedy V, Telford N. Who are the young people choosing web-based mental health support? Findings from the implementation of Australia's National Web-based Youth Mental Health Service, eheadspace. JMIR mental health. 2016;3(3).
28. Reyes-Portillo JA, Mufson L, Greenhill LL, Gould MS, Fisher PW, Tarlow N, Rynn MA. Web-based interventions for youth internalizing problems: a systematic review. Journal of the American Academy of Child & Adolescent Psychiatry. 2014;53(12):1254–70.
29. O'Dea B, Calear AL, Perry Y. Is e-health the answer to gaps in adolescent mental health service provision? Curr Opin Psychiatry. 2015;28(4):336–42.
30. Ebert DD, Zarski AC, Christensen H, Stikkelbroek Y, Cuijpers P, Berking M, Riper H. Internet and computer-based cognitive behavioral therapy for anxiety and depression in youth: a meta-analysis of randomized controlled outcome trials. PLoS One. 2015;10(3):e0119895.
31. Spence SH, Holmes JM, March S, Lipp OV. The feasibility and outcome of clinic plus Internet delivery of cognitive-behavior therapy for childhood anxiety. J Consult Clin Psychol. 2006;74(3):614.
32. Spence SH, Holmes J, Donovan CL, Kenardy J. BRAVE for Teenagers-ONLINE: an Internet based program for adolescents with anxiety. Brisbane: University of Queensland; 2006.
33. March S, Spence SH, Donovan CL. The efficacy of an Internet-based cognitive-behavioral therapy intervention for child anxiety disorders. J Pediatr Psychol. 2008;34(5):474–87.
34. Stasiak K, Merry SN, Frampton C, Moor S. Delivering solid treatments on shaky ground: feasibility study of an online therapy for child anxiety in the aftermath of a natural disaster. Psychother Res. 2016:1–11.
35. Spence SH, Donovan CL, March S, Gamble A, Anderson RE, Prosser S, Kenardy J. A randomized controlled trial of online versus clinic-based CBT for adolescent anxiety. J Consult Clin Psychol. 2011;79(5):629.
36. Khanna MS, Kendall PC. Computer-assisted cognitive behavioral therapy for child anxiety: results of a randomized clinical trial. J Consult Clin Psychol. 2010;78(5):737.
37. Wuthrich VM, Rapee RM, Cunningham MJ, Lyneham HJ, Hudson JL, Schniering CA. A randomized controlled trial of the Cool Teens CD-ROM computerized program for adolescent anxiety. J Am Acad Child Adolesc Psychiatry. 2012;51(3):261–70.
38. Tillfors M, Andersson G, Ekselius L, Furmark T, Lewenhaupt S, Karlsson A, Carlbring P. A randomized trial of Internet-delivered treatment for social anxiety disorder in high school students. Cogn Behav Ther. 2011;40(2):147–57.
39. Abeles P, Verduyn C, Robinson A, Smith P, Yule W, Proudfoot J. Computerized CBT for adolescent depression ("Stressbusters") and its initial evaluation through an extended case series. Behav Cogn Psychother. 2009;37(2):151–65.
40. Richardson T, Stallard P, Velleman S. Computerised cognitive behavioural therapy for the prevention and treatment of depression and anxiety in children and adolescents: a systematic review. Clin Child Fam Psychol Rev. 2010;13(3):275–90.
41. Smith P, Scott R, Eshkevari E, Jatta F, Leigh E, Harris V, Robinson A, Abeles P, Proudfoot J, Verduyn C, Yule W. Computerised CBT for depressed adolescents: randomised controlled trial. Behav Res Ther. 2015;73:104–10.
42. Gerrits RS, van der Zanden RA, Visscher RF, Conijn BP. Master your mood online: a preventive chat group intervention for adolescents. Aust E J Adv Mental Health. 2007;6(3):152–62.

43. van der Zanden R, Kramer J, Gerrits R, Cuijpers P. Effectiveness of an online group course for depression in adolescents and young adults: a randomized trial. J Med Internet Res. 2012;14(3):e86.
44. Gladstone T, Marko-Holguin M, Henry J, Fogel J, Diehl A, Van Voorhees BW. Understanding adolescent response to a technology-based depression prevention program. J Clin Child Adolesc Psychol. 2014;43(1):102–14.
45. Gladstone TG, Marko-Holguin M, Rothberg P, Nidetz J, Diehl A, DeFrino DT, Harris M, Ching E, Eder M, Canel J, Bell C. An Internet-based adolescent depression preventive intervention: study protocol for a randomized control trial. Trials. 2015;16(1):203.
46. Van Voorhees BW, Fogel J, Reinecke MA, Gladstone T, Stuart S, Gollan J, Bradford N, Domanico R, Fagan B, Ross R, Larson J. Randomized clinical trial of an Internet-based depression prevention program for adolescents (Project CATCH-IT) in primary care: 12-week outcomes. J Dev Behav Pediatr. 2009;30(1):23–37.
47. Ip P, Chim D, Chan KL, Li TM, Ho FK, Voorhees BW, Tiwari A, Tsang A, Chan CW, Ho M, Tso W. Effectiveness of a culturally attuned Internet-based depression prevention program for Chinese adolescents: a randomized controlled trial. Depress Anxiety. 2016;33(12):1123–31.
48. Robinson J, Hetrick S, Cox G, Bendall S, Yuen HP, Yung A, Pirkis J. Can an Internet-based intervention reduce suicidal ideation, depression and hopelessness among secondary school students: results from a pilot study. Early Interv Psychiatry. 2016;10(1):28–35.
49. Robinson J, Hetrick S, Cox G, Bendall S, Yung A, Yuen HP, Templer K, Pirkis J. The development of a randomised controlled trial testing the effects of an online intervention among school students at risk of suicide. BMC Psychiatry. 2014;14(1):155.
50. Calear AL, Christensen H, Mackinnon A, Griffiths KM, O'Kearney R. The YouthMood Project: a cluster randomized controlled trial of an online cognitive behavioral program with adolescents. J Consult Clin Psychol. 2009;77(6):1021.
51. Neil AL, Batterham P, Christensen H, Bennett K, Griffiths KM. Predictors of adherence by adolescents to a cognitive behavior therapy website in school and community-based settings. J Med Internet Res. 2009;11(1):e6.
52. Calear AL, Christensen H, Mackinnon A, Griffiths KM. Adherence to the MoodGYM program: outcomes and predictors for an adolescent school-based population. J Affect Disord. 2013;147(1):338–44.
53. Sportel BE, de Hullu E, de Jong PJ, Nauta MH. Cognitive bias modification versus CBT in reducing adolescent social anxiety: a randomized controlled trial. PLoS One. 2013;8(5):e64355.
54. Staugaard SR. Threatening faces and social anxiety: a literature review. Clin Psychol Rev. 2010;30(6):669–90.
55. Salemink E, van den Hout M. Validation of the "recognition task" used in the training of interpretation biases. J Behav Ther Exp Psychiatry. 2010;41(2):140–4.
56. Santucci LC, McHugh RK, Elkins RM, Schechter B, Ross MS, Landa CE, Eisen S, Barlow DH. Pilot implementation of computerized cognitive behavioral therapy in a university health setting. Adm Policy Ment Health. 2014;41(4):514–21.
57. Knaevelsrud C, Brand J, Lange A, Ruwaard J, Wagner B. Web-based psychotherapy for posttraumatic stress disorder in war-traumatized Arab patients: randomized controlled trial. J Med Internet Res. 2015;17(3).
58. Spence J, Titov N, Dear BF, Johnston L, Solley K, Lorian C, Wootton B, Zou J, Schwenke G. Randomized controlled trial of Internet-delivered cognitive behavioral therapy for posttraumatic stress disorder. Depress Anxiety. 2011;28(7):541–50.
59. Lovell K, Bower P, Gellatly J, Byford S, Bee P, McMillan D, Arundel C, Gilbody S, Gega L, Hardy G, Reynolds S. Low-intensity cognitive-behaviour therapy interventions for obsessive-compulsive disorder compared to waiting list for therapist-led cognitive-behaviour therapy: 3-arm randomised controlled trial of clinical effectiveness. PLoS Med. 2017;14(6):e1002337.
60. Wantland DJ, Portillo CJ, Holzemer WL, Slaughter R, McGhee EM. The effectiveness of Web-based vs. non-Web-based interventions: a meta-analysis of behavioral change outcomes. J Med Internet Res. 2004;6(4):e40.
61. Rees CS, Anderson RA, Finlay-Jones A. OCD? Not Me! Protocol for the development and evaluation of a web-based self-guided treatment for youth with obsessive-compulsive disorder. BMJ Open. 2015;5(4):e007486.
62. Rees CS, Anderson RA, Kane RT, Finlay-Jones AL. Online obsessive-compulsive disorder treatment: preliminary results of the "OCD? Not Me!" Self-guided Internet-based cognitive behavioral therapy program for young people. JMIR Ment health. 2016;3(3):e29.
63. Enander J, Andersson E, Mataix-Cols D, Lichtenstein L, Alström K, Andersson G, Ljótsson B, Rück C. Therapist guided Internet based cognitive behavioural therapy for body dysmorphic disorder: single blind randomised controlled trial. BMJ. 2016;352:i241.
64. Taylor CB, Bryson S, Luce KH, Cunning D, Doyle AC, Abascal LB, Rockwell R, Dev P, Winzelberg AJ, Wilfley DE. Prevention of eating disorders in at-risk college-age women. Arch Gen Psychiatry. 2006;63(8):881–8.
65. Kass AE, Trockel M, Safer DL, Sinton MM, Cunning D, Rizk MT, Genkin BH, Weisman HL, Bailey JO, Jacobi C, Wilfley DE. Internet-based preventive intervention for reducing eating disorder risk: a randomized controlled trial comparing guided with unguided self-help. Behav Res Ther. 2014;63:90–8.
66. Gosling JA, Glozier N, Griffiths K, Ritterband L, Thorndike F, Mackinnon A, Hehir KK, Bennett A, Bennett K, Christensen H. The GoodNight study—online CBT for insomnia for the indicated prevention of depression: study protocol for a randomised controlled trial. Trials. 2014;15(1):56.

67. de Bruin EJ, Bögels SM, Oort FJ, Meijer AM. Efficacy of cognitive behavioral therapy for insomnia in adolescents: a randomized controlled trial with Internet therapy, group therapy and a waiting list condition. Sleep. 2015;38(12):1913–26.
68. Davidson TM, Yuen EK, Felton JW, McCauley J, Gros KS, Ruggiero KJ. Feasibility assessment of a brief, web-based behavioral activation intervention for adolescents with depressed mood. Int J Psychiatry Med. 2014;48(1):69–82.
69. Pinto MD, Hickman RL, Clochesy J, Buchner M. Avatar-based depression self-management technology: promising approach to improve depressive symptoms among young adults. Appl Nurs Res. 2013;26(1):45–8.
70. Manicavasagar V, Horswood D, Burckhardt R, Lum A, Hadzi-Pavlovic D, Parker G. Feasibility and effectiveness of a web-based positive psychology program for youth mental health: randomized controlled trial. J Med Internet Res. 2014;16(6):e140.
71. Burckhardt R, Manicavasagar V, Batterham PJ, Miller LM, Talbot E, Lum A. A web-based adolescent positive psychology program in schools: randomized controlled trial. J Med Internet Res. 2015;17(7).
72. Matthews A, Naran N, Kirkby KC. Symbolic online exposure for spider fear: habituation of fear, disgust and physiological arousal and predictors of symptom improvement. J Behav Ther Exp Psychiatry. 2015;47:129–37.
73. Carper MM, McHugh RK, Barlow DH. The dissemination of computer-based psychological treatment: a preliminary analysis of patient and clinician perceptions. Administration and Policy in Mental Health and Mental Health Services Research. 2013;40(2):87–95.
74. Crutzen R, De Nooijer J, Brouwer W, Oenema A, Brug J, De Vries NK. Internet-delivered interventions aimed at adolescents: a Delphi study on dissemination and exposure. Health Educ Res. 2008;23(3):427–39.
75. Van Voorhees BW, Fogel J, Pomper BE, Marko M, Reid N, Watson N, Larson J, Bradford N, Fagan B, Zuckerman S, Wiedmann P. Adolescent dose and ratings of an Internet-based depression prevention program: a randomized trial of primary care physician brief advice versus a motivational interview. Journal of cognitive and behavioral psychotherapies: the official journal of the International Institute for the Advanced Studies of Psychotherapy and Applied. Ment Health. 2009;9(1):1.
76. Eisen JC, Marko-Holguin M, Fogel J, Cardenas A, Bradford N, Fagan B, Wiedmann P, Van Voorhees BW. Pilot study of implementation of an Internet-based depression prevention intervention (CATCH-IT) for adolescents in 12 US primary care practices: clinical and management/organizational behavioral perspectives. Prim Care Companion CNS Disord. 2013;15(6).
77. DeFrino DT, Marko-Holguin M, Cordel S, Anker L, Bansa M, Van Voorhees B. "Why Should I Tell My Business?": an Emerging Theory of Coping and Disclosure in Teens. Res Theory Nurs Pract. 2016;30(2):124–42.
78. Bansa M, Brown D, DeFrino D, Mahoney N, Saulsberry A, Marko-Holguin M, Fogel J, Gladstone TR, Van Voorhees BW. A little effort can withstand the hardship: fielding an internet-based intervention to prevent depression among urban racial/ethnic minority adolescents in a primary care setting. J Natl Med Assoc. 2017.; https://doi.org/10.1016/j.jnma.2017.02.006.
79. Rochlen AB, Zack JS, Speyer C. Online therapy: review of relevant definitions, debates, and current empirical support. J Clin Psychol. 2004;60(3):269–83.
80. Goodwin BC, Ford DE, Hsiung RC, Houston TK, Fogel J, Van Voorhees BW. First, do no harm: referring primary care patients with depression to an Internet support group. Telemed J E Health. 2017. https://doi.org/10.1089/tmj.2017.0004.
81. Saulsberry A, Marko-Holguin M, Blomeke K, Hinkle C, Fogel J, Gladstone T, Bell C, Reinecke M, Corden M, Van Voorhees BW. Randomized clinical trial of a primary care Internet-based intervention to prevent adolescent depression: one-year outcomes. J Can Acad Child Adolesc Psychiatry. 2013;22(2):106.
82. Christensen H, Petrie K. State of the e-mental health field in Australia: where are we now? Aust N Z J Psychiatry. 2013;47(2):117–20.
83. Kanuri N, Newman MG, Ruzek JI, Kuhn E, Manjula M, Jones M, Thomas N, Abbott JA, Sharma S, Taylor CB. The feasibility, acceptability, and efficacy of delivering Internet-based self-help and guided self-help interventions for generalized anxiety disorder to indian university students: design of a randomized controlled trial. JMIR Res Protoc. 2015;4(4):e136.
84. Abuwalla Z, Kadhem Z, Gladstone T, Mikhael E, Bishay A, Van Voorhees BW. Proposed model for the cultural adaptation of an Internet-based depression prevention intervention (CATCH-IT) for Arab adolescents. Int J Adolesc Med Health. 2017. https://doi.org/10.1515/ijamh-2016-0147.
85. Sobowale K, Zhou AN, Van Voorhees BW, Stewart S, Tsang A, Ip P, Fabrizio C, Wong KL, Chim D. Adaptation of an Internet-based depression prevention intervention for Chinese adolescents: from "CATCH-IT" to "grasp the opportunity". Int J Adolesc Med Health. 2013;25(2):127–37.
86. Gerhards SA, De Graaf LE, Jacobs LE, Severens JL, Huibers MJ, Arntz A, Riper H, Widdershoven G, Metsemakers JF, Evers SM. Economic evaluation of online computerised cognitive–behavioural therapy without support for depression in primary care: randomised trial. Br J Psychiatry. 2010;196(4):310–8.
87. Gehring ND, McGrath P, Wozney L, Soleimani A, Bennett K, Hartling L, Huguet A, Dyson MP, Newton AS. Pediatric eMental healthcare technologies: a systematic review of implementation foci in research studies, and government and organizational documents. Implement Sci. 2017;12(1):76.
88. May J, Kazee N, Castillo S, Bahroos N, Kennedy S, Castillo A, Frese W, Marko-Holguin M, Crawford TJ, Van Voorhees BW. From silos to an innovative health care delivery and patient engagement model for

children in Medicaid. Healthc (Amst). 2017. https://doi.org/10.1016/j.hjdsi.2016.
89. Van Voorhees BW, Mahoney N, Mazo R, Barrera AZ, Siemer CP, Gladstone TR, Muñoz RF. Internet-based depression prevention over the life course: a call for behavioral vaccines. Psychiatr Clin North Am. 2011;34(1):167–83.
90. Van Voorhees BW, Hsiung RC, Marko-Holguin M, Houston TK, Fogel J, Lee R, Ford DE. Internal versus external motivation in referral of primary care patients with depression to an Internet support group: randomized controlled trial. J Med Internet Res. 2013;15(3):e42.
91. Van Voorhees BW, Watson N, Bridges JF, Fogel J, Galas J, Kramer C, Connery M, McGill A, Marko M, Cardenas A, Landsback J. Development and pilot study of a marketing strategy for primary care/Internet–based depression prevention intervention for adolescents (The CATCH-IT Intervention). Prim Care Companion J Clin Psychiatry. 2010;12(3). https://doi.org/10.4088/PCC.09m00791blu.
92. Van Voorhees BW. Pilot study of Internet-based early intervention for combat-related mental distress. J Rehabil Res Dev. 2012;49(8):1175.
93. Van Voorhees BW, Gladstone T, Cordel S, Marko-Holguin M, Beardslee W, Kuwabara S, Kaplan MA, Fogel J, Diehl A, Hansen C, Bell C. Development of a technology-based behavioral vaccine to prevent adolescent depression: a health system integration model. Internet Interventions. 2015;2(3):303–13.
94. Saulsberry A, Corden ME, Taylor-Crawford K, Crawford TJ, Johnson M, Froemel J, Walls A, Fogel J, Marko-Holguin M, Van Voorhees BW. Chicago Urban Resiliency Building (CURB): an Internet-based depression-prevention intervention for urban African-American and Latino adolescents. J Child Fam Stud. 2013;22(1):150–60.

17 Video Games and Their Impact on Teens' Mental Health

Melissa E. DeRosier and James M. Thomas

Current Trends in Video Gaming

Though it is hard to believe, video gaming is a relatively new phenomenon. While the first computerized games were introduced in the early 1970s, it has only been in the past two decades that video gaming has truly become embedded in American culture [1]. The advent of affordable computerized hardware, high-speed Internet connectivity, and an expanding array of efficient distribution models for games have revolutionized the way Americans spend their leisure time. As of today, practically every teenager uses video games for entertainment, estimated at 97% of all teens ages 13–17 years, and the gender gap among teen gamers continues to narrow with a reported 94% of females and 99% of males playing video games [2]. And, while disparities have existed in the past, rates of video game usage by teens are now much more universal, with high consistency in the numbers of video game players across racial and ethnic subgroups and across different income levels.

In the USA, about 60% of those teens who play video games do so regularly, meaning for 3 or more hours per week. On average, adolescents spend 6.5 hours per week playing video games, and this time is spent across a variety of different devices that support gaming. The particular platforms and devices used for gaming have evolved tremendously in recent years, and we should expect innovations in video gaming hardware and software to continue to evolve into the future. For example, advancements in mobile technologies have led to a drastic increase in the number of teens who engage with video games on mobile platforms (e.g., cell phones, tablets), increasing from just 8% in 2009 to more than 50% in 2016 [3, 4]. As shown in Fig. 17.1, of the many different options for playing video games, the top most frequently used devices are computers (desktop or laptop), dedicated game consoles (e.g., Wii, PlayStation, Xbox), smart phones, wireless

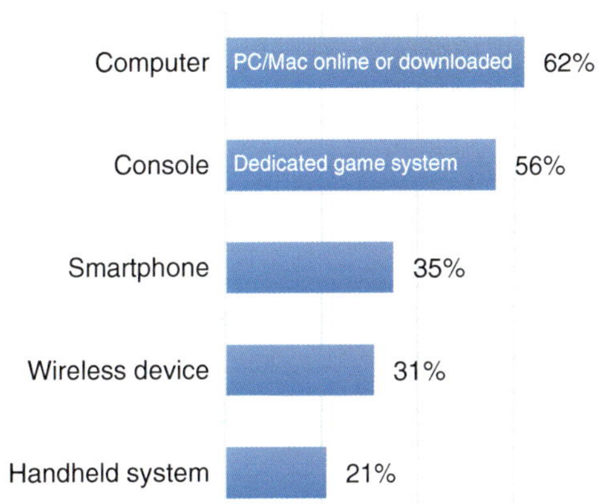

Fig. 17.1 Top five device gamers use to play video games

M.E. DeRosier, Ph.D. (✉) • J.M. Thomas, Ph.D.
3C Institute, Durham, NC, USA
e-mail: derosier@3cisd.com

M.A. Moreno, A. Radovic (eds.), *Technology and Adolescent Mental Health*,
https://doi.org/10.1007/978-3-319-69638-6_17

devices (e.g., iPad, Kindle Fire), and dedicated handheld systems (e.g., Nintendo DS, PlayStation Portable) [5].

Types of Video Games

With the ever-increasing number of game titles and the constantly evolving nature of technology, it is impossible to construct a definitive and unchanging list of the most popular video games among adolescents. However, any given game is likely to represent one or more **genres**, and having a basic understanding of these genres, including the game experience and what it takes to be successful as a player, can be very useful to the practitioner when talking with teens about their video gaming behavior. To this end, Fig. 17.2 graphically illustrates several common video game genres—and combinations of genres—along with examples of popular game titles within each, and Table 17.1 summarizes the type of gameplay involved for each genre and some of the skills required to successfully play a game within that genre. While a discussion of technical specifications is beyond the scope of this chapter, it is important to note that, irrespective of genre type, any given game title can be presented via 2D or 3D graphics and from first-person (i.e., virtual world is seen through the eyes of the player's character) or third-person (i.e., player's character is visible on the screen, and camera angle is from behind and slightly above the character) perspective. Some subgenres, such as shooter games, tend to be first person, but this tendency is not universal, and games often include the ability for the player to switch perspectives between first and third during the course of gameplay.

Practitioner Tip
There is no definitive taxonomy of video game genres, and people may hold very different views of what genres exist and what genre(s) a given game title falls within. When talking with a teen patient about their video gaming behavior, it might be useful to show him/her Fig. 17.2 as a springboard for discussion. If, for example, a teen tends to play open world games, perhaps she could share how Fig. 17.2's representation is correct or incorrect in her opinion. This discussion would likely open up lines of communication with the teen, demonstrate the practitioner's interest in the teen's interests, and give the teen an opportunity to be the expert in a discussion.

Action is by far the most popular video game genre (see Fig. 17.2). The primary focus of action games is on accomplishing physical feats within a virtual world. To be successful, players must make selections (e.g., what tool or special ability to use) and purposefully act on the virtual environment (e.g., objects and characters). The gameplay is fast-paced with the player being required to make and enact decisions quickly or risk defeat in the game world. Action genre games can involve a variety of different types of action. For example, Platform games, such as the popular *Super Mario Bros* series, require the player to navigate increasingly complex landscapes with obstacles by using special tools and abilities and avoiding dangerous objects and characters. In combat-oriented games, players may participate in the action using a variety of weapons (shooter games) or physical combat techniques, such as martial arts (fighting games). In challenge-oriented games, players may use vehicles (racing games) or virtual sports equipment (sports) to compete against other characters.

Games within the **adventure** genre require players to solve a series of puzzles by interacting with other characters and the environment, often in a nonconfrontational manner. Adventure games provide a rich story world where the narrative and interactive story elements drive gameplay and the player enacts a role (often as the hero) to achieve long-term objectives (often with

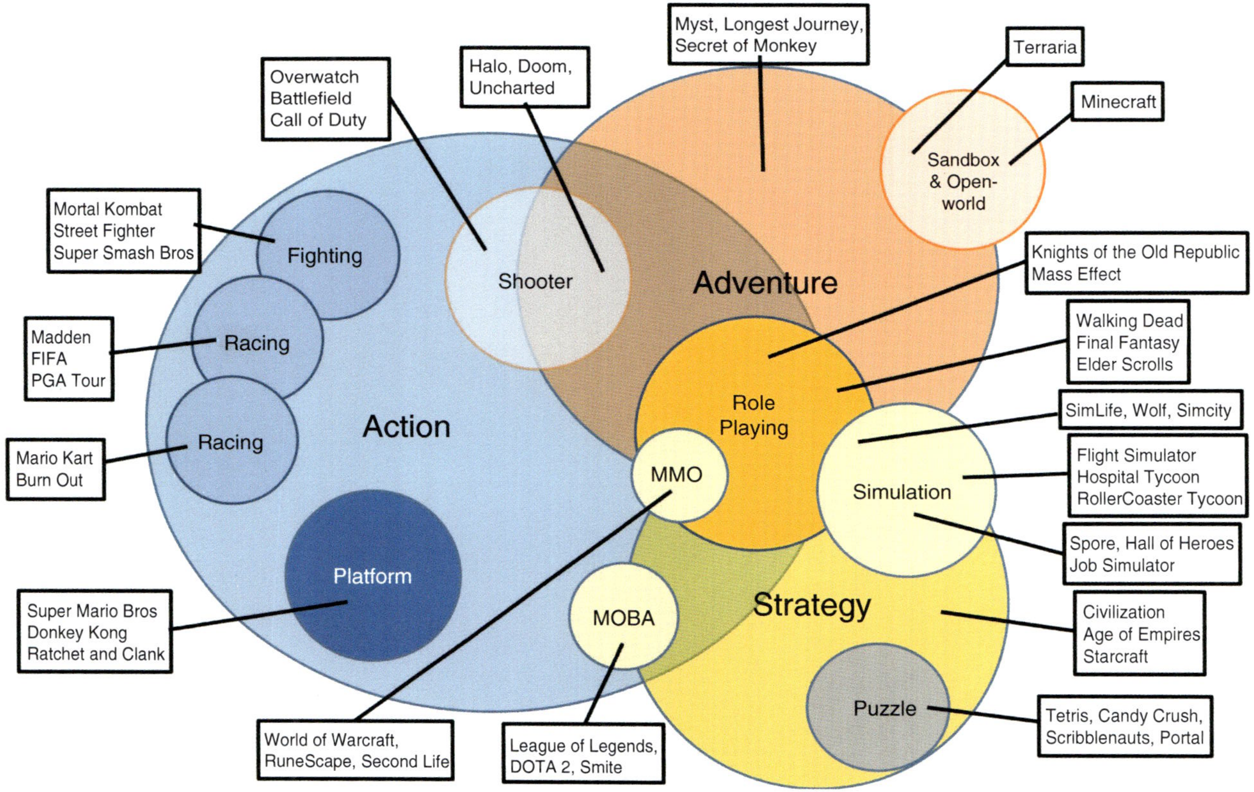

Fig. 17.2 Graphic illustration of video game genres and sub-genres with exemplar video game titles. *Note*. MMO = Massive Multi-player Online; MOBA = Multi-player Online Battle Arena

Table 17.1 Gameplay and skills involved in different types of video game genres

Genre	Focus of gameplay	Skills required
Action	Physical challenges where the player guides a character through a series of obstacles	• Eye-hand coordination • Motor skills • Concentration
Adventure	Puzzle solving where the player navigates a virtual world and solves story-based puzzles by interacting with other characters and the environment	• Deductive reasoning • Problem solving • Creativity • Spatial reasoning
Open-world and Sandbox	Free-roaming exploration and influence in an open virtual world where players can build, create, interact, and otherwise progress through the game as they choose	• Curiosity • Critical thinking • Planning • Self-awareness
Strategy	Planning and applying specific strategies and tactical problem solving, alone or in coordination with other human players, in order to progress through challenges and achieve victory	• Strategic thinking • Tactical reasoning • Cognitive flexibility • Decision-making • Communication • Collaboration
Role playing	Assuming the role of a specified character (or character class) and engaging with other virtual or human players to complete story-based quests or missions and strengthen one's character	• Cooperation • Negotiation • Conflict management • Planning • Imagination
Simulation	Experiencing virtual situations that simulate real-life, often in order to build the player's skills for enacting those activities in parallel real-world situations	• Problem solving • Self-awareness • Perspective taking • Perseverance

smaller objectives along the way). The focus of gameplay is on exploration, item gathering (e.g., tools, weapons, treasure), puzzle solving, and, in the case of action-adventure games, combat.

A newer, and growing, genre is **open-world** games which provide a large and rich virtual world where players have considerable freedom in what they do and where they go within that world. Gameplay is largely exploratory where the player generates their own objectives and determines their own course. **Sandbox** games are a subgenre of open-world games that allow the player full autonomy to develop their character and change the game world as they choose, often with no concrete goal or end to the game. The quintessential example of a pure Sandbox game is the wildly popular *Minecraft*, where players have the power to change every cubic foot of the game landscape into whatever architectural, artistic, or functional forms they can imagine. Increasingly, new releases of popular adventure games (such as *Grand Theft Auto V*) are offering more open and less linear game experiences, allowing players to more freely explore the story world.

Strategy games focus on thinking and strategic planning in order to achieve missions, solve problems, and/or defeat opponents, similar in many ways to board games. On the purely strategic end of this genre are puzzle games, including the highly popular "casual games" of *Candy Crush* and *Tetris*, which involve applying a set of strategies to solve game-based puzzle boards. However, many games within this genre are militaristic, involving a high level of both strategic and tactical decision-making to defeat opponents and achieve victory. Militaristic strategy games may be turn-based (such as *Chess*) where each player has a period of time by which to make a choice or progress in real time with play advancing in a continuous manner (such as *Starcraft*). The most complex and fast-paced militaristic strategy games are **Multiplayer online battle arenas** (MOBAs) where players interact online in real time with other human players, coordinating their actions as a team in direct competition with other teams of human players.

Role-playing games (RPGs) typically combine action, adventure, and/or strategy elements into gameplay, but what differentiates RPGs is that the player assumes a particular role and acts out that role within the story world's narrative. Each role (or class) has a defined set of abilities, skills, and characteristics, and a primary focus of gameplay is on character development, including the collection of objects and experience points that will strengthen and advance one's character. For example, in *Dungeons and Dragons*, a player within the rogue class will be particularly good at sneaky combat, finding traps, and stealthy tricks, such as lock picking, whereas a player within the bard class will be capable of magic and particularly good at intuition and healing. RPGs are typically multiplayer where players, each in their own role, engage with one another to progress through a storyline, working together to solve mysteries, achieve quests, and defeat enemies.

RPGs which involve a very large world with a very large number of players participating simultaneously are called **massively multiplayer online role-playing games** (MMORPGs). The classic example of an MMORPG is *World of Warcraft* (WoW), a multifaceted fantasy world with numerous quests, challenges, and character types which currently is played by more than 5.6 million people across the world. As Internet speed and accessibility increase, game titles within this genre are likely to continue to increase as well.

Simulations commonly intermix adventure and strategy gameplay elements and may also include a role-playing component. Simulations are designed to closely emulate real-life activities so that players may experience what it would be like to engage in that activity in real-life. Simulations can be purely experiential, such as *RollerCoaster Tycoon* which is a construction and management simulation game where players custom build amusement parks and rides or the *SimCity* series where players use a given budget to expand and build their own custom city. But most simulations include educational or training objectives, and the majority of learning games are simulations where the intent is for players to learn and practice specific skills so they will be better prepared and able to enact those skills within parallel real-life situations. While most simulation games continue to be 2D, advancements in 3D technology, including more affordable hardware, mean that this genre is likely to see an increasing number of immersive 3D virtual environments into the future.

Motivations to Play Video Games

In addition to understanding the types of video games that teens play, it is also helpful to clarify the underlying motivation(s) that may drive a teen's video gaming behavior. Most game titles include an array of gameplay elements that could satisfy a variety of different motivations. In working with teen patients, and trying to determine the impact of their video gaming behavior on mental health functioning, practitioners would benefit from exploring **why** a teen selects to play a given video game title or games within a given genre. While the theoretical and empirical work in this area is still in its infancy, some research-based models of video gaming motivation do exist and may help guide practitioners in discussing the motivational pull(s) of video gaming with their teen patients. The following briefly summarizes this work with the goal of providing practitioners with possible talking points for discussing video gaming behavior with their teen patients.

A portion of the research into video gaming motivation has focused on formulating classification systems. As early as 1996, Bartle presented his *taxonomy of player types* [6] which classifies players as **killers**, **achievers**, **socializers**, or **explorers** (see Fig. 17.3) based on video gaming preferences (Bartle's original work focused on multiplayer online games, though his system has since been applied more broadly) [7]. Conceptually, Bartle defines a given player type across two dimensions of in-game behavior: (1) the degree to which the player prefers to act on versus interact with game elements, including objects and other characters, and (2) the degree to which the player focuses his/her actions on peo-

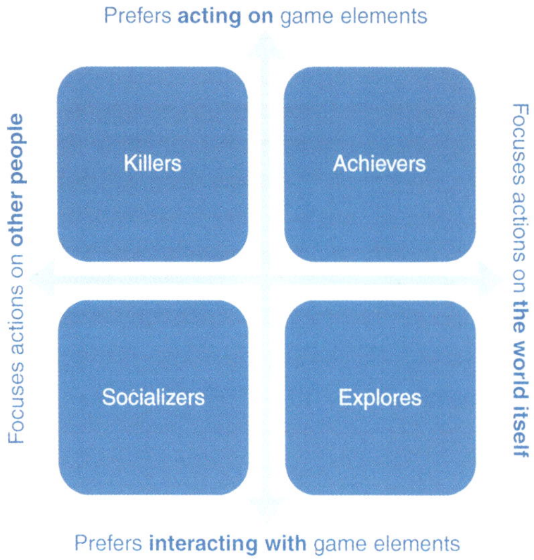

Fig. 17.3 Bartle's *Taxonomy of Game Players*

ple in the game world versus on the world itself. For example, both killers and socializers prefer gameplay that engages other people (virtual characters or other human players) in the game world, but killers prefer to act on (e.g., kill) those people, whereas socializers prefer to talk, work with, or otherwise develop in-game relationships with them. Both achievers and explorers prefer gameplay that involves the virtual world itself, but actions by achievers focus on overcoming obstacles, collecting objects, completing quests, and otherwise acting on the virtual world, whereas explorers prefer to explore, manipulate, discover, and otherwise learn about the virtual world. While Bartle's work provides an interesting framework and has informed subsequent research and theory into video game motivation, [8] there is **no** research to indicate differences in psychological or behavioral adjustment as a function of such classification systems. Further, it's important to keep in mind that most video game players will not fall cleanly into only one particular category. While there may be general tendencies to prefer one genre over another, video game players will often rotate their play among various different game titles, and game genres, as their interests shift during the course of a given day or week. Thus, trying to categorize teens into different types of players is likely of **limited utility**.

Rather than trying to derive psychological states from video gaming preferences, more recent work has taken the alternative approach to directly examine the psychological states and needs that drive players to engage in video games. In other words, for whichever video game(s) a teen plays, this research explores questions like "What motivates you to want to play that game?", "What do you get out of playing that game?", and "What need does playing that game satisfy?". While these theoretical models of video gaming motivation are still evolving, two examples may be useful for practitioners to help frame discussions with their teen patients.

First, Sherry and colleagues [9] found that players are motivated to play video games in order to attain one or more of the following psychological states: (1) **competition**, the experience of defeating others; (2) **challenge**, the experience of success following effort; (3) **diversion**, the ability to escape and distract oneself from stressful real-life events; (4) **fantasy**, the experience of novel or unrealistic stimuli; (5) **social interaction**, the ability to interact socially with others; and (6) **arousal**, the experience of activated positive emotions, such as joy, interest, and excitement. Of these six, Sherry et al. found that challenge is the top motivation for playing video games. Across age groups and genders, video games that enable players to experience mastery through cognitive effort (e.g., solving cognitive puzzles) were the most motivating [10], and the researchers hypothesized that this may be because game-based challenges can result in the highly pleasurable altered state called "flow." In 1990, Csikszentmihalyi [11] labeled "flow" as an intrinsically rewarding state of highly focused concentration leading to a decreased sense of time and self-awareness and a perception of seamless control between thought and action.

A second example of recent work on video gaming motivation is that of Ryan and colleagues [12, 13] who found that, regardless of video game title or genre, motivation to play a video game was predicted by the degree to which that video game satisfied three basic psychological needs: (1) **autonomy**, game provides flexibility over

Table 17.2 Examples of game-based features that satisfy basic psychological needs

Autonomy
• Able to customize their game world, such as creating their own character
• Able to make meaningful choices and there are consequences to those choices
• Multiple ways for players to reach a goal
Competence
• Decisions need to be made frequently to move the game forward
• Performance measured in multiple ways
• Progression in the game linked to player performance
• Feedback on performance given frequently with the ability to replay or redo
Relatedness
• Mechanisms for players to talk with one another
• Opportunities for collaboration among players (e.g., to complete quests)
• Opportunities for competitive group play (e.g., competing guilds or clans)

movement and strategies, choice over tasks and goals, and rewards that give feedback without being controlling; (2) **competence**, game provides ongoing challenges and tasks with opportunities for achievement and feedback; and (3) **relatedness**, game provides interactions among players. Table 17.2 provides a sampling of features that games can offer to help satisfy these three basic psychological needs. Research by Ryan et al. [12] demonstrated that when video game play was psychologically satisfying—particularly when the game satisfied the needs of autonomy and competence—a player's post-game sense of well-being was significantly higher, and this finding held across gender and age groups and across different game genres.

Currently, the research literature does not provide sufficient evidence to link video game player types nor video gaming motivational theories to mental health symptoms or behavioral adjustment in teens. However, these taxonomies and motivational theories can provide useful frameworks for engaging in discussions with teen patients. For any given teen, video gaming is likely to consume some, if not a considerable, portion of their leisure time, and for many, playing video games will be a significant component of their social experiences. Practitioners who have a greater understanding of what the various video game genres entail, and why teens may be motivated to play them, will be in a better position to engage with their teen patients to explore and understand this influential aspect of their lives.

Practitioner Tip

In addition to talking with teens about the specific video game titles, and genres, they play, engaging teens in a discussion about what motivates them to play those games will help build rapport as well as a greater understanding of the psychological needs that the teen's gaming behavior may be satisfying. It may be that these psychological needs may also be driving real-world behaviors by the teen.

Commercial Video Games and Mental and Behavioral Health

The research literature connecting exposure to video games (or video game genres) and the mental and behavioral health of teens is continually evolving. The early research on video gaming largely focused on identifying its negative impacts. Studies investigated the potentially addictive nature of video games, and the concomitant negative outcomes of excessive video gaming, such as social isolation (see Chap. 10). Efforts were made to identify healthy versus unhealthy levels of "**screen time**," similar to the earlier generation of research investigating excessive television watching. Findings from such studies were used to inform healthcare guidelines, such as the American Academy of Pediatrics' *Recommendations for Children's Media Use* [14]. These guidelines have changed over time, and will likely continue to change, as the research on exposure time to video games also continues.

As it became increasingly evident that **solely** considering time spent video gaming was insufficient for predicting negative outcomes, concern-based research studies began to shift to also investigate the type of video game being played, with particular focus on **violent video games** (i.e., shooter and fighting subgenres). Considerable research was undertaken in the examination of violent video gaming and its impact on health and well-being. A recent meta-analysis by the American Psychological Association (APA) *Task Force on Media Violence* concluded that exposure to violent video games is a significant risk factor in the prediction of negative outcomes among children, teens, and young adults [15]. These negative outcomes included increased antisocial behavior, thoughts, and emotions, decreased prosocial behavior, lower empathy for others, and desensitization to aggression. However, as noted in the APA report, no single risk factor can determine whether a given person will engage in criminal violence or develop a mental health disorder. A myriad of other factors, such as socioeconomic status, ethnicity, and social supports, may also contribute, and it is the cumulative risk across factors that tends to result in violent incidents toward self or others. Therefore, violent video gaming should be considered one of many possible contributing factors in a teen's life.

Over the past decade, there has been a shift in the research literature on video gaming. While research continues on the potentially negative impacts of commercial video games, a new scientific field has emerged which focuses on understanding how **video games can be used for good**. Increasingly, researchers have begun to recognize that video gaming can have significant and lasting positive benefits for health and well-being and that video games offer a potentially powerful tool for mental and behavioral health intervention. Part of this power comes from the inherently engaging nature of video games, and the strong preference for technologies in society at large, but particularly among youth and young adults [16]. As the research regarding the positive impacts of video gaming continues to mature, parents and mental health practitioners will be progressively better able to leverage video games to help foster mental and behavioral health outcomes for children and adolescents.

Practitioner Tip
While much has been said about the particularly harmful nature of first-person shooter games, it is important to note that the APA report did not cite a significant difference in the impact of violent video gaming based on the perspective of the player. Thus, one's viewpoint during the violence of a video game may be less important than participation in the virtual violence itself.

Positive Impacts of Commercial Video Games

Mounting evidence supports that playing commercial video games **can** result in significant social, emotional, and cognitive benefits. In the following discussion, we provide a sample of studies showing such positive impacts. However, debate continues in the research literature regarding whether and how commercial video games can have a positive influence on teen mental and behavioral health. In particular, while not the sole predictive factor, the dosage of, or time spent, video gaming should be considered a **mediating** factor where, as in many things, moderation is key. For example, occasionally engaging with others within a multiplayer online virtual world may yield meaningful friendships and decrease feelings of loneliness, but when most of your social interactions take place online, real-world friendships suffer, and feelings of loneliness and isolation can actually increase [17]. Therefore, it is important to keep in mind that the potential for positive impact on teens' health and well-being will likely be undermined if video gaming is excessive or restricted to violent or antisocial video games.

With regard to **social impacts**, commercial video games that provide opportunities for teens to work cooperatively and communicate with one another online (such as multiplayer Sandbox games, MOBAs, and MMORPGs) have been found to build social connections and decrease social isolation [18–22]. For example, in a study of over 30,000 MMORPG players, Yee [20] found that interacting with others in the virtual world resulted in meaningful, socially supportive relationships in which there was real emotional investment. Players reported that the relationships they formed in the online virtual world, and the interactions within that world, were equivalent to real-life friendships and that these interactions helped them practice prosocial skills for the real-world, such as leadership skills.

For teens who suffer from social anxiety, and therefore may avoid social interactions or withdrawal from others in the real-world, a multiplayer video game can provide a less anxiety-provoking place to engage with others. Virtual social interactions are at a distance, which can effectively reduce social anxiety and increase social risk-taking. For example, in a study of MMORPG players across 45 different countries, Cole and Griffith [23] reported that the game world was attractive to many players because they were able to express themselves in the virtual world in ways that they would not feel comfortable doing in real-life (e.g., due to their appearance, gender, sexuality, or age).

Practitioner Tip

The sociology of gaming has shifted tremendously over the past few decades with the **remote** multiplayer aspect becoming the dominant mode of gaming. Whereas the majority of games in the 1980s and 1990s featured a single player, in a room alone, going into a private world, the majority of gaming now involves people using games to connect and interact with other people in a semipublic world. Thus, gaming has evolved from a technology that fosters social isolation to one that can actually **promote** social integration. It is important to consider how empowering video gaming can be for teens with barriers to socialization, such as appearance, age, geographic isolation, and physical mobility issues. Games can serve as a common socialization space for teens who would otherwise be unable or unlikely to interact.

In effect, the safer, freer online social environment facilitates social connections and social interactions, which in turn, provide meaningful opportunities for teens to practice social skills with others. Multiplayer online games frequently involve collaboration, communication, and social problem solving among players, and these social learning opportunities can translate into social skills gains for improved real-world relationships. For example, in a study of adolescents with autism spectrum disorder (ASD)—a disorder marked by social challenges and often isolation—Gallup and colleagues [18] found that playing MMORPGs decreased social barriers and assisted in building social relationships and social interactions, both within the virtual world and in real-life (e.g., interacting with other MMORPG players outside of the game).

There is also some evidence that playing prosocial commercial video games can increase real-world prosocial behavior. For example, a study by Gentile and colleagues [22] found that undergraduate students who played prosocial games (i.e., *Super Mario Sunshine* and *Chibi-Robo*) were more likely to engage in cooperative and helpful behavior with others in real-life. The authors also found, in a longitudinal study with adolescents in Japan, that playing these prosocial video games significantly predicted prosocial behavior 3–4 months later [22]. Importantly, this work also provided evidence of bidirectionality in these effects whereby not only did playing prosocial video games tend to increase prosocial behavior, but also those with higher prosocial tendencies tended to select to play prosocial video games.

With regard to possible **emotional benefits** of playing commercial video games, there is evidence that increased social connectedness from involvement in multiplayer online games (when used in moderation) can reduce feelings of loneliness, anxiety, and depression [24–27]. In addition, there is a growing literature demonstrating the positive emotional benefits of what are called "**casual video games**" (CVGs). CVGs are very simple games with clear, straightforward rules and gameplay, do not require special or advanced gaming skills, and can be played in short spurts with no lengthy time commitment. While CVGs can be from any video game genre, they tend to be puzzle-strategy games. Highly popular examples include *Candy Crush*, *Bejeweled*, *Peggle*, *Angry Birds*, and *Tetris*.

Several studies have demonstrated significant mood elevation as a result of playing CVGs. For example, in the study of clinical **depression**, Russoniello and colleagues [28] conducted a randomized clinical trial to investigate the impact of playing popular smartphone CVGs, such as *Bejeweled* or *Bookworm*. They found that 30 min of CVG gameplay three times per week over a 1-month period resulted in significant declines in depressive symptoms, above and beyond any positive impact of anti-depressant medication. In a separate clinical trial, Russoniello and colleagues [29] found evidence that playing CVGs resulted in mood-lifting brain wave activity patterns (e.g., decreased left and increased right alpha brain waves) and heart rate variability changes consistent with a relaxed state. Participants in this research also reported significant declines in feelings of tension, anxiety, anger, and depression following just 20 min of CVG gameplay. In both trials, the control group (which did not play CVGs) did not exhibit these physiological and emotional changes.

Along with mood elevation, CVGs may hold particular potential for alleviating **anxiety and stress**. For example, in a follow-up study by Russoniello and colleagues, [30] CVG exposure over a 1-month period resulted in significantly greater declines in both state and trait anxiety symptom severity compared to the control group. And, in a study of preoperative anxiety in pediatric patients about to undergo outpatient surgery, Patel [31] found that playing CVGs significantly lowered youth's level of anxiety to an extent comparable with medication (i.e., oral midazolam). It may be that CVGs are particularly effective for satisfying the psychological need of diversion or the ability to escape and distract oneself from stressful real-life events (see Sherry et al. discussion above). Engaging in simple, straightforward gameplay may facilitate entering an "absorption-dissociation" state whereby CVG players are able to focus their attention on a small set of easily manageable, low frustration cognitive tasks and block out extraneous stress-inducing thoughts [32, 33]. An experimental study by Holmes and colleagues using a Trauma Film Paradigm seems to provide some support for this hypothesis. Following viewing a traumatic film, subsequent incidents of flashbacks (sensory perceptive, visuospatial memories of disturbing scenes presented in the film) were compared for participants who did and did not engage with *Tetris* for 10 min following the film [34, 35]. Those who played *Tetris* experienced significantly fewer flashbacks than those who did not play this CVG. In this research, playing *Tetris* seems to have distracted participants from the traumatic visual imagery of the film and interfered with the typical consolidation of traumatic memories which fuel experiences of subsequent flashbacks (a core symptom of post-traumatic stress disorder or **PTSD**).

In addition to potential benefits for teens' social and emotional well-being, evidence suggests that commercial video games may also enhance **cognitive functioning** in the areas of **attention and memory**. For example, in a study of adolescents and young adults, Moisala and colleagues [36] investigated behavioral performance and brain activity during working memory tasks and found a significant association between time spent gaming (in participants' daily lives) and better performance, accuracy, and speed, particularly as the task became more demanding. fMRI (functional magnetic resonance imaging) findings provided further support for this association, showing that the link between gaming experience and brain activity in areas associated with attention and memory (i.e., frontoparietal network) was particularly strong during more challenging working memory tasks. These patterns of results held regardless of the genre of video game played by participants. Moisala hypothesized that video gaming may enhance a player's ability to attend to relevant items, efficiently remove irrelevant items, and recover more quickly from attentional shifts during working memory tasks.

However, it is important to note that the research literature is inconsistent regarding whether video gaming increases or decreases attentional skills. Chan and Rabinowitz, [37] for example, found that playing video games was associated with symptoms of attention-deficit/ hyperactivity disorder (ADHD) in high school students. This discrepancy in findings may reflect the specific type of attention being studied [38]. Specifically, studies showing a negative association for gaming tend to assess attention in terms of focusing on a single object/task and controlling behavioral impulses, whereas studies showing a positive association tend to assess attention in terms of being able to filter audiovisual stimuli, rapidly shift attention, and ignore distractions. While no causal research has linked video gaming with the former type of attention, there does appear to be causal evidence that video gaming can improve the visual spatial attention and reasoning. For example, Subrahmanyam and Greenfield [39] found that fifth graders showed significant improvement in their dynamic spatial skills (ability to perceive, track, and process objects in movement) after playing the action video game *Marble Madness*, whereas the control group which played a word game (*Conjecture*) did not. In related research, there is also evidence that video gaming can enhance eye-hand coordination, motor planning, and rapid mental processing. For example, Middleton and colleagues [40] randomly assigned young adults to play *Wii Play* minigames (*Shooting Range*, *Pose Mii*, and *Table Tennis*) for 2–4 hours or play no video games over several days. Participants' performance before and after a 2-week period was measured using a virtual reality surgical simulator (*Simbionix LapMentor*). Those who played the Wii games consistently performed better than the control group, including significantly greater improvement in hand-eye coordination and speed of completion.

Impactful Video Games for Mental and Behavioral Health

The previous sections of this chapter underscore how video games and video gaming experiences cannot be considered homogenous. Commercial video games cover a broad array of genres, and different video gaming experiences offer different affordances for different mental and behavioral health issues. And, in a positive trend, studies are beginning to reveal the ways in which commercial video games—which were built primarily just to entertain—can actually produce a variety of health benefits. Now, we turn our attention from the accidental behavioral health benefits of commercial video games to discussion of "impactful video games" which are **intentionally** developed to foster positive mental and behavioral health.

In recent years, innovators have leveraged the prodigious technical advances commercial games have produced in realistic graphics, gameplay mechanics, and personalization to create video games that offer the potential to effectively alleviate targeted mental health problems and/or improve psychosocial functioning. In this section, we provide a brief review of a sampling of these impactful video games along with evidence, where available, that supports their use for therapeutic purposes. In the coming years, we should expect the number and range of offerings of impactful video games to grow substantially, in conjunction with a growing research literature demonstrating the ways by which these games can augment, accelerate, and amplify mental and behavioral health treatments. As a result, knowledgeable practitioners will be increasingly able to incorporate these innovative technologies into their treatment planning with teen patients. In the following paragraphs, we highlight examples of games that specifically target depression, anxiety disorders, attention disorders, and social-emotional skills.

A number of impactful games have been developed for the treatment of **depression**. A recent meta-analysis examined the relative impact of four different types of video games for alleviating depressive symptoms—psychoeducation/training, exercising, virtual reality exposure therapy, and entertainment—in studies that included randomized control groups [41]. With the caveats that only eight studies were included in the meta-analysis, and that these studies involved both adults and teens, findings indicated that exposure games resulted in the greatest decline in depressive symptoms (Cohen's *d* effect size of −.67), with psychoeducation/training and entertainment games being next most impactful (Cohen's *d* = −.41 and −.41, respectively) and exercising games being least impactful (Cohen's *d* = −.24).

Exposure games for depression focus on providing an immersive simulation of the experience of being depressed in an effort to increase empathy, understanding, and normalization of these experiences. For example, *Depression Quest* is an adventure-simulation game which allows the player to experience the life of a depressed person (www.depressionquest.com). A second example is *Elude* which is an adventure game that allows the player to move through a series of landscapes to metaphorically experience emotional states, including depression (http://gambit.mit.edu/loadgame/elude.php). While these specific exposure games were not included in the above meta-analysis, their value as psychoeducational tools has been noted, particularly for fostering greater understanding of depression for significant others who support those who are depressed.

Research-based **psychoeducation and training video games for depression** include *SPARX* (*Smart, Positive, Active, Realistic, X-factor thoughts*), an adventure game that delivers cognitive-behavioral therapy techniques as the teen navigates challenges within a fantasy world [42]. For example, in the first realm of the story world, players encounter GNATS (Gloomy Negative Automatic Thoughts) and must use cognitive restructuring to combat their negative messages (e.g., "you're a loser") and proceed to the next realm. A randomized clinical trial with 187 adolescents seeking treatment for depression in New Zealand found that *SPARX* was as effective as treatment-as-usual (i.e., in-person psychotherapy) for alleviating depressive symptoms, both immediately and at 3-month follow-up. In addition, teen patients reported enjoying *SPARX*, and adherence to the video game treatment was high.

Another example of an adventure video game for combating depression is *Maya* which emulates a hero's quest akin to some commercial video games, while integrating cognitive-behavioral and interpersonal therapy strategies into the problem-solving aspects of gameplay [43]. The player engages in the game as *Maya*, a depressed teen who must overcome her depressive affect, cognitions, and behavior to enter into and achieve in-game objectives. An acceptability trial with adolescent girls diagnosed with depression found that teen patients reported *Maya* helped them learn useful social and mental health related behaviors.

In the treatment of **anxiety disorders** (e.g., phobias, PTSD, obsessive-compulsive disorder), impactful video games can thoughtfully use the virtual environment and gameplay mechanics to implement effective in-person treatment strategies for lowering anxiety and avoidant behaviors, specifically relaxation training and exposure-and-response-prevention training. An example of a pure **relaxation training** game is *Deep* which uses the virtual reality headset Oculus Rift to lead players through breathing exercises within an underwater world (www.exploredeep.com). As the player successfully engages in relaxed breathing, the virtual world responds by becoming more calm and peaceful. A second example is *Personal Zen* which is more akin to a casual game in functionality, is commercially available for free, and is based in research to reduce anxiety and stress (www.personalzen.com).

In vivo relaxation practice can also be combined with **biofeedback techniques** (e.g., real-time information about heart rate) as well as psychoeducation (e.g., identifying one's triggers or signs of anxiety) to further enhance the therapeutic benefits. For example, *Relax to Win* is a two-player competitive game where feedback from a galvanic skin response (GSR) sensor is used to control the speed of the player's dragon during a virtual race [44]. The better the player is able to relax, the faster his/her dragon flies. There is evidence that game-based virtual relaxation training combined with biofeedback can result in significant declines in anxiety symptoms. For example, in a randomized clinical trial with teens, researchers found that use of two relaxation video games—*Freeze-Framer* and *Journey to the Wild*

Devine—with biofeedback (i.e., skin electrodes for heartrate variability and skin conductance level) resulted in significant reductions in anxiety compared to wait-list control [45]. And recently, a randomized clinical trial with 138 adolescents which used an active control condition (i.e., played the commercial action-adventure game *Rayman 2: The Great Escape*) found that playing the biofeedback game *Dojo* resulted in a more rapid decline in personalized anxiety symptoms compared to control [46]. In the *Dojo* game, players learn to recognize changes in their physiology and emotional states in order to regulate their emotions within a variety of virtual scenarios (e.g., gather items while avoiding the Fear Monster in the catacombs).

Turning now to the **treatment of attention problems**, considerable research has investigated how video gaming experiences combined with biofeedback methods may be able to reduce symptoms of ADHD and improve attention. As early as 1996, Pope and Bogart [47] found that increasing the difficulty of a video game based on brainwave activity that indicated waning attention was effective for increasing the attention span of youth diagnosed with ADHD. A more recent review of the literature by Butnik [48] summarized evidence that providing biofeedback to the form of a video game (e.g., whereby performance in the game is determined by the player's ability to modulate target brainwave activity) has empirical support for reductions in core ADHD symptoms for adolescents and young adults diagnosed with ADHD. Examples of impactful video games with biofeedback for the treatment of attention problems include *Project Evo* (currently undergoing clinical trial) and *Captain's Log* [49–51].

A novel recent application of video gaming in the treatment of ADHD by Weerdmeester and colleagues [52] tested the full-body *Adventurous Dreaming Highflying Dragon* game with children and young adolescents with ADHD. In this study, youth in both conditions interacted with a full-body video game using the Xbox Kinect (i.e., player's body acts as the game controller), but those in the treatment condition completed *Adventurous* which specifically included tasks that require attention and self-control. Results showed that those who interacted with the ADHD-training-specific game realized greater improvements in teacher-rated ADHD symptoms compared to active control participants.

Beyond the treatment of mood disorders and ADHD, there are relatively fewer available options for impactful video games, and the evidence for efficacy is largely missing. For more **serious mental health disorders**, such as schizophrenia, the therapeutic focus of video gaming has primarily been on brain training to improve cognitive functioning, such as episodic memory deficits. For example, Bellack and colleagues [53] created a computer-assisted cognitive remediation program for patients with significant cognitive impairments, including those with schizophrenia and traumatic brain injury. Use of the game-like computerized exercises to engage patients in cognitive training, **combined** with training and support by an in-person therapist, was found to be a feasible treatment approach, but clinical trial results on its efficacy remain pending. Similarly, Shrimpton and Hurworth [54] created an adventure game entitled *Pogo's Pledge* to provide psychoeducational messages to youth who had experienced their first episode of psychosis. While initial review by an expert panel was largely positive, the complex, difficult to navigate game mechanics were found to significantly undermine usability of this game by patients.

Another category of impactful video games does not target specific mental health disorders per se but rather addresses specific **social-emotional and behavioral skills** which are concomitant with an array of mental health disorders as well as psychosocial adjustment more generally. These video games may be tested with specific patient populations, but their use is not intended to be restricted to those populations. For example, *Let's Face It* is an impactful video game designed to teach facial recognition skills (e.g., identifying the emotions of others from facial expressions) which has been shown to produce measurable improvements in facial recognition skills for preadolescents and adolescents with autism spectrum disorder (ASD) who played the

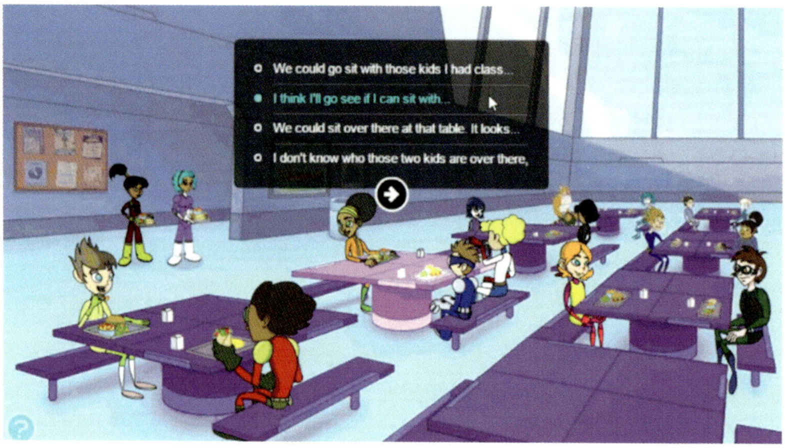

Fig. 17.4 Screenshot from *Hall of Heroes* SEL game. Developed by the authors of this chapter (and distributed separately by www.centervention.com)

game, whereas wait-list control youth did not [55]. While individuals with ASD have particular difficulty recognizing facial cues, facial recognition skills are a universal component in communication and empathy for all social relationship, making *Let's Face It* (and games like it) more broadly applicable.

A second example of a generally applicable impactful video game for social-emotional learning (SEL) is *Hall of Heroes* (see Fig. 17.4) [56]. *Hall of Heroes* is an immersive adventure game designed to enhance the social and emotional functioning of early adolescents across six core skill areas: communication, cooperation, emotion regulation, empathy, impulse control, and social initiation. *Hall of Heroes* engages teens in social problem solving as they navigate a virtual school for students with special powers and complete story-based social situations and challenges (e.g., responding to teasing, managing peer pressure). The in-game social challenges were built on social learning theory in late elementary and middle school years, as well as cognitive-behavioral social skills training methods for custom gameplay mechanics. The game world is intended to provide teens with safe and engaging virtual simulations through which they can learn and practice social emotional skills applicable to real-life social situations. A randomized clinical trial demonstrated that youth who completed *Hall of Heroes* showed significant improvements in their social, emotional, and behavioral health compared to the wait-list control condition.

Integrating Impactful Video Games into Treatment

Many impactful video games are designed to be used as **self-help tools**, and there is evidence that these games can result in positive benefits when used independently by teens. Given that negative mental health stereotypes and stigma associated with seeking mental health treatment still exist in our society, making impactful video games more broadly accessible could have significant positive public health benefits [57]. In particular, we know that many youth who experience significant mental health symptoms never seek or receive treatment. The safe and private virtual environment offered through a video game could lower fear and stigma barriers to teens' seeking help [58]. In addition, game-based therapeutic programs could lower cost, time, and other logistical barriers (e.g., travel, scheduling), compared to in-person treatment methods, so that more teens could more easily access treatment for mental and behavioral health issues. In effect, availability of impactful video games for self-help could result in more teens realizing the benefits of effective mental health treatment.

However, beyond their use for self-help, practitioners should consider how impactful video games could be used to augment in-person treatment with teens. As part of a larger treatment plan, impactful video games could be integrated in several manners. First, impactful video games could be used in a "preparation for learning" model whereby teens complete a portion of gameplay prior to an in-person session. If, for example, the game was psychoeducational, teens could be more ready to explore topics or practice techniques because they would come into the in-person session with foundational learning. Second, practitioners and teen patients could engage in an impactful video game together during the in-person session. Much as practitioners would use board or other games during sessions, observing as the teen interacts with the virtual game world would provide concrete opportunities to engage with the youth to explore thought processes, examine decision-making, and consider alternatives and consequences. Third, gameplay at home, following in-person sessions, can be used to reinforce those therapeutic methods and strategies learned in therapy. As with other "homework" reinforcement methods, video gameplay could provide teens with direct application and practice experiences but do so in a manner more engaging than paper-and-pencil worksheets (or other traditional methods) and therefore be more likely to be completed by teens. In the end, integrating impactful video games into the treatment plan for patients provides practitioners with innovative and engaging methods to augment, enhance, and accelerate therapeutic benefits for teens.

Practitioner Tip

Integrating video gameplay into in-person sessions can provide teen patients and their practitioners with concrete examples and a shared language to facilitate discussion and processing of difficult emotions or experiences, particularly for teens who struggle with self-expression.

Conclusion

This chapter proposed to assist mental health practitioners who work with teens to better understand the increasingly widespread and varied roles video games can play in their lives. Furthermore, we described how entertainment games have demonstrated positive effects on adolescent mental health and how a newer impactful video games, built with explicit goals for improving mental health, are showing even more promise. We explored an array of different impactful video games that have been developed to address mental and behavioral health issues pertinent to teens. Clearly, this trend is likely to only grow stronger over the coming years, as the evidence supporting the therapeutic benefits of integrating video games (commercial and impactful) into treatment with teens continues to grow as well. Our hope is that those who work with teens can bring a deeper understanding of video gaming to their practice and by doing so, foster positive mental and behavioral health for their patients.

Acknowledgments The authors would like to thank their three sons—Jefferson Thomas, Benjamin Thomas, and Lincoln Thomas—who provided considerable input (and fact-checking) for this chapter regarding popular commercial video games, video game genres, and video gaming experiences. Their feedback and sharing were integral in helping the authors conceptualize teens' gameplay experiences when writing the first section of this chapter. The authors would also like to thank Mary Whatley who aided considerably in conducting a literature search and compiling the citations included in this chapter.

References

1. Yi M. They got game: stacks of new releases for hungry video game enthusiasts mean it's boom time for an industry now even bigger than Hollywood. San Francisco Chronicle [Internet]; 2004 Dec [cited 2017 Apr 26]. http://www.sfgate.com/news/article/THEY-GOT-GAME-Stacks-of-new-releases-for-hungry-2663371.php
2. Lenhart A, Kahne J, Middaugh E, MacGill A, Evans C, Vitak J. Teens, video games, and civics. Pew Research Center [Internet]; 2008 Sep [cited 2017 Apr 26]. http://www.pewinternet.org/2008/09/16/teens-video-games-and-civics/#.
3. Statista: The Statistics Portal. Statistics and facts on mobile gaming [Internet]. Hamburg, Germany: Statista; [cited 2017 Apr 26]. https://www.statista.com/topics/1906/mobile-gaming/
4. NPD Group. Average time spent playing games on mobile devices has increased 57 percent since 2012 [Internet]; 2014 [cited] 2017 Apr 27. https://www.npd.com/wps/portal/npd/us/news/press-releases/2015/

average-time-spent-playing-games-on-mobile-devices-has-increased-57-percent-since-2012/
5. Entertainment Software Association. Essential facts about the computer and video game industry [Internet]. Washington, DC: ESA; 2015 Apr [cited 2017 Apr 27]. 20 p. http://www.theesa.com/wp-content/uploads/2015/04/ESA-Essential-Facts-2015.pdf
6. Bartle R. Hearts, clubs, diamonds, spades: players who suit MUDS. J MUD Res [Internet]. 1996 [cited 2017 Apr 26];1(1). http://mud.co.uk/richard/hcds.htm.
7. Bartle RA. Designing virtual worlds. New Riders: Berkely; 2004.
8. Yee N. Motivations for play in online games. Cyberpsychol Behav. 2006;9(6):772–5.
9. Sherry JL, Lucas K, Greenberg BS, Lachlan K. Video game uses and gratifications as predictors of use and game preference. In: Bryant J, Vorderer P, editors. Playing video games: motives, responses, and consequences. Mahwah: Lawrence Erlbaum; 2006. p. 213–24.
10. Boyan A, Sherry JL. The challenge in creating games for education: aligning mental models with game models. Child Dev Perspect. 2011;5(2):82–7.
11. Csikszentmihalyi M. Flow: the psychology of optimal experience. New York: Harper & Row; 1990.
12. Ryan RM, Rigby CS, Przybylski AK. The motivational pull of video games: a self-determination theory approach. Motiv Emot. 2006;30:347–64.
13. Przybylski AK, Rigby CS, Ryan RMA. motivational model of video game engagement. Rev Gen Psychol. 2010;14(2):154–66.
14. American Academy of Pediatrics [Internet]. Elk Grove Village, IL: AAP; 2017 [cited 2017 Apr 27]. https://www.aap.org/en-us/advocacy-and-policy/aap-health-initiatives/Pages/Media-and-Children.aspx
15. APA Task Force on Violent Media. Technical report on the review of the violent video game literature [Internet]. Washington, DC: American Psychological Association; 2015 [cited 2017 Apr 27]. 31 p. http://www.apa.org/pi/families/review-video-games.pdf
16. Gee JP. What video games have to teach us about learning and literacy. New York: St. Martin's Press; 2003.
17. Smyth JM. Beyond self-selection in video game play: an experimental examination of the consequences of Massively Multiplayer Online Role-Playing Game play. Cyberpsychol Behav. 2007;10(5):717–21.
18. Gallup J, Serianni B, Duff C, Gallup A. An exploration of friendships and socialization for adolescents with autism engaged in Massively Multiplayer Online Role-Playing Games (MMORPG). Educ Train Autism Dev Disabil. 2016;51(3):223–37.
19. Olson CK, Kutner LA, Warner DE. The role of violent video game content in adolescent development. J Adolesc Res. 2008;23(1):55–75.
20. Yee N. The demographics, motivations, and derived experiences of users of massively multi-user online graphical environments. Presence. 2006;15(3):309–29.
21. Zhong Z. The effects of collective MMORPG (Massively Multiplayer Online Role-Playing Games) play on gamers' online and offline social capital. Comput Human Behav. 2011;27(6):2352–63.
22. Gentile DA, Anderson CA, Yukawa S, Ihori N, Saleem M, Ming LK, et al. The effects of prosocial video games on prosocial behaviors: international evidence from correlational, longitudinal, and experimental studies. Pers Soc Psychol Bull. 2009;35:752–63.
23. Cole H, Griffiths MD. Social interactions in massively multiplayer online role-playing gamers. Cyberpsychol Behav. 2007;10(4):575–83.
24. Belozerov SA. Virtual worlds of MMORPG. Part II. Remedy for social and psychological ill-being. Psychology: Journal of Higher School of Economics. 2015;12(1):71–89.
25. LaRose R. Eastin MS, Gregg J. Reformulating the Internet paradox: social cognitive explanations of Internet use and depression. J Online Behav. 2001;1(2).
26. Shaw LH, Grant LM. defense of the internet: the relationship between internet communication and depression, loneliness, self-esteem, and perceived social support. Cyberpsychol Behav. 2002;5(2):157–71.
27. Snodgrass JG, Lacy MG, Francois Dengah HJ 2nd, Fagan J. Enhancing one life rather than living two: playing MMOs with offline friends. Comput Human Behav. 2011;27(3):1211–22.
28. Russoniello CV, Fish M, O'Brien K. The efficacy of casual video game play in reducing clinical depression: a randomized controlled study. Games Health J. 2013;2(6):341–6.
29. Russoniello CV, O'Brien K, Parks JM. The effectiveness of casual video games in improving mood and decreasing stress. J Cyber Ther Rehabil. 2009;2(1):53–66.
30. Fish MT, Russoniello CV, O'Brien K. The efficacy of prescribed casual videogame play in reducing symptoms of anxiety: a randomized controlled study. Games Health J. 2014;3(5):291–5.
31. Patel A, Schieble T, Davidson M, Tran MC, Schoenberg C, Delphin E, et al. Distraction with a hand-held video game reduces pediatric preoperative anxiety. Paediatr Anaesth. 2006;16(10):1019–27.
32. Colwell J. Needs met through computer game play among adolescents. Personal Individ Differ. 2007;43:2072–82.
33. Snodgrass JG, Lacy M, Francois Dengah HJ 2nd, Fagan J, Most D. Magical flight and monstrous stress: technologies of absorption and mental wellness in Azeroth. Cult Med Psychiatry 2011;35(1):26–62.
34. Holmes EA, James EL, Coode-Bate T, Deeprose C. Can playing the computer game "Tetris" reduce the build-up of flashbacks for trauma? A proposal from cognitive science. PLoS One. 2009;4(1):e4153.
35. Holmes EA, James EL, Kilford EJ, Deeprose C. Key steps in developing a cognitive vaccine against traumatic flashbacks: visuospatial Tetris versus Verbal Pub Quiz. PLoS One. 2010;5(11):e13706.

36. Moisala M, Salmela V, Hietajarvi L, Carlson S, Vuontela V, Lonka K, et al. Gaming is related to enhanced working memory performance and task-related cortical activity. Brain Res. 2017;1655:204–15.
37. Chan PA, Rabinowitz TA. cross-sectional analysis of video games and attention deficit hyperactivity disorder symptoms in adolescents. Ann Gen Psychiatry. 2006;5(16):5–16.
38. Barlett CP, Anderson CA, Swing EL. Video game effects—confirmed, suspected, and speculative. Simul Gaming. 2009;40(3):377–403.
39. Subrahmanyam K, Greenfield PM. Effect of video game practice on spatial skills in girls and boys. J Appl Dev Psychol. 1994;15(1):13–32.
40. Middleton KK, Hamilton T, Tsai PC, Middleton DB, Falcone JL, Hamad G. Improved nondominant hand performance on a laparoscopic virtual reality simulator after playing the Nintendo Wii. Surg Endosc. 2013;27(11):4224–31.
41. Li J, Theng Y, Foo S. Game-based digital interventions for depression therapy: A systematic review and meta-analysis. Cyberpsychol Behav Soc Netw. 2014;17(8):519–27.
42. Merry SN, Stasiak K, Shepherd M, Frampton C, Fleming T, Lucassen MF. The effectiveness of SPARX, a computerised self help intervention for adolescents seeking help for depression: randomised controlled non-inferiority trial. BMJ. 2012;344:e2598.
43. Carrasco AE. Acceptability of an adventure video game in the treatment of female adolescents with symptoms of depression. Res Psychother. 2016;19(1):10–8.
44. Sharry J, McDermott M, Condron J. 'Relax To Win'—treating children with anxiety problems with a biofeedback video game. Eistach. 2003;2:22–6.
45. Knox M, Lentini J, Cummings TS, McGrady A, Whearty K, Sancrant L. Game-based biofeedback for paediatric anxiety and depression. Ment Health Fam Med. 2011;8(3):195–203.
46. Scholten H, Malmberg M, Lobel A, Engels A, Granic IA. randomized controlled trial to test the effectiveness of an immersive 3D video game for anxiety prevention among adolescents. PLoS One. 2016;11(1):e0147763.
47. Pope AT, Bogart EH. Extended attention span training system: video game neurotherapy for attention deficit disorder. Child Study Journal. 1996;26(1):39–50.
48. Butnik SM. Neurofeedback in adolescents and adults with Attention Deficit Hyperactivity Disorder. J Clin Psychol. 2005;61(5):621–5.
49. Nodell B. Game your brain to treat depression, studies suggest. News Beat: UW Health Sciences [Internet]. 03 Jan 2017 [cited 28 Apr 2017]; Research [about 3 screens]. http://hsnewsbeat.uw.edu/story/studies-suggest-gaming-your-brain-treat-depression
50. Anguera JA, Gunning FM, Arean PA. Improving late life depression and cognitive control through the use of therapeutic video game technology: a proof-of-concept randomized trial. Depress Anxiety. 2016 Dec [cited 28 Apr 2017]. https://doi.org/10.1002/da.22588
51. Rabiner DL, Murray DW, Skinner AT, Malone PSA. randomized trial of two promising computer-based interventions for students with attention difficulties. J Abnorm Child Psychol. 2010;38(1):131–42.
52. Weerdmeester J, Cima M, Granic I, Hashemian Y, Gotsis M. A feasibility study on the effectiveness of a full-body videogame intervention for decreasing attention deficit hyperactivity disorder symptoms. Games for Health. 2016;5(4):258–69.
53. Bellack AS, Dickinson D, Morris SE, Tenhula WN. The development of a computer-assisted cognitive remediation program for patients with schizophrenia. Isr J Psychiatry Relat Sci. 2005;42(1):5–14.
54. Shrimpton B, Hurworth R. Adventures in evaluation: reviewing a CD-ROM based adventure game designed for young people recovering from psychosis. J Educ Multimed Hypermedia. 2005;14(3):273–90.
55. Tanaka JW, Wolf JM, Klaiman C, Koenig K, Cockburn J, Herlihy L, et al. Using computerized games to teach face recognition skills to children with autism spectrum disorder: the Let's Face It! program. J Child Psychol Psychiatry. 2010;51(8):944–52.
56. Brown ER, Craig AB, DeRosier ME. Hall of Heroes: a social skills training game to prepare students for the transition to middle school. Forthcoming: J Early Adolesc; 2017.
57. Corrigan PW, Druss BG, Perlick DA. The impact of mental illness stigma on seeking and participating in mental health care. Psychol Sci Public Interest. 2014;15(2):37–70.
58. Shandley K, Austin D, Klein B, Kyrios M. An evaluation of 'Reach Out Central': an online gaming program for supporting the mental health of young people. Health Educ Res. 2010;25(4):563–74.

18 Apps for Mental Health

Oliver Lindhiem and Jordan L. Harris

History of Mental Health Apps

Even before the advent of modern smartphones, early mental health apps were developed for personal digital assistants (PDAs) such as the PalmPilot which was introduced in 1997. PDAs were viewed as an ideal tool to assist in treatment delivery of skill-based therapies such as cognitive-behavioral treatments [1]. Examples include the facilitation of self-statements, breathing control practice, and exposure exercises, for the treatment of panic disorder [2], support for adolescents with autism spectrum disorder [3], and monitoring PTSD symptoms [4]. Apple's first iPhone came to market in 2007. From 2008 to 2009, the creation of the BlackBerry App World, Apple's App Store, and Google's Android Market (later called Google Play Store) allowed users to download mobile application software (apps) directly onto their smartphones. Mental health apps began being developed almost immediately, entering the market around this time [5]. With a rapidly growing market for downloadable apps, the sophistication of apps grew very quickly. By late 2010, over 300,000 apps were available across numerous platforms. Of these, about 8000 were health related with only a small portion of those focused on mental health [6]. A 2015 survey found that the number of health-related apps had almost doubled to 15,000 with one-third of that number being specific to mental health [7]. Although mental health apps can vary greatly from one another, in general a mental health app is a mobile application that aims to reduce symptoms for either a specific diagnosis or transdiagnostic symptoms through the use of app features and can be used as a stand-alone treatment or an add-on to treatment. Although many apps are unique in design and content, there are typical features that can be found in most mental health apps (Fig. 18.1).

Typical Features Common to Most Mental Health Apps

Content. Therapeutic content can be housed in mental health apps in various ways including modules or chapters (e.g., a digital book) on various topics and digital "libraries" or "dictionaries" organized by topic with definitions of various CBT and other therapeutic skills and techniques. Content can also include videos and/or audio files that explain or model various skills or techniques. Some apps even include a feature to

O. Lindhiem, Ph.D. (✉)
Department of Psychiatry, University of Pittsburgh, Pittsburgh, PA, USA
e-mail: lindhiemoj@upmc.edu

J.L. Harris
University of Pittsburgh Medical Center, Pittsburgh, PA, USA

M.A. Moreno, A. Radovic (eds.), *Technology and Adolescent Mental Health*,
https://doi.org/10.1007/978-3-319-69638-6_18

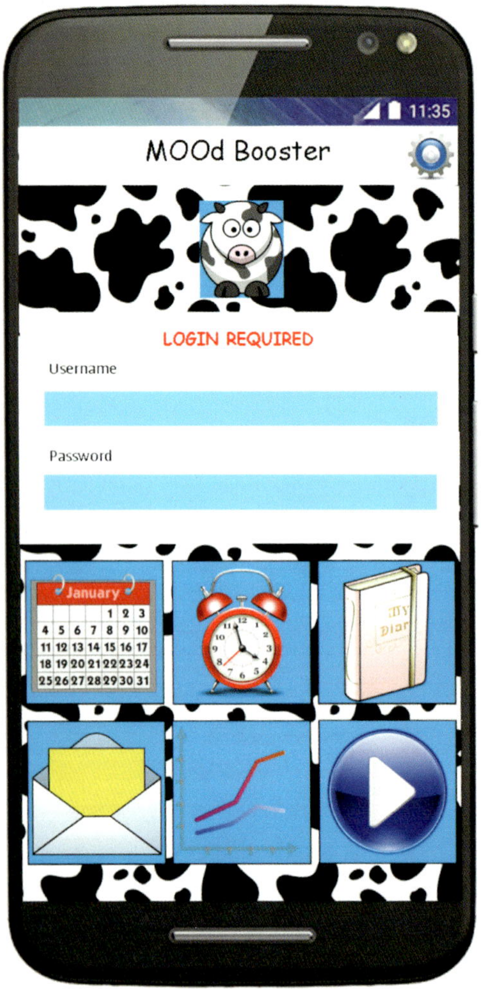

Fig. 18.1 A mock-up of a typical mental health app that highlights many of the features that are commonly available: calendar, alarm, mood diary, message system, symptom tracker, and video library

record a therapy session so that it can be reviewed again later by the patient [8]. The ways that apps organize their content make each app unique and provide the user with an experience that may differ from app to app (even those that are focused on the same specific disorder).

Diaries and symptom tracking. Many mental health apps include a diary feature to track mood, daily activities, or problem behaviors. There is evidence that diaries can give useful insight into behaviors, depressive symptoms, and emotional self-awareness [9, 10]. Digital diaries can also collect data on between-session treatment adherence and skills practice. Such methods have numerous advantages over traditional retrospective diaries including the sequencing of data and the ability to estimate individual variability in responses over time [11, 12]. Another advantage of a digital diary over a traditional pen-and-paper diary is that real-time contextual factors can also be assessed (e.g., GPS location, time, weather). Real-time diary entries can also eliminate the problem of recall bias resulting in data with greater reliability and validity compared to retrospective reports. Numerous studies have documented the poor correspondence between real-time data and retrospective reports making this an important advantage [13, 14]. Diary entries can be event-based (e.g., after an interpersonal interaction) or time-based (e.g., every 2 hours or electronic prompts given at random intervals), and because phones are much more portable than pen-and-paper diaries, compliance rates are higher on digital diaries [15]. Apps that are linked to a clinician portal can also transmit the data to be viewed by a clinician before or during a treatment session. Finally, diary data can be used to track treatment progress over the course of treatment.

Alarms and appointment reminders. Alarm features are common and can be used for several different purposes, including reminders to practice a skill, make a diary entry (e.g., mood tracking), take a medication, or complete a therapist-assigned homework activity. For apps that are linked to a clinician portal, the clinician can set an alarm at any time between treatment sessions. Alarms can also be used as appointment reminders. For cases of PTSD, an appointment reminder feature can be especially helpful given that PTSD avoidance symptoms can lead to a decrease in session attendance. To assist in recall of scheduled treatment sessions, some apps have calendars that are populated with appointment reminders and alarms to reduce the cases of PTSD avoidance symptoms [8]. Overall, alarms can help to normalize routine and create patterns in behavior.

Messaging. Messaging features can be found on many mental health apps and can be helpful in delivering content to the adolescent quickly and easily. These systems can allow one-way messaging (clinician to adolescent; adolescent to clinician) or two-way messaging. One-way messaging from the clinician to adolescent can be used for appointment reminders, encouragement, skill tips, or reminders to complete therapeutic "home practice" activities. One-way messaging from the adolescent to the clinician can be used to send progress updates or "in the moment" observations that can be addressed at the next therapy session. Two-way messaging can be used therapeutically in various ways such as coaching a patient in real time through an in vivo exposure exercise or delivering brief therapeutic content. Content of a message can fall into a variety of categories such as asking/answering questions or providing positive reinforcement [16–18]. The volume of messages sent/received can vary from user to user, and messages can be tailored to each user to fit their particular needs [18]. In our experience, clinicians tend to prefer one-way messaging systems to two-way messaging systems because this reduces user perceptions and expectations that the clinician is "on call" and available to respond to messages in real time. Messaging systems, particularly two-way messaging, can also introduce complications around insurance billing and reimbursement of clinician time.

Videos. Mental health apps occasionally include videos that can serve several functions such as instructional behavioral modeling guides or prerecorded affirmative messages of support. The use of videos for education is not a new concept to the mental health field, but the widespread access to mental health apps has opened up new and exciting possibilities for the use of videos as modeling or support tools. If ever a task or topic covered in session is difficult to explain in words or could be better learned through observation, videos can be used as an alternative method of conveying or reinforcing a topic covered in session with an adolescent. If done well, videos can deliver useful and functional knowledge to the viewer while also being fun. Use of video modeling as educational tools has been researched over the past two decades. One such study was on the use of mental health apps as an assistive technology for adults with autism spectrum disorder which found that the use of video-based instructions and behavioral modeling was an effective substitute for a job support aid. In addition, the sooner they began using the apps, the more effective it was as a substitute for a vocational aid [19]. Video-messaging has also been used effectively in studies of smoking cessation [20].

Special Features Available on Some Mental Health Apps

Connectivity/synchronization with a clinician web portal. Some mental health apps have been developed to communicate with a clinician web portal. The web portal often includes a dashboard that displays diary data or symptom trajectories from the patient app. The portal can also be used to send appointment reminders and messages or set alarms to remind the adolescent to practice skills or techniques that were learned during a therapy session. Some clinician web portals offer visual information feedback that graphs summary information or session-by-session change to track changes in symptoms in different contexts, self-efficacy, coping thoughts, etc. [21]. Although not always a common feature, a connected clinician web portal can be an efficient way to track adolescent data over the course of treatment.

Interactive features (e.g., troubleshooting guide). Interactive features give the user the opportunity to seek guidance or opportunities to develop useful skills in a way that is hands-on and often fun. Some mental health apps have interactive features that, when used in the moment of anxiety or distress, can generalize learned skills to new settings, thus encouraging practice of behaviors to improve symptoms [22]. In vivo features such as a troubleshooting guide can be used to apply coping strategies in a more valid context than in the office during sessions. An alternative to a written troubleshooting guide is an audio/audiovisual virtual coaching feature. A feature such as this one provides a real-time instruction meant to remind and encourage skill use (e.g., relaxation breathing techniques) [6]. At the moment there are not many mental health apps on the market that have videos integrated into the system. By 2012 only 6% of studies done on mental health apps included apps with videos as a feature [23].

Games. Games are the most frequently downloaded items on smartphone app markets such as Google Play. Increasingly, mental health apps are beginning to incorporate games into their platform [6]. Games often provide the player with motivation to achieve a certain goal, often resulting in a virtual reward or sense of achievement. By incorporating mental health topics and evidence-based interventions into the framework of the game design, the player is motivated by the game itself to engage in desired behavior. In addition to patient motivation and education games incorporated into mental health apps, games are also designed to be a distraction during times of intense emotion or stress [24, 25]. It can be difficult to find a playable game that incorporates psychotherapy topics, which is why some apps have turned to "gamification" of the apps as a method of making the apps feel like games. Gamification is a method of increasing motivation to perform existing goals through the use of rewards and feedback, without the use of a game itself [22]. A gamified app based on measures of anxiety and stress reactivity was found to be helpful for the user even after a single use of the app [25]. Examples are apps that offer reinforcement and rewards (e.g., points, unlockable, etc.) that make intrinsic rewards more tangible for the user. Gamification can make any feature of a mental health app work like a game with the use of narrative feedback and/or a reward that aims to contribute toward the overall goal, which in most cases is reduction of symptoms.

Avatars/customization. Avatars are included in some mental health apps to make them more fun, particularly in apps designed for children. They can vary from a selectable picture from a small catalogue of options to a fully customizable figure that in some cases may resemble a person. A 2015 study found that participants found a virtual coach avatar to be relatable and helpful [26]. Although it may be difficult to find mental health apps that have avatars, there is some evidence suggesting that the autonomy to customize an avatar (often resembling the users' ideal state) increases the likelihood of behavior modification over time, viewing the avatar as a model whom they strive to resemble [22].

Potential Benefits of Mental Health Apps

The pace of innovation in the technology sector is far more rapid than the pace of scientific investigation. Although mental health apps can be developed and programmed within a matter of days, it can take years to conduct a randomized controlled trial (RCT) designed to evaluate their efficacy. It is therefore not surprising that there are far more mental health apps than there are studies evaluating their efficacy. Many mental health apps that are on the market have little or no empirical support as to any immediate- or long-term benefit [23, 27]. However, of the apps that have been tested, some have been found to use techniques such as relaxation and calming audio which may only reduce mild symptoms [28]. Until very recently, there were very few studies on the therapeutic utility of mental health apps [29]. This is gradually beginning to change, with more and more clinical trials being published every year. Many of the more rigorous clinical trials to date have evaluated behavioral health apps for behaviors related to weight loss [30], smoking cessation [31], and treatment adherence for chronic medical conditions such as diabetes [32], rather than mental health apps per se. The results of clinical trials for mental health apps are beginning to appear in the literature for conditions such as social anxiety disorder [33] and depression [34] with promising results. As more apps are developed and health consumerism grows, it will become increasingly challenging to sort through apps to find ones that are evidence-based [35]. A recent meta-analysis identified 25 clinical trials designed to test the utility of mobile technologies (smartphone apps, personal digital assistants, or text messaging systems) for enhancing treatment outcome for psychotherapy or other behavioral health interventions [36]. Mobile technologies were found be effective both as stand-alone interventions compared to no treatment (11 studies) and as adjunctive devices (10 studies), with effect sizes falling in between the "small" and "medium" ranges.

Improved motivation. Mental health apps also have the potential to improve clinical outcome *indirectly* by enhancing motivation, increasing show rates for appointments, and reducing dropout. This can happen in several ways. First, the ability to track symptoms over time can be motivating. Second, some apps included motivational messages or videos. Third, some apps allow clinician contact or automated alarms designed to enhance the utilization of therapeutic content or practice. Finally, some apps include features designed specifically to enhance motivation using principles or reinforcement (e.g., points, digital rewards) to encourage patients to stick with treatment.

Enhanced access to care. There are numerous barriers (both perceived and real) that prevent patients from accessing mental health services. These barriers include the availability of local services, transportation, cost, and perceived stigma. Structural barriers such as distance and reimbursement for travel may deter adolescents from attending sessions [24]. Mental health apps have tremendous potential to overcome these barriers. Utilizing many of the features listed previously in this chapter, mental health apps can enhance access to care for adolescents by providing them with free screening tools for depression [37] and supporting those who may have difficulties making it to sessions as often as needed. Some mental health apps utilize features such as GPS to help make access to care easier [6]. In some cases mental health apps incorporate GPS mapping of nearby clinics. This tool could be the difference between engaging and not engaging in clinical treatment. Physical location is only one of the problems; for many the primary barriers are attitude and stigma about treatment [24]. Adolescents who feel depressed (and may even search the Internet for "depression") do not always seek treatment. Mobile apps have the potential of reaching these individuals and motivating them to find and engage with treatment [28]. Some mobile apps address the issue of stigma of receiving mental health care which may prove to be a key to improving access to care given the high rates of smartphone ownership across all races, ethnicities, and socioeconomic groups.

Considerations in Selecting an App

There are numerous things to consider when selecting a mental health app including cost, training requirements, evidence of efficacy, usability, connectivity requirements, and security features. Figure 18.2 shows a checklist of questions to consider in selecting a mental health app to use with (or assign to) an adolescent. There are also other rating scales such as the *Mobile Application Rating Scale (MARS)* [38].

Are there any restrictions on using the app? Restrictions on using a mental health app include cost, compatibility with a device, and training requirements. There is some variability in pricing of mental health apps. While many are free, others range in price from $0.99 to $4.99 (a very small percentage tend to be more expensive). Some free apps are connected to a service that has a weekly/monthly/yearly charge that may also vary in price. Apps like this can often be identified by signifying that they contain "in-app purchases" sometimes costing hundreds of dollars. Outside of cost, the other barrier tends to be device compatibility. Some apps have been developed for cross-platform use and can be installed on either Apple (iPhone) or Android devices, although most can only be used with one or the other.

Is there evidence for the app's efficacy? As noted earlier in this chapter, the speed of app development outpaces researchers' abilities to conduct clinical trials. A 2013 review identified more than 1500 apps available for download on one or more of the app stores that focused on depression, but only 32 published research papers associated with these apps [39]. However, even apps that have not formally been evaluated in a clinical trial often rely on content that has decades of empirical support. One can therefore look for apps with empirically supported content (e.g.,

Fig. 18.2 A sample checklist to aid clinicians in selecting a mental health app

App Selection Checklist	YES	NO
Are there any restrictions on using the app?	☐	☐
Is there evidence for the app's efficacy?	☐	☐
Is the app intuitive/easy to use?	☐	☐
Does the app require internet connectivity?	☐	☐
Is the app designed to be used as a supplement to therapy?	☐	☐
Is the app designed to be used with a particular "brand name" treatment?	☐	☐
Is the app private, secure, and HIPAA compliant?	☐	☐
Is the app compatible with the user's device?	☐	☐

cognitive-behavioral skills, behavioral activation, mindfulness, exposure principles) even if the app itself has not been formally evaluated in a clinical trial.

Is the app intuitive/easy to use? Developers of some mental health apps are careful to use principles of user-centered design to ensure that apps are intuitive and easy to use. This is particularly important for apps that are designed for use by individuals with severe psychiatric conditions, cognitive impairments, or low literacy. For example, careful usability testing has gone into the development of FOCUS, a smartphone system for enhancing self-management skills for individuals with schizophrenia [40]. This system which targets medication adherence, symptom management, sleep and mood regulation, and social functioning was designed with testing and feedback from consumers at each stage of development.

Web app versus native app? Most mental health apps can be downloaded directly from Google Play or the Apple App Store onto a mobile device. Once downloaded, some features may work without further connectivity (e.g., videos, symptom tracking, games), but other features may require ongoing connectivity in order to function (e.g., messaging features, clinician-initiated alarms). Limited access to an internet connection serves as the primary barrier when selecting an app that utilizes internet connection for certain features.

Is the app designed as a stand-alone intervention or adjunctive device? Because of direct-to-consumer marketing, many people download and use mental health apps in much the same way as consumers of self-help books. However, there is limited research on mental health apps as effective self-help tools. There has been some exploratory research done on the use of mental health apps as a stand-alone therapy. Some of the features available on mental health apps (e.g., mood/behavior tracking, troubleshooting guide, library, etc.) can be used for self-discovery and skill learning. In some cases, the concepts from the apps may not only help people understand their own mood or emotions but may also help individuals coach other people as well [41].

In contrast, other mental health apps are designed to augment therapy sessions. Many specialized apps have been created due to the need to reinforce materials outside of sessions. Apps designed to supplement treatment can range from apps with a broad focus and numerous features to apps with a specific aim (e.g., mood tracking). Mental health apps as an add-on to treatment can function as a useful tool to identify and regulate behaviors or emotions that occur outside of sessions. Often mental health apps are equipped with mood- or behavior-tracking diaries. Assessments can also be administered via an app in the form of a homework assignment after session. The results of these assessments can be analyzed during the next session, helping to bridge the gap between therapy sessions and improving adherence to treatment [5].

Is the app designed to be used with a particular "brand name" treatment? When selecting an app to use with an adolescent, it is important to be mindful that some apps are designed with a particular treatment in mind (often an evidence-based CBT). From 2007 to 2012, evidence-based treatments made up 73% of studies done on mental health apps that were developed around an intervention. Only 16% were not centered around a theory nor an evidence-based treatment [23]. Although an app may have been developed and tested using one type of "brand name" treatment, it may have generalizable features that can be used with a different type of treatment that has similar aims and goals. It may be useful to do a literature search on an app to see with which type of treatment it was designed to be used. If published articles are not available, the App Store or Google Play Store often has the email address of the developer who may be able to answer questions.

Privacy/security/HIPAA compliance. A major consideration in selecting an app is whether it poses a risk to the therapeutic relationship, adolescent privacy, or confidentiality. Integrated messaging features that send or receive messages between the clinician and patient have the potential to blur the line of the therapeutic boundary [6]. Data security may also be important to consider, particularly if the patient enters data into the app such as mood, daily activities, or other symptom information. It is important to understand whether the data is stored on the device or on a remote server, whether the data is encrypted, and other security features to ensure data security. All features in the app that store protected health information (PHI) should comply with Health Insurance Portability and Accountability Act (HIPAA) requirements. The security features of mental health apps should be carefully evaluated before they are recommended to adolescents. There are resources available at *healthit.gov* that provide guidelines for security rules and tips [42].

Device ownership and compatibility issues. Although the rate of smartphone ownership is rising rapidly in the United States, not all patients will own a mobile device that is compatible with the ability to download mental health apps. Furthermore, many apps are only designed for a single platform (e.g., Apple, Android). A patient who owns an iPhone, for example, will not be able to use a mental health app that has been developed for Android devices (e.g., Galaxy). Apps that have been developed for cross-platform use will have the greatest potential for utilization by a wider population.

Billing. Finally, issues around billing may need to be considered, particularly if using an app system will increase clinical work for the clinician (e.g., logging into a clinical portal, sending alerts and reminders). In most cases, these activities are likely not reimbursable. Ideally, a clinician and patient will jointly decide on an app that will have clinical value without additional burden to the therapist (e.g., a simple and intuitive system that requires no more than a few minutes of attention from the clinician at the beginning and/or end of a treatment session).

Clinical Case Example

Mia is a 15-year-old female with moderate depression who has recently started seeing a therapist. She was referred for therapy by her school guidance counselor after teacher concerns that she seemed withdrawn and her grades were slipping. Her therapist has been able to establish a good working alliance with her and has started a course of cognitive-behavioral therapy (CBT) for depression. Her therapist has asked Mia to start completing a mood diary three times a day, but Mia has found the pen-and-paper forms to be a hassle and frequently forgets to complete her assignments. During a session, her therapist notices that Mia has a new Android smartphone and suggests that a mood-tracking app might be a good way to increase the rate of diary completion. They take the last few minutes of session to look for an app on the Google Play Store. At first they are a bit overwhelmed by the choices but work their way through the checklist described earlier in this chapter (see Fig. 18.2). Mia and her therapist settle on the "Mood Booster" app which includes a mood-tracking feature. Although the app itself has not been tested in a clinical trial, all of its features and content include traditional cognitive-behavioral techniques with decades of empirical support. All the data on the app is encrypted and links to a HIPAA compliant clinician portal. Mia finds using the app fun and easy, and her compliance with mood tracking increases markedly. Her therapist is able to track Mia's mood ratings on the clinician portal and review them with Mia during session. Use of the app and clinician portal does not take up any additional time for Mia's clinician, and so billing considerations are not an issue. In her free time between sessions, Mia has also explored some of the additional features on the app such as a video library with demonstrations of cognitive-behavioral techniques. Over the next 3 months, Mia and her therapist begin to see gradual improvements in her daily mood.

Conclusion and Caution

Although mental health apps have great potential to enhance clinical practice, it is important to exercise caution when selecting an app to use with an adolescent. Currently, there is very little regulation surrounding the distribution of mental health apps. As a result, there is tremendous variability in the quality of mental health apps available in app stores. In 2013, the UK National Health Service (NHS) formally endorsed a selection of mental health apps by creating a "Health Apps Library" on the "NHS Choices" website [7] only to remove them in 2015 [43] after concerns were expressed about the security of the apps and little evidence for the efficacy of their content. Without endorsing any specific apps, the World Health Organization (WHO) recently recommended "the use of electronic and mobile health technologies" for "the promotion of self-care" in their Mental Health Action Plan 2013–2020 [7]. Mental health apps will likely continue to see a growing trend as they become more sophisticated and individual apps gain research support.

References

1. Piasecki TM, Hufford MR, Solhan M, Trull TJ. Assessing clients in their natural environments with electronic diaries: rationale, benefits, limitations, and barriers. Psychol Assess. 2007;19(1):25–43.
2. Kenardy JA, Dow MGT, Johnston DW, Newman MG, Thomson A, Taylor CBA. comparison of delivery methods of cognitive-behavioral therapy for panic disorder: an international multicenter trial. J Consult Clin Psychol. 2003;71(6):1068–75.
3. Ferguson H, Smith Myles B, Hagiwara T. Using a personal digital assistant to enhance the independence of an adolescent with asperger syndrome. Educ Train Dev Disabil. 2005;40(1):60–7.
4. Pederson ER, Kaysen DL, Lindgren KP, Blayney J, Simpson TL. Impact of daily assessments on distress and PTSD symptoms in trauma-exposed women. J Interpers Violence. 2014;29(5):824–45.
5. Giota KG, Kleftaras G. Mental health apps: innovations, risks and ethical considerations. E-Health TelecommunicationSystemsandNetworks.2014;3(3):19–23.
6. Luxton DD, McCann RA, Bush NE, Mishkind MC, Reger GM. mHealth for mental health: integrating smartphone technology in behavioral health-

care. Professional Psychology: Research & Practice. 2011;42(6):505–12.
7. Anthes E. Pocket psychiatry: mobile mental-health apps have exploded onto the market, but few have been thoroughly tested. Nature. April 2016;2016(7):20–3.
8. Reger GM, Hoffman J, Riggs D, Rothbaum BO, Ruzek J, Holloway KM. The "PE Coach" smartphone application: an innovative approach to improving implementation, fidelity, and homework adherence during prolonged exposure. Psychol Serv. 2013;10(3):342–9.
9. Torous J, Staples P, Shanahan M, Lin C, Peck P, Keshavan MS, et al. Utilizing a personal smartphone custom app to assess the Patient Health Questionnaire-9 (PHQ-9) depressive symptoms in patients with major depressive disorder. JMIR Metal Health. 2015;2(1):1–11.
10. Reid SC, Kauer SD, Hearps SJ, Crooke AH, Khor AS, Sanci L, et al. A mobile phone application for the assessment and management of youth mental health problems in primary care: a randomised controlled trial. BMC Fam Pract. 2011;12(131):1–13.
11. Bolger N, Davis A, Rafaeli E. Diary methods: capturing life as it is lived. Annu Rev Psychol. 2003;54:579–616.
12. Ebner-Priemer UW, Trull TJ. Ecological momentary assessment of mood disorders and mood dysregulation. Psychol Assess. 2009;21(4):463–75.
13. Stone AA, Broderick JE. Real-time data collection for pain: appraisal and current status. Pain Med. 2007;8:85–93.
14. Stone AA, Broderick JE, Shiffman S, Schwartz JE. Understanding recall of weekly pain from a momentary assessment perspective: absolute agreement between- and within-person consistency, and judged change in weekly pain. Pain. 2004;107:61–9.
15. Matthews M, Doherty G, Sharry J, Fitzpatrick C. Mobile phone mood charting for adolescents. British Journal of Guidance & Counseling. 2008;36(2):113–29.
16. Kirwan M, Vandelanotte C, Fenning A, Duncan MJ. Diabetes self-management smartphone application for adults with type 1 diabetes: randomized controlled trial. J Med Internet Res. 2013;15(11):53–66.
17. Haug S, Schaub MP, Venzin V, Meyer C, John U. Efficacy of a text message-based smoking cessation intervention for young people: a cluster randomized controlled trial. J Med Internet Res. 2013;15(8):e171.
18. Louch G, Dalkin S, Bodansky J, Conner M. An exploratory randomised controlled trial using short messaging service to facilitate insulin administration in young adults with type 1 diabetes. Psychol Health Med. 2013;18(2):166–74.
19. Gentry T, Kriner R, Sima A, McDonough J, Wehman P. Reducing the need for personal supports among workers with autism using an iPod touch as an assistive technology: delayed randomized control trial. J Autism Dev Disord. 2014;45(3):669–84.
20. Whittaker R, Dorey E, Bramley D, Bullen C, Denny S, Elley CR, et al. A theory-based video messaging mobile phone intervention for smoking cessation: randomized controlled trial. J Med Internet Res. 2011;13(1):e10.
21. Pramana G, Parmanto B, Kendall PC, Silk JS. The SmartCAT: an mHealth platform for ecological momentary intervention (EMI) in child anxiety treatment. Telemedicine and e-Health. 2014;20(5):1–9.
22. Bakker D, Kazantzis N, Rickwood D, Rickard N. Mental health smartphone apps: review and evidence-based recommendations for future developments. JMIR Metal Health. 2016;3(1):e7.
23. Fiordelli M, Diviani N, Schulz PJ. Mapping mHealth research: a decade of evolution. J Med Internet Res. 2013;15(5):e95.
24. Price M, Yuen EK, Goetter EM, Herbert JD, Forman EM, Acierno R, et al. mHealth: a mechanism to deliver more accessible, more effective mental health care. Clin Psychol Psychother. 2014;21(5):427–36.
25. Dennis TA, O'Toole LJ. Mental health on the go: effects of a gamified attention-bias modification mobile application in trait-anxious adults. Clinical Psychological Science. 2014;2(5):576–90.
26. Pinto MD, Greenblatt AM, Hickman RL, Rice HM, Thomas TL, Clochesy JM. Assessing the critical parameters of eSMART-MH: a promising avatar-based digital therapeutic intervention to reduce depressive symptoms. Perspect Psychiatr Care. 2015;52(3):157–68.
27. Larsen ME, Nicholas J, Christensen H. Quantifying App Store dynamics: longitudinal tracking of mental health apps. JMIR Mhealth Uhealth. 2016;4(3):e96.
28. Radovic A, Vona PL, Santostefano AM, Ciaravino S, Miller E, Stein BD. Smartphone applications for mental health. Cyberpsychol Behav Soc Netw. 2016;19(7):465–70.
29. Boschen MJ. Mobile telephones and psychotherapy: II a review of empirical research. Behavior Therapist. 2009;32(8):175–81.
30. Burke LE, Conroy MB, Sereika SM, Elci OU, Styn MA, Acharya SD, et al. The effect of electronic self-monitoring on weight loss and dietary intake: a randomized behavioral weight loss trial. Obesity. 2011;19(2):338–44.
31. Buller DB, Borland R, Bettinghaus EP, Shane JH, Zimmerman DE. Randomized trial of a smartphone mobile application compared to text messaging to support smoking cessation. Telemedicine and e-Health. 2014;20(3):206–14.
32. Cafazzo JA, Casselman M, Hamming N, Katzman DK, Palmert MR. Design of an mHealth App for the self-management of adolescent Type 1 Diabetes: a pilot study. J Med Internet Res. 2012;14(3):e70.
33. Dagoo J, Persson Asplund R, Andersson Bsenko H, Hjerling S, Holmberg A, Westh S, et al. Cognitive behavior therapy versus interpersonal psychotherapy for social anxiety disorder delivered via smartphone and computer: a randomized controlled trial. J Anxiety Disord. 2014;28(4):410–7.
34. Watts S, Mackenzie A, Thomas C, Griskaitis A, Mewton L, Williams A, et al. CBT for depression: a pilot RCT comparing mobile phone vs. computer. BMC Psychiatry. 2013;13(1):49.

35. Shen N, Levitan M-J, Johnson A, Bender JL, Hamilton-Page M, Jadad AR, et al. Finding a depression app: a review and content analysis of the depression app marketplace. JMIR mHealth uHealth. 2015;3(1):e16.
36. Lindhiem O, Bennett CB, Rosen DK, Silk JS. Mobile technology boosts the effectiveness of psychotherapy and behavioral interventions: a meta-analysis. Behav Modif. 2015;39(6):785–804.
37. BinDhim NF, Shaman AM, Trevena L, Basyouni MH, Pont LG, Alhawassi TM. Depression screening via a smartphone app: cross-country user characteristics and feasibility. J Am Med Inform Assoc. 2015;22(1):29–34.
38. Stoyanov SR, Hides L, Kavanagh DJ, Zelenko O, Tjondronegoro D, Mani M. Mobile app rating scale: a new tool for assessing the quality of health mobile apps. JMIR mHealth uHealth. 2015;3(1):e27.
39. Martinez-Perez B, de la Torre-Diez I, Lopez-Coronado M. Mobile health applications for the most prevalent conditions by the World Health Organization: review and analysis. J Med Internet Res. 2013;15(6):e120.
40. Ben-Zeev D, Kaiser SM, Brenner CJ, Begale M, Duffecy J, Mohr DC. Development and usability testing of FOCUS: a smartphone system for self-management of schizophrenia. Psychiatr Rehabil J. 2013;36(4):289–96.
41. Morris ME, Kathawala Q, Leen TK, Gorenstein EE, Guilak F, Labhard M, et al. Mobile therapy: case study evaluations of a cell phone application for emotional self-awareness. J Med Internet Res. 2010;12(2):e10.
42. HealthIT.gov. Managing mobile devices in your health care organization. 2013.
43. Misra S. NHS Health Apps Library closing amid questions about app security & quality: what can we learn?: iMedical Apps; 2015 http://www.imedicalapps.com/2015/10/nhs-health-apps-library-closing-commentary/.

Comprehensive Approaches Using Technology to Address Mental Health

19

Scottye J. Cash, Stephanie Craig Rushing, and David Stephens

Comprehensive Approaches Using Technology to Address Mental Health

Ensuring adolescents have the resources and skills they need to have positive mental health is critically important but challenging [1–4]. Untreated mental health needs can lead to suicidal behaviors, substance use, academic problems, and impaired development. Getting treatment for mental health issues, however, is difficult with this population, as many adolescents do not seek help for a mental health issue [2, 3, 5–8]. Some of the reasons for not seeking help include feeling stigmatized, not fully understanding what it means to have a mental health issue, not fully appreciating the implications of not getting treatment, and being unsure about how to obtain treatment [2, 3, 5–8]. Research has also shown that adolescents tend to turn to their friends or family when they need mental health support rather than relying on health-care professionals or hotlines [9, 10]. Given the significant consequences of not obtaining mental health support when needed, finding ways to support adolescents to get this help is critical [1, 9]. Technology may provide a unique set of approaches to help adolescents obtain support for mental health issues in ways that make sense to them.

The access and use of mobile technology has grown exponentially over the past 10 years [11]. The Pew Research Center found that 88% of adolescents have access to a smartphone and 94% of these adolescents go online at least one time a day [12]. Ninety percent of adolescents text at least once a day and send and receive an average of 30 texts per day. Even among teens who don't have access to a smartphone, 68% of these teens go online every day. Seventy-one percent of teens use Facebook, 52% use Instagram, and 41% use Snapchat. Seventy-one percent of teens reported that they use multiple social networking sites. The data on adolescent's technology use provides support that harnessing the power of technology combined with evidence-based mental health support can provide a critical linkage between mental health need and seeking help.

The following section provides information on websites and corresponding organizations that use social media and technology to improve adolescent well-being and mental health. The research on many of these initiatives is in its beginning stages; however, when research is available, the research will be presented. While

S.J. Cash, M.S.S.W., Ph.D. (✉)
The Ohio State University, Columbus, OH, USA
e-mail: cash.33@osu.edu

S.C. Rushing, Ph.D., M.P.H. • D. Stephens, B.S.N., R.N.N., R.N.
Northwest Portland Area Indian Health Board, Portland, OR, USA
e-mail: SCraig@npaihb.org; dstephens@npaihb.org

M.A. Moreno, A. Radovic (eds.), *Technology and Adolescent Mental Health*,
https://doi.org/10.1007/978-3-319-69638-6_19

there are many examples on the Internet, those chosen for this chapter meet the following criteria:

1. The organization specifically targets well-being and/or mental health for adolescents.
2. The organization uses multimedia tools (videos, text, chat, fact sheets) to engage with and provide information to adolescents.
3. The organization's materials are provided free of charge.
4. Usage data, at a minimum, are collected by the organization on their various approaches to present material.
5. Materials were developed based on empirical evidence.

Innovative sites and organizations are highlighted below and include sites in the United States and Australia. Given that Australia is at the forefront of using technology to deliver mental health services, it is believed that the methods and materials they have to offer are worthwhile and can be translated to US populations. While there are some differences in word usage and dialects between Australia and the United States, the materials are still applicable across time and space. One caveat to note is that Australia has universal health care, which provides them with some flexibility to provide services based on need rather than insurance. Using technology though to support people going through difficult times or have mental health problems is one way to overcome the barriers of limitations of insurance and geographical location. The We R Native site was developed for Native American adolescents and in collaboration with ReachOut.com and au.reachout.com. While there are cultural components to the We R Native site, the materials are appropriate for clinicians to recommend and use in their practice.

The information on the sites and resources provided in this chapter can be used by clinicians in different settings (e.g., hospitals, mental health clinics, pediatrician offices, primary care physicians, etc.). While some of the organizations and sites may not initially appear to be conducive to use in a clinical setting, specific examples on how they can be used are provided. Some sites have more components than others as well as a more substantial evidence base. When available, the evidence on the sites will be provided. The goal of the chapter is to provide a user-friendly set of resources that will engage the adolescent, support the adolescent in ways that make sense to them, and provide them with resources that are of interest to them.

Inspire Foundation and au.reachout.com (Australia) and ReachOut.com (United States)

Background

In 1997, Jack Health launched the Inspire Foundation and au.reachout.com in Australia to serve as the world's first online approach to help youth who were struggling with mental health issues [13]. Research on mental health and help seeking in Australia has shown that 25% of all youth have a mental health issue; however, 70% of those do not seek help from mental health providers [14]. Data from 2016 showed that 110,000 unique visitors access the site each month, with over 1.31 million visitors each year. Given the availability of technology and the increasing uptake of youth accessing the Internet, they decided to harness the power of the Internet to reach more youth in a space that youth would be most likely to use.

In 2010, Inspire Foundation launched ReachOut.com in the United States, to help meet this gap in online mental health services for adolescents. There are three key tenets of the ReachOut.com model that differentiate it from others. First, all of the materials presented and the medium in which they are presented are vetted by youth prior to being released. Second, the materials are also designed so that youth can drive what kind of information and support they want to receive; in essence, meet the youth where they are. Third, they operate from a strength perspective framing mental health issues as "tough times" not as illnesses. The discussion on ReachOut.com will be divided into two parts, the Australia model and the United States model. Each website has unique features which are important to highlight.

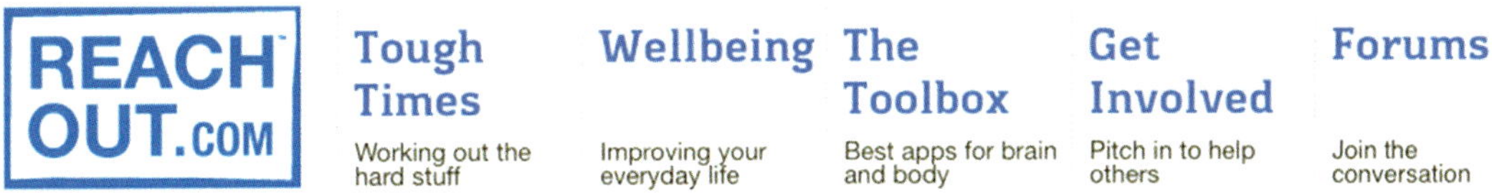
REACH OUT.COM
Tough Times
Working out the hard stuff
Wellbeing
Improving your everyday life
The Toolbox
Best apps for brain and body
Get Involved
Pitch in to help others
Forums
Join the conversation

Fig. 19.1 Australia's au.reachout.com main page (Source: http://au.reachout.com/)

Australia au.reachout.com

au.reachout.com has six main components to achieve the goals of increasing mental health literacy, decreasing mental health stigma, and increasing help-seeking behaviors. Collins and colleagues (2011) identify the core elements "research supported information created by young people and professionals delivered through over 25 factsheets; an online community forum and blog; an online game based on cognitive behavioural therapy; digital and social media including podcasts, digital stories and video; and use of social networking services to deliver content and build community." (p. 41) [15]. The organization also focuses on helping youth build their skills related to help seeking and managing tough times. The model was designed as an action research model that connects professionals to the material that can then be delivered in the community or in educational settings.

Australia's ReachOut.com has three key components in their website: the main website, Reachout Professionals, and Reachout Parents. The first is the main site au.reachout.com which provides the user with the opportunity to explore and receive support and facts related to "Tough Times," "Well-being," "The Toolbox," "Get Involved," and "Forums" (Fig. 19.1).

Tough Times

The Tough Times section provides users with a mix of fact sheets, videos, and audio clips dealing with a range of issues. Some of the specific issues include mental health, bullying, self-harm, eating disorders, and stress and anxiety. As noted previously, all of the content that is posted has been vetted by youth, to ensure that the materials are in language and mediums that the youth understand and are developmentally appropriate. Evidence-based information is also used when developing the fact sheets and recommended resources.

A new feature, ReachOut Next Steps, was added in 2016 that was co-developed with the Young and Well Centre's (http://www.youngandwellcrc.org.au/) grant from the Australian Research Council. Next Steps is a powerful tool that helps the youth identify issue(s), via an online quiz, and they are then guided to specific recommendations to obtain support. The types of support they receive include connections to local agencies, mobile apps, and websites. The user is then able to download a pdf that has a listing of all of the recommended resources.

Well-being

The Well-being pages provide users with a list of actions and information to help the user implement new strategies that support well-being. Some of the topics on the Well-being page include information and techniques on mental fitness (e.g., relaxation, coping, strengths, etc.), personal identity (e.g., body image, sexual identity, disability, etc.), school and "Uni" (university) studying (e.g., managing studying stress, sleeping issues, etc.), goals and motivations (e.g., setting goals and motivation), social skills (e.g., meeting new people and communication skills), and sex and relationships.

The Toolbox

The Toolbox asks users to take a short quiz on what areas the user would like to work on, including Health and Fitness, Being Independent, Relationships & Helping Others, Thoughts & Emotions, and Dealing with Tough Times (Fig. 19.2). Once they decide which area(s) they would like to work on are then guided to develop specific goals that address the issues identified in

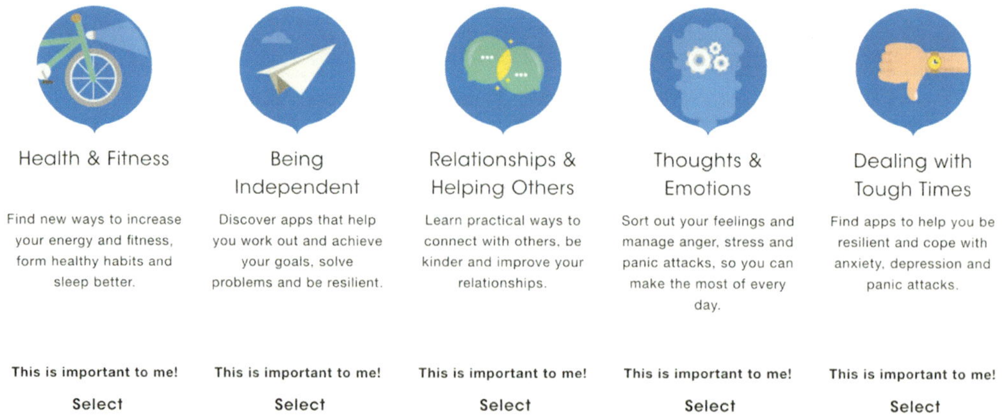

Fig. 19.2 Australia's au.reachout.com Toolbox site (Source: http://au.reachout.com/sites/thetoolbox/)

the quiz. Once goals are set, the users are provided with goal-specific and prescreened apps. au.reachout.com was also responsible for developing three apps "Breathe," "Recharge," "eScape," and "Worry Time." The Toolbox also provides users with the option to Receive Free SMS/Text Tips from their different campaigns. A few examples of the types of SMS tip categories include "Stress Tips," "Problem Solving Attempts," and "Random Acts of Kindness."

An example is presented below.

The Toolbox goal chosen was Thoughts & Emotions and "Relax," and these were three of seven different apps that were suggested to help reach this goal. ReachOut.com "Breathe" provides a user-friendly interface where users are directed to place their finger on the screen and breathe in and out. eScape is a music-driven app where users give the app permission to access their music. The app then maps the different songs to different moods. Users are prompted to identify their current mood and then identify the type of mood the user would like to achieve. Headspace is an app that guides users through different types of meditations related to the users' specific goals (Fig. 19.3).

Get Involved

Users are encouraged to get involved in the promotion of ReachOut.com. The different mechanisms for getting involved include volunteering to serve on the Youth Advisory Board, moderating the forum, distributing promotional materials, wearing ReachOut.com merchandise, and donating.

Forums

The Forums provide users with an opportunity to network with other individuals who may be going through similar tough times. The Forums are peer moderated, and moderators receive training to assist them in identifying alarming posts (e.g., self-harm) and inappropriate posts. In 2016, they incorporated a new tool, Moderator Assistant, that uses machine learning in the moderating process. Moderator Assistant uses "natural language process techniques to highlight key information and automatically classify and prioritise high-risk posts for moderators, driving faster response times for people in great need." (http://about.au.reachout.com/moderation-tool-boosts-efficiency-of-mental-health-forums-2016/). Moderator Assistant also provides a chat function, behind the scenes, to help moderators discuss potential responses to chats. The forum is a very popular feature of au.reachout.com. In the screenshot below, the number of posts in the "Tough Times/Somethings not Right" forum is significant (20,723 posts).

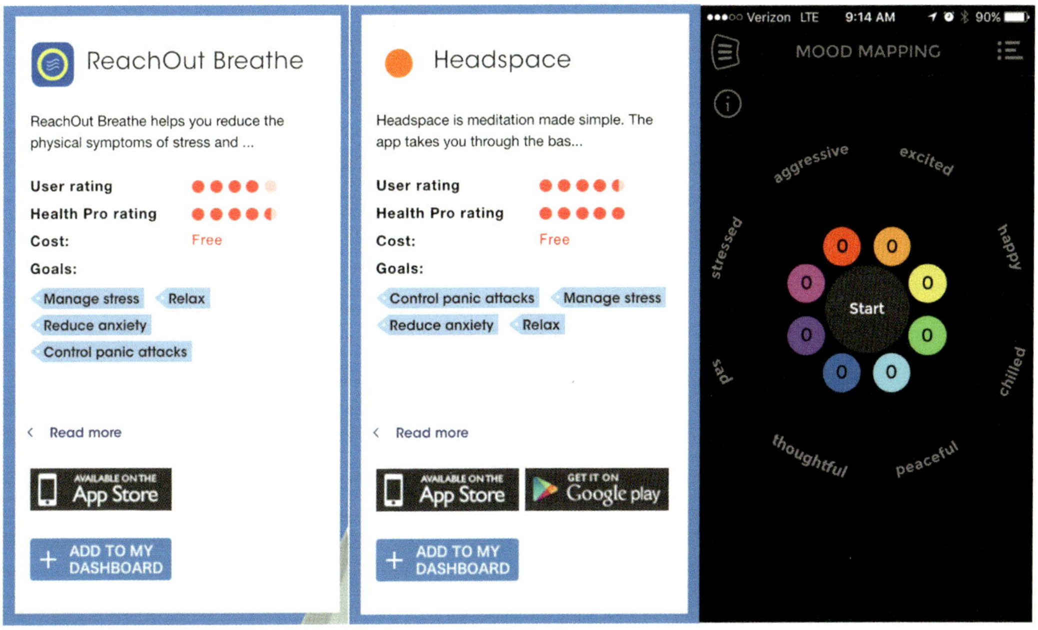

Fig. 19.3 Australia au.reachout.com App Suggestions based on Toolbox Quiz (Source: http://au.reachout.com/sites/thetoolbox/goals/relax)

au.reachout.com Parent and Professionals Companion Websites

Professionals

The ReachOut.com Professionals page was developed to support professionals working with youth who were struggling with mental health issues (Fig. 19.4). The professionals targeted include those working in schools, mental health clinics, and general youth-serving organizations. The information on the site includes a variety of resources including mental health fact sheets, how to work parents, mobile technology apps to suggest to patients that support mental health, professional development, and resources and ideas for teachers.

Parents

The au.reachout.com Parent page was designed to help parents initiate and carry out conversations with their children about mental health issues (Fig. 19.5). The site includes fact sheets, tips for how to have tough conversations, forums, and a coaching module. The coaching module is for parents who have 12–18-year-olds and want to help with identifying what they need, what is working with their youth, and what is getting in the way. The service is free and is individually tailored.

Evidence on au.reachout.com

Collins and colleagues (2011) conducted a mixed methodology study to determine how au.reachout.com was used, level of psychological distress (K-10; [16]), impact of au.reachout.com on mental health literacy and stigma, and help-seeking behaviors. The most frequently accessed pages included "Depression: types, causes, and symptoms, *Mental health difficulties*, and *Mood Disorders*" (p. 44) [15]. The level of psychological distress was significant. Almost 20% of users scores in the high range and 51.8% scores in the very high range. The participants noted that the content on au.reachout.com contributed to their understanding of mental health issues and the options that were available to address mental

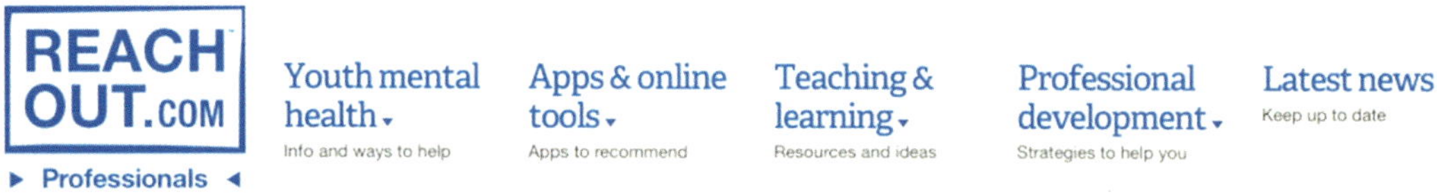

Fig. 19.4 Australia's au.reachout.com Professionals site (Source: http://au.professionals.reachout.com/)

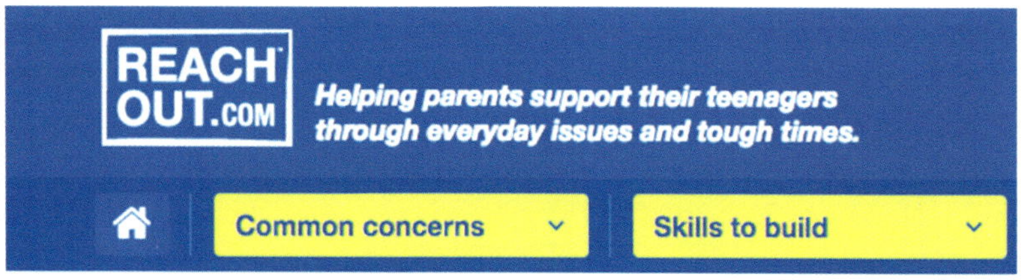

Fig. 19.5 Australia's au.reachout.com Parent website (Source: https://parents.au.reachout.com/)

health issues. The website also helped users to gain an understanding of how other people experienced mental health issues. The participants also reported that they would make friends with someone with a mental health issue (84%), would work with them on a job (68.8%), and would attend a party with them (70.8%).

The impact of au.reachout.com on help-seeking behaviors was mixed. Thirty-five percent of participants said that au.reachout.com helped the person ask for professional help with 43.3% saying that au.reachout.com provided them with information that increased their knowledge of skills to seek help. The participants were more likely to seek help from friends or family; unless their psychological distress was high, then they were less likely to seek help from them. Overall, participants were, however, less likely to seek help from traditional and face-to-face services.

Metcalf and colleagues (2016) [17] conducted a longitudinal study (participants completed surveys at Times 1 and 2; $n = 573$) to determine how au.reachout.com promoted mental health literacy and increased help seeking. The top three reasons that users visited au.reachout.com were to look for help when going through a tough time (54%), look for general info (15%), and look for tips on improving well-being (10%). The two highest categories of information that participants were looking for included information on depression (18%) and anxiety (12%). The data, from the DASS-21 Scores, showed that the participants' level of depression, anxiety, and stress at baseline was alarming. Forty-two percent of participants had extremely severe depression, 37% had extremely severe anxiety, and 16% had extremely severe stress. The data on help-seeking behaviors showed the top four sources of support individuals were likely to use: friends (61%), search engine (50%), parent (45%), and partner/girlfriend/boyfriend/spouse (40%). Thirty-three percent were likely to talk face-to-face with a mental health provider, and 24% were likely to talk with their doctor.

The participants reported high levels of personal stigma toward mental health issues. Researchers explored how a specific, hypothetical diagnosis was associated with how the participant viewed the stigma associated with them. For example, if the person had depression with substance misuse, 39% of respondents said that if they had this diagnosis, they wouldn't tell anyone. For depression, 28% of respondents said that people with depression are unpredictable. If the respondent had psychosis, 25% believed they could snap out of this problem and believed that the problem is not a real medical illness, and people with this problem are unpredictable.

Overall, the sample in this study had high levels of psychological distress. Even with these high levels of psychological distress, their willingness to seek professional help was low, but their willingness to seek help from informal sources was high. Their knowledge of mental health diagnoses was on par with youth from general Australian surveys; however, they showed higher levels of mental health stigma compared to the same population. au.reachout.com shows significant promise in providing youth with opportunities to learn more about mental health and help-seeking opportunities as was evidenced in the change in views about mental health and help-seeking resources used. au.reachout.com continues to develop website components and applications to help support young people going through tough times.

ReachOut.com (United States)

The US version of ReachOut.com is similar to the Australian website, however with fewer features. As with the Australian website, the site targets 13–24-year-olds and includes fact sheets on mental health issues and other issues that adolescents encounter. The site is diverse as it includes information presented on fact sheets, as well as multimedia information presented through videos and audio stories.

The main page of ReachOut.com is presented below (Fig. 19.6).

Evidence on ReachOut.com (United States)

In a study conducted by Keyes and Cash (2012) [10], data were collected, via an online survey, among Californians who visited the site ($n = 95$). Data were collected on why the person was visiting ReachOut.com, time spent on the site, help seeking, mental health stigma, and knowledge of mental illness. The primary reasons for visiting the site were to look for help when they were going through a tough time (26.3%), check out what was new (17.9%), look for information (16.8%), and hear about others' stories (14.7%). Fifty-seven percent of participants reported that

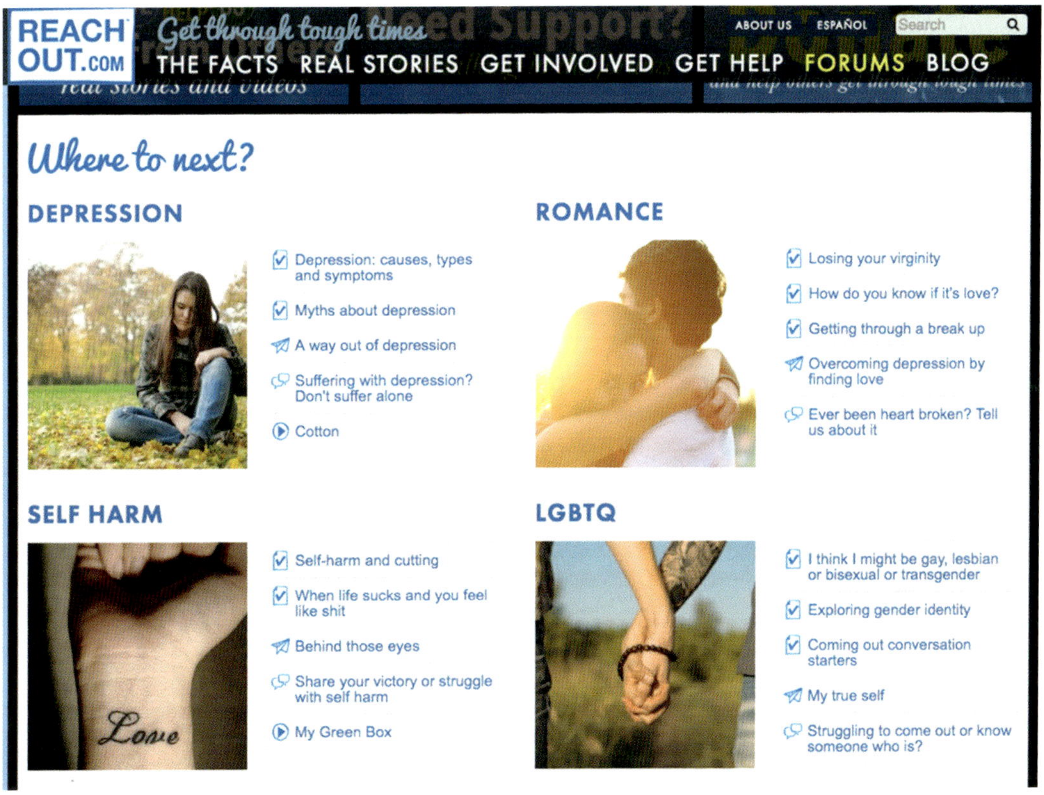

Fig. 19.6 USA ReachOut.com main page (Source: http://us.ReachOut.com/)

they spent more than 10 min on the site that day. When a participant needed help to get through a tough time, they were most likely to speak to a friend (75%) or family member (64.9%). They were least likely to use a phone hotline (12.3%) or a medical doctor (22.2%).

Forty-five percent of participants identified they had good to very good knowledge of mental illness, and 83.3% said they believed that anyone can experience a mental illness. However, 51% agreed that they would not want anyone to know if they, themselves, had a mental illness.

ReachOut.com provides a unique platform for helping youth through difficult times. While the site doesn't have as many features as the Australian site, it does have varied methods for educating and supporting youth during their times of need. Both the Australian and US ReachOut sites embrace the idea that the website will only be good and relevant if youth are included as leaders in the organization. Youth are involved in the planning, creation of the materials, implementation, and evaluation. The Youth Advisory Boards vet all materials that go on the sites. The sites also employ participatory research designs that are co-created with the staff. Youth also participate in the implementation of the methods, analyses, and write-up of the results.

The sites also appear to have good face validity as the site provides materials that cover a wide range of topics that directly affect adolescents. The forums are engaging, and as reported above, the Australian Forum has a large number of users.

How Clinicians Can Use These Sites

ReachOut.com in both Australia and the United States are resources that can help with increasing mental health literacy, reducing mental health stigma, and increasing help seeking. While there are some language differences, the Australian site has the most features and has the most amount of empirical evidence to support its use. However, it is recommended that clinicians look to see what is available on both sites and let their patient know what options are available.

Ideally, the ReachOut.com sites can be used for prevention, education, and early intervention. From a prevention and educational approach, clinicians can post flyers and pamphlets around the waiting rooms and/or in their offices to get their attention in a way that isn't confrontational. See, for example, http://au.reachout.com/get-involved/order-reachout-merchandise. As part of an intervention, a clinician, who recently diagnosed a patient with a mental health issue, can show the site to their patient in an effort to help educate the adolescent on their specific mental health issue. The language and materials that are used on the site about mental health issues have all been vetted through their Youth Advisory Boards, so using the website to help provide additional information is a unique approach.

For example, a 16-year-old adolescent is diagnosed with depression. He isn't sure what depression is and what this new diagnosis means, so the clinician provides him with some information. Using a simple Google search, for the information from the National Institute of Mental Health is informative, however, may not be engaging to an adolescent and/or be written in terms that adolescents may engage with (see Fig. 19.7 below).

If the clinician, however, referred the adolescent to ReachOut.com, the site first discusses "Going Through Tough Times," which can be a less intimidating approach to discussing mental health issues. Second, the site is graphically pleasing and has language that has been vetted by other youth (Figs. 19.8 and 19.9).

Finally, each au.reachout.com page has a "Listen" button to be able to hear the content that is being presented on the page. ReachOut.com provides the patient with a web-based framework to look up other material and possibly engage with other youth who are going through similar issues.

Example poster or pamphlet (Fig. 19.10).

From an intervention approach, the clinician could use the site in multiple ways. From the example above, the information could be used to help provide information and optimally reduce or remove the stigma associated with having a mental illness. The clinician could point the patient to the main site and specific resources and encour-

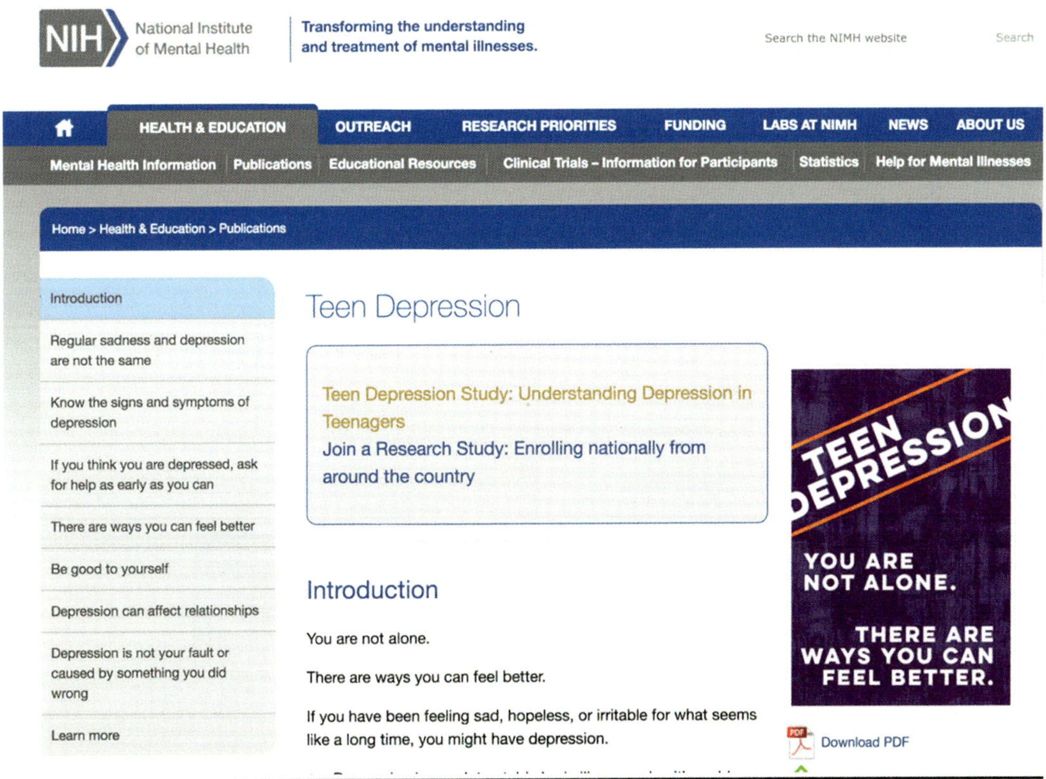

Fig. 19.7 Comparative web page by NIH on teen depression (Source: https://www.nimh.nih.gov/health/publications/teen-depression/index.shtml)

age the adolescent to check out the site. At future meetings, the site could be used to discuss any thoughts or feelings the adolescent had while looking at the material. The clinician could probe further to see if the information was helpful and had changed his/her mind about having a mental health issue. The clinician could also use the information on the websites about help seeking to determine if this information was likely to increase the likelihood that the adolescent would want to seek additional help. The site may also provide the clinician and adolescent with a starting point to continue having conversations about mental health and any other life issues that are causing them difficulties.

The clinician could also access materials and resources from the ReachOut.com Professionals site (au.professionals.reachout.com). Finally, the clinician could also provide the adolescent's parent and/or guardian with the parent version of the site (https://parents.au.reachout.com/).

The resources available on the US and Australian version of ReachOut.com are comprehensive and engaging. They aim to provide a safe space for adolescents to learn more about mental health and life issues (e.g., sexuality, bullying, etc.) and seek help if needed.

We R Native

According to the Center for Native American Youth, the American Indian and Alaska Native (AI/AN; Native) population is young and swiftly growing [18]. Youth 25 years old and younger make up 41% of the 5.4 million AI/AN population. Between 2000 and 2010, the AI/AN population grew 27%, compared to less than 10% for the total US population [19].

AI/AN Adolescent Mental Health. Despite immense cultural resilience and pride, AI/AN youth are one of the most at-risk populations in

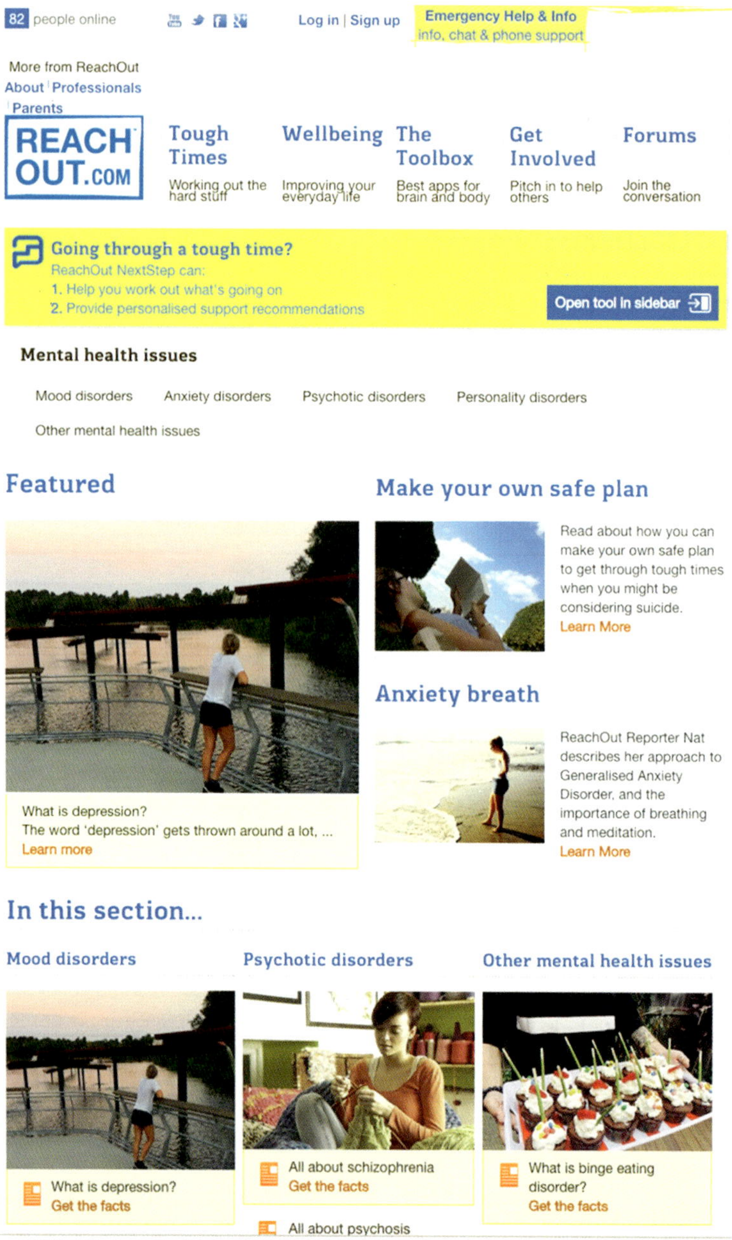

Fig. 19.8 USA ReachOut.com comparative web page for teen depression (Source: http://au.reachout.com/tough-times/mental-health-issues

the United States, caused, in part, by enduring intergenerational trauma, forced relocation and assimilation, the boarding school system, and other devastating US policies [18]. Native youth today often live in communities that are disproportionately affected by high rates of poverty, unemployment, health disparities, substance abuse, low education attainment, family violence, and crime [20]. As a result, AI/AN youth are disproportionally impacted by high rates of stress, depression, and suicide. Over 21% of AI/AN high school students seriously considered suicide, and 14.7% attempted suicide in 2010 (national averages 15.8% and 7.8%, respectively) [21]. Moreover, 78% of AI/AN high school students have consumed alcohol (national average, 71%), and 22.3% have been bullied at school (national average, 20.1%). As a result, suicide

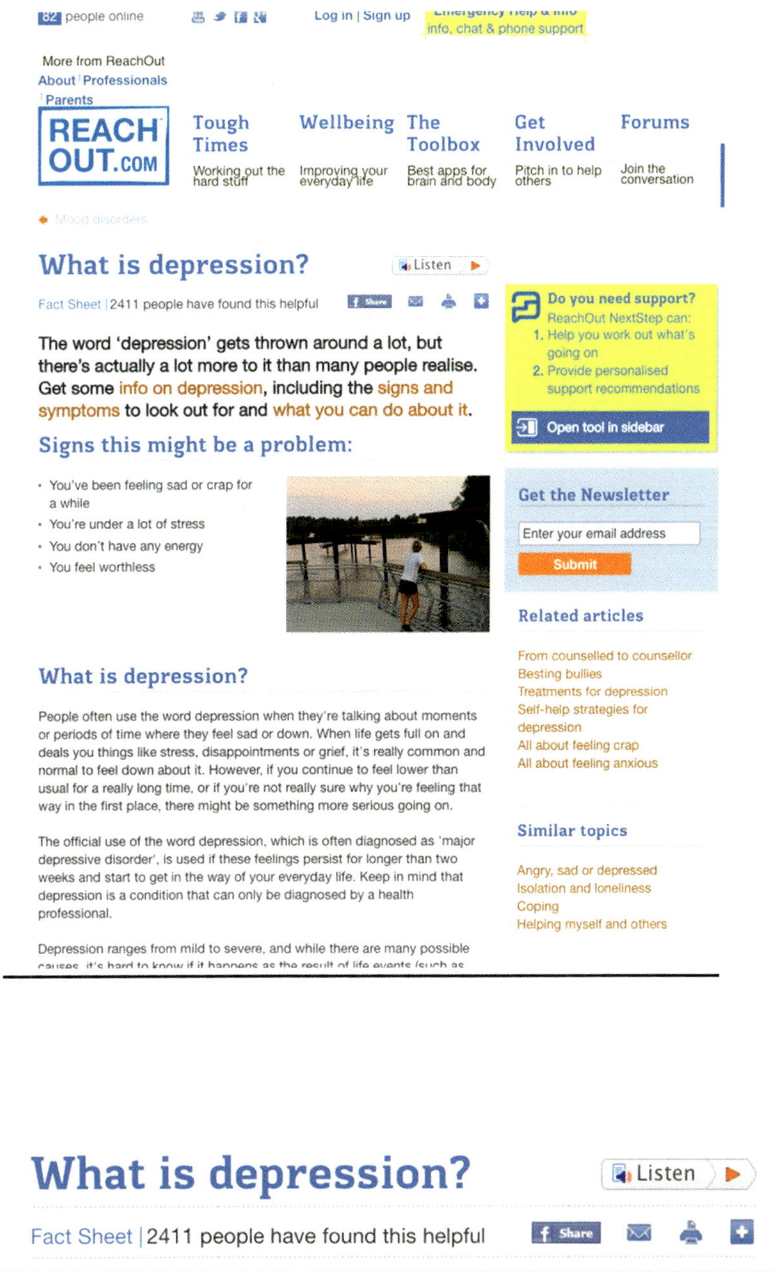

Fig. 19.9 Additional material for comparisons between NIH and ReachOut.com web page (Source: http://au.reachout.com/depression)

remains the second leading cause of death for AI/AN teens and young adults [22].

To raise awareness and reverse these concerning trends, Native youth across the United States are stepping up and getting actively involved in mental health and suicide prevention efforts [23]. Harnessing the power of peer education, technology, and social media, AI/AN youth are leading the way—promoting cultural pride, community connectedness, and cultural teachings in suicide prevention efforts—all protective factors for physical, mental, and spiritual health [18].

Tech Use in Indian Country. While the speed and quality of Internet access and cell phone coverage are highly variable in tribal communities across the United States, it is swiftly

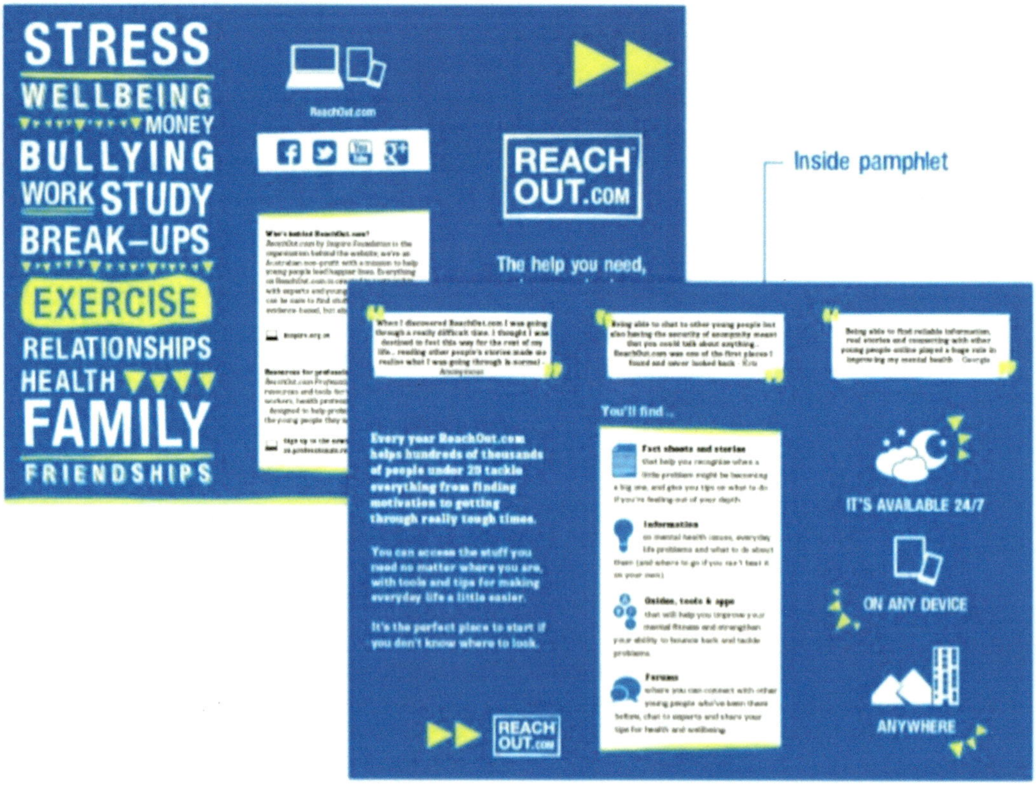

Fig. 19.10 Example posters and pamphlets from Australia's au.reachout.com (Source: https://au.reachout.com/get-involved/order-reachout-merchandise)

and steadily improving. In 2009, urban and rural AI/AN youth (13–21 years old) in the Pacific Northwest reported frequent media technology use, mirroring patterns reported by teens in the general population [24]. In 2016, in a national survey of over 675 AI/AN teens and young adults, 78% had regular access to a smartphone, and 46% had regular access to a computer. Over 92% reported accessing the Internet from a phone on a daily or weekly basis, and 50% reported going online from a computer as often (Rushing PI, report pending).

Online Health Information Seeking. In 2009, over 75% of urban and rural AI/AN youth in the Pacific Northwest reported ever going online to get health information [24]. By 2016, online health seeking was the norm for AI/AN youth. In a national survey of over 675 AI/AN youth, over 62% of AI/AN teens and young adults reported getting health information from the Internet on a weekly or monthly basis, and 66% received health information from social networking sites as often; 45% reported having searched for "stress or anxiety" and 40% for "depression or suicide" on the Internet (Rushing PI, report pending). When asked about sensitive health topics like depression or birth control, respondents reported feeling *most* comfortable going online (39%), talking to a friend or sibling (37%), or talking to a clinician (26%), trusted adult (24%), or parent (27%) about their questions or concerns.

We R Native Development

Recognizing that a broad, multimedia health service was needed to compete for Native youth's time and attention online, *We R Native* was jointly designed by the Northwest Portland Area Indian Health Board's suicide prevention project (THRIVE) and its sexual health promotion project (Project Red Talon).

Partners and Roles. The Northwest Portland Area Indian Health Board (NPAIHB) is a tribal nonprofit organization that serves the 43 federally recognized tribes in ID, OR, and WA (Pacific Northwest or NW). The NPAIHB has collaborated with the NW tribes, states, federal agencies, and community partners on AI/AN health research, surveillance, and policy change for over 35 years.

THRIVE project (Tribal Health: Reaching out InVolves Everyone) has worked with the NW tribes to prevent suicide since 2009; and Project Red Talon has provided training and technical assistance to tribes and tribal organizations throughout the United States on implementing and evaluating culturally appropriate sexual health and STI/HIV prevention programs since 1988. Both projects seek to promote protective factors among AI/AN youth (i.e., health seeking, cultural identification, community connections through community service, etc.), connect youth to teen-friendly health resources, and build resilience and coping skills.

To generate a wireframe and content for the *We R Native* website, NPAIHB staff worked in close collaboration with ReachOut USA: us.ReachOut.com. All of *We R Native*'s mental health pages were provided by ReachOut and then reviewed and edited by AI/AN youth and Indian Health Service mental health staff to improve cultural relevance. To create the *We R Native* brand and website, the NPAIHB hired a media firm (Indig), who helped design the name, logo, site imagery, and interactive features, with substantial iterative input from AI/AN youth across the United States along the way.

We R Native: A Multimedia Health Resource. Guided by this formative research, the Northwest Portland Area Indian Health Board launched *We R Native* in 2011, as a multimedia health resource for Native youth, by Native youth [24, 25]. The service includes an interactive website (www.weRnative.org), a text messaging service (Text NATIVE to 97779), a Facebook page, a YouTube channel, Instagram, Twitter, and print marketing materials. Special features include monthly contests, community service grants ($475), and an interactive "Ask Auntie" Q&A service. The service includes content on social, emotional, physical, sexual, and spiritual health, as well as on AI/AN culture, the environment, and health activism.

The website contains over 330 health and wellness pages, all reviewed by Native youth and experts in public health, mental health, community engagement, and activism. By holistically covering a variety of topics important to Native youth, the service delivers sensitive health messages within and between popular and trending topics. For example, messages promoting STD testing can be imbedded in content on dating in social media posts, blending popular and AI/AN culture, with important facts on how youth can protect themselves (Fig. 19.11).

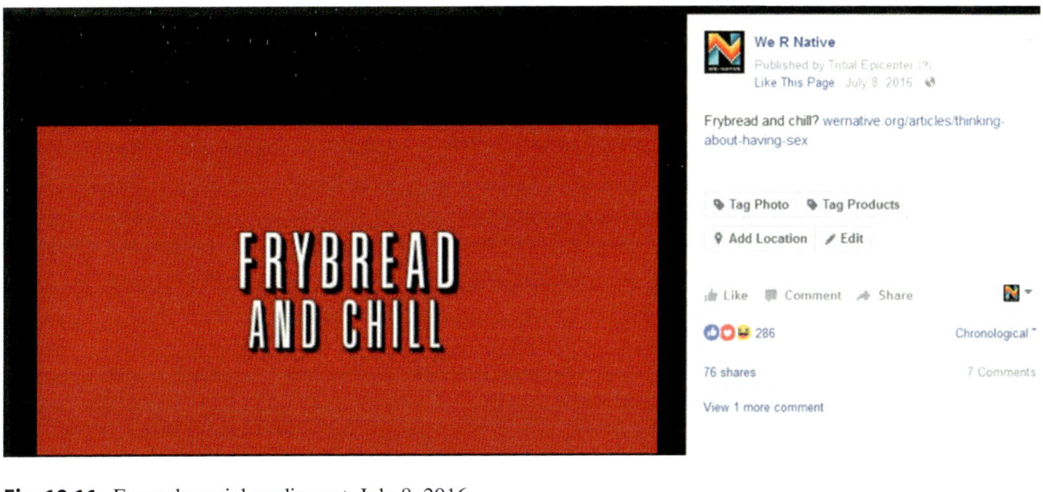

Fig. 19.11 Example social media post, July 8, 2016

We R Native Goals and Strategies. *We R Native* strives to address the health and social issues important to Native youth, while promoting holistic health and positive identity. Building upon the core principles of positive youth development, *We R Native*:

- Provides age-appropriate health information addressing physical, mental, social, and spiritual health
- Promotes education, community engagement, and community service
- Promotes cultural identity and pride
- Highlights youth-friendly media and current events that reflect healthy social norms
- Offers safe "spaces" where Native youth can feel comfortable, empowered, and connected to other AI/AN youth, regardless of their age, race, gender, cultural identity, language, sexual orientation, disability, or literacy

Collectively, their overarching goals are to connect AI/AN youth to culturally appropriate tools and resources that promote healthy behaviors and peer norms and build protective factors against suicide and substance abuse at the individual, family, and community level.

Use, Reach, and Demographics. *We R Native* collects and monitors digital metrics recommended by www.digitalgov.gov. Since its launch, the website has received over 367,000 page views. Roughly 2/3 of the website's users are female; 1/3 are male. The average user visits three pages per visit and stays on the site 3:00 min. Similar user demographics and mobile technology use rates have been observed within our other *We R Native* communication channels. By February 2016, *We R Native*'s YouTube channel had 450 health and wellness videos with over 77,300 video views. The *We R Native* text messaging service delivers weekly text messages to over 4400 subscribers located across the United States.

To date, the *We R Native* Facebook page has over 42,000 likes and over 4200 Twitter followers. Altogether, *We R Native* reaches over 32,000 users per week through its various channels, a growing number of whom are accessing the content from mobile devices.

Mental health topics account for approximately 15% of the site's total traffic, and culture accounts for nearly 20% of the site's traffic.

Messaging Campaigns. To design health promotion messages and campaigns that resonate with AI/AN youth, the NPAIHB uses social marketing, an evidence-based planning process that has been shown to improve the impact of health promotion messages. The framework uses formative research to identify priority populations; segment the community into distinct audiences; pretest messages, materials, and strategies with the appropriate audience; and monitor the campaign to assess its effectiveness [26]. Iterative phases of review and community feedback ensure that resultant campaign products reflect the preferred language, tone, attitudes, norms, and values of the target audience.

Every month, *We R Native* disseminates messaging campaigns that promote healthy norms and behaviors, aligning campaign topics with national health observances. Two recent examples include a campaign to address concerning social media posts and a suicide prevention campaign:

- **Concerning Post Campaign:** In 2015, tribal health educators in the Pacific NW expressed concern about the prevalence of "concerning posts" on social media and links between mental health, cyberbullying, and suicide. To better understand AI/AN adolescents' perspectives on concerning content viewed on social media, the NPAIHB partnered with the Social Media Adolescent Health Research Team at Seattle Children's Hospital to carry out focus groups with AI/AN youth. Most youth participating in the focus groups reported that they'd seen concerning posts by their peers on social media, and Facebook was their preferred platform to intervene (Fig. 19.12).

THRIVE then partnered with *We R Native* to deliver a series of campaign messages directly to Native youth about how to respond to concerning posts on social media. The messages were delivered in January 2015 and again in 2016, reaching over 178,600 viewers in 2016, with an average reach of 44,673 people per day. An ongoing study

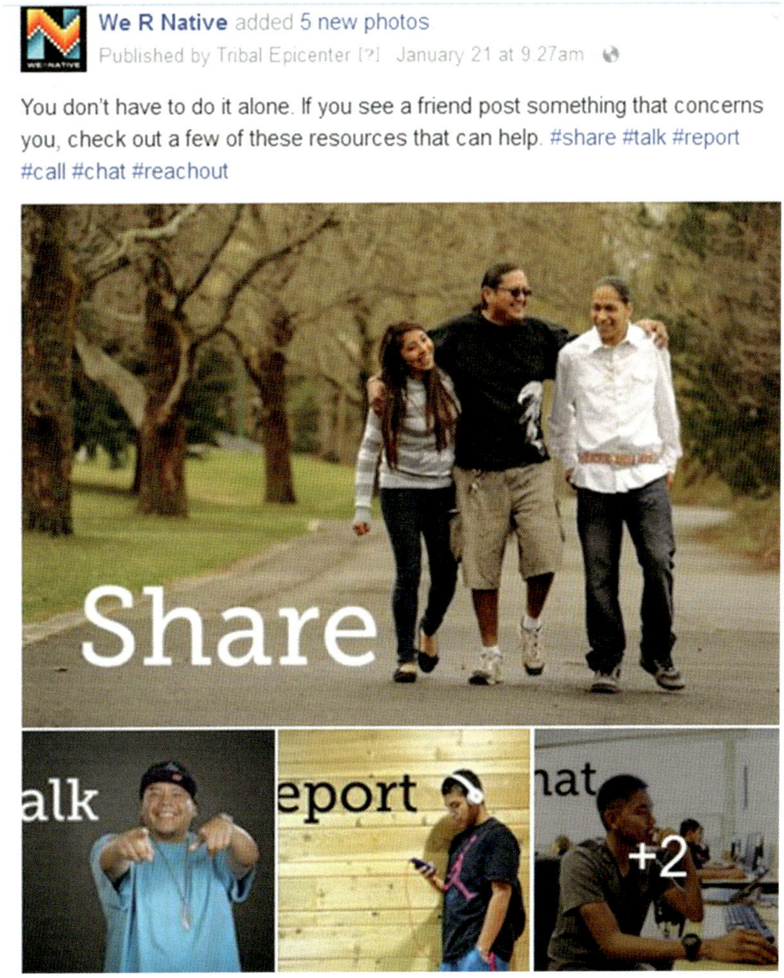

Fig. 19.12 Facebook Post

is now evaluating whether an educational training video for parents and adults who work with Native youth—that offers proactive ways to address concerning social media posts, including intervention and referral skills—will improve the identification of high-risk youth, linking them to timely, appropriate care.

- **We Are Connected. #WeNeedYouHere:** In 2015, THRIVE launched a campaign that encourages youth to identify suicide warning signs and seek help; and in 2016, a sister campaign for LGBT and Two-Spirit youth: *Loved and Accepted. #WeNeedYouHere.* The campaign's images, lived-experience videos, and blog posts were promoted via *We R Native*'s media channels (website, Facebook, YouTube, Instagram, Text Message). Together, the campaign and the *#WeNeedYouHere* hashtag were included on over 150 posts, reaching over 1.4 million people from September 2015 to September 2016.

Altogether, *We R Native*'s messages addressing mental health, suicide, bullying, and drug and alcohol abuse reached nearly 2.5 million viewers last year and helped promote cultural pride, resilience, leadership skills, and youth empowerment. These messages are further amplified by a cadre of 100+ Youth Ambassadors, who help generate multimedia content for the site, host outreach and awareness events in their local communities, and represent *We R Native* at national youth conferences.

Conclusion

Many AI/AN youth receive insufficient mental health education and clinical health services, and technology-based interventions can help bridge this gap in ways that are familiar and inviting. Social marketing and formative research activities can make technology-based health interventions more meaningful and relevant for AI/AN youth. Much work remains to be done, however, to adapt and rigorously evaluate mental health interventions in AI/AN communities. Fortunately, exciting progress is being made in the field. By providing mental information across multiple media platforms, we hope to reach the greatest number of AI/AN youth, when and where each young person is ready.

How Clinicians Can Use This Site:

- Visit *We R Native*'s "Gear" page to access health fact sheets, tip cards, posters, and other free promotional items. Order online or print these materials to connect AI/AN patients to the service.
- Visit *We R Native*'s sister site for adults—HealthyNativeYouth.org—a one-stop shop for health advocates who want to expand learning opportunities for Native youth. The site contains guides and tools to deliver effective, age-appropriate health curricula.

beyondblue

beyondblue started in Australia in October 2000 to raise awareness, through media campaigns, on depression and stigma. In 2011, beyondblue added a campaign around anxiety and recently added suicide prevention to their purpose. Their goal is to equip "everyone in Australia with the knowledge and skills to protect their own mental health…support those around them….making anxiety, depression, and suicide part of everyday conversation" [27]. In regard to adolescents, they target schools and universities to promote mental health literacy, reduce stigma, and increase help seeking. Two initiatives for adolescents are Brains can have a mind of their own (The Brain) and MindMatters. The Brain and MindMatters provide tools to help promote mental health literacy, assist with safety planning, and provide a framework for schools. The focus of beyondblue centers around mental health promotion and awareness to help teenagers seek support.

Youth beyondblue

The Brain or Brains can have a mind of their own [28] was developed as a mechanism to educate young people (12–18 years old) on identifying symptoms of anxiety, depression, and suicide and then promote help-seeking behaviors. A brain, with the slogan "a mind of its own," was used as the main character to help people realize that depression and anxiety aren't caused by something they personally did wrong, but rather, the brain operates, in layperson's term, on its own (Fig. 19.13).

The campaign is intended to normalize depression and anxiety. The website provides guidance on how to access to The Brain videos and with the intended goal that youth are intrigued to learn more about the symptoms (Fig. 19.14). Once

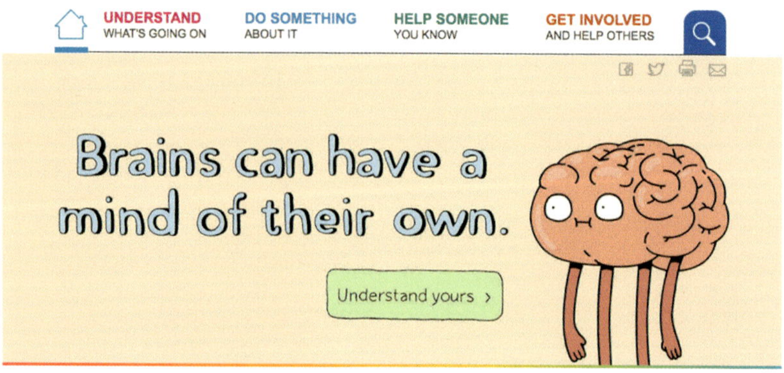

Fig. 19.13 Brains can have a mind of their own quiz page (Source: https://www.youthbeyondblue.com/understand-what's-going-on/the-brain-quiz/)

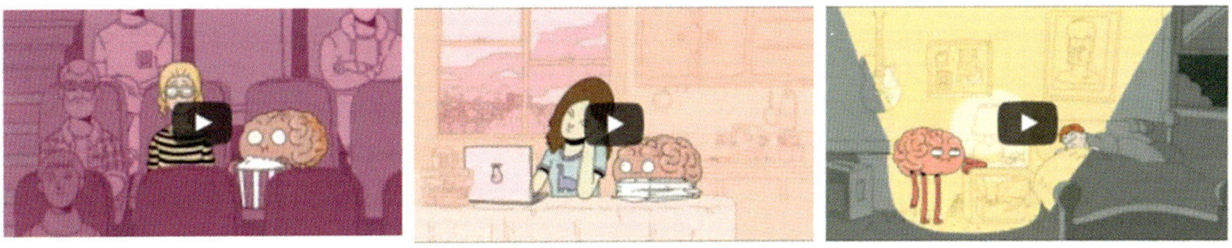

Fig. 19.14 Brains can have a mind of their own videos (Source: https://www.youthbeyondblue.com/)

they visit the website, they are then guided to a set of mental health resources that are age specific and have been vetted for use with this population. The pictures below show three videos that focus on depression symptoms: (1) no longer enjoying activities, (2) difficulty concentrating, and (3) having difficulties sleeping.

While The Brain campaign isn't a direct intervention, research has shown that there is power in reducing mental health stigma so the person is willing to seek help [5]. The campaign is situated in Australia; however, the messages can be translated to the United States.

How Clinicians Can Use This Site

The Brain videos can be used by clinicians to help introduce the concepts of depression, anxiety, and suicide in a "quirky" way that may seem to be less threatening or uncomfortable. If a clinician believes an adolescent has depression and/or anxiety, the clinician can watch these videos with the adolescent and start the conversation there.

Optimally, these videos and the other beyondblue materials can serve as a starting point to educate the adolescents on mental health with the goal of reducing the stigma associated with mental health.

MindMatters

MindMatters.edu.au is a free, evidence-based program provided in secondary schools in Australia to help improve the well-being of adolescents and address mental health. Their central tenets are to promote, prevent, intervene early, and improve resilience and relationships. The approach focuses on well-being of the entire school, including students, staff, and administration. MindMatters is a framework that schools can adopt, where the school is provided with planning tools, structure for implementing programs, curriculum, evaluation tools, and ongoing support to promote mental health strategies in their school. They believe that "the best mental health strategy is one that prevents issues from arising in the first place."

MindMatters provides planning materials that guide the school through the process of creating an environment that supports well-being and positive mental health. The framework is comprised of four key components: positive school community, student skills for resilience, parents and families, and support for students experiencing mental health difficulties. Professional learning modules are provided through online videos, the MindMatters expert panel, and downloadable resources for each module.

Evidence

MindMatters was developed based on evidence from the KidsMatter Primary and KidsMatter Early Childhood programs and was adapted to secondary school (middle to high school) populations. Dix and colleagues' (2012) [29] study on KidsMatter found that schools that had high implementation of the program had a significantly positive effect on a student's academic achievement. Specifically, the quality of the implementation of the program was "equivalent to 6 months more schooling by Year 7, over and above any influence of socioeconomic background" (p. 45). Evidence on how the MindMatters program affects school and/or mental health outcomes is currently not available. However, statistics are available on the usage of

MindMatters across Australia: 1433 participating schools across the territories, with 35 schools in the Australian Capital Territory, 504 in New South Wales, 64 in the Northern Territory, 267 in Queensland, 166 in South Australia, 62 in Tasmania, 201 in Victoria, and 134 in Western Australia. There have also been 68,720 modules completed, 9145 event attendees, and 31,572 people signed up for MindMatters [30].

How Clinicians Can Use This Site

MindMatters was developed as a school-based system in Australia, which may not initially seem as a useful resource for clinicians here in the United States. The MindMatters can be used in at least two ways: resources and modules can be shared with clinical staff and other health-care professionals and as a framework to engage the local school system in understanding and supporting mental health in their schools. While not all of the MindMatters planning and materials may be useful, there are specific parts of the curriculum that can be shared and utilized by multiple stakeholders. The MindMatters materials are comprehensive, structured, free, and can be shared.

The mental health system has more demand than supply in many communities. MindMatters could possibly be used as a framework to engage local schools or the school district to promote mental health and well-being. The entire curriculum may not be possible to implement; however, there are numerous resources that could be adapted to facilitate use among clinicians and the community.

That'sNotCool.com

That'sNotCool.com was developed to help adolescents learn more information about digital dating abuse and develop strategies about how to prevent dating violence. Similar to the other youth-based initiatives, the content is developed with youth. The content was developed in conjunction with Futures Without Violence, Office on Violence Against Women, and The Advertising Council. The content also includes information from groups that are marginalized including Native youth, LGBTQI, youth with disabilities, and youth of color. The website also includes content for adults including educators, advocates, and ambassadors. The site was awarded a Webby Award and The Communicator Award. Currently, the site does not provide any information on the effectiveness of the site on reducing dating violence. There are also no materials on any ongoing studies on the site.

The website uses a number of techniques to help adolescents understand more about digital dating issues, positive dating behaviors, and strategies to address digital dating abuse. The main components of the website are the videos, quizzes, and knowledge building. Their components include video on how to "Delete Digital Abuse," Cool Not Cool Quiz Cards, Statistics on Digital abuse, Adult Ally Tools, Social Hub, the TNC video channel, Ambassador stories, and social networking. They have content on Facebook, Tumblr, Twitter, YouTube, Instagram, and Pinterest. An example of one of the quiz modules is presented in Fig. 19.15.

How Clinicians Can Use This Site

That's not cool can provide clinicians with another youth-friendly mechanism to discuss issues that the adolescent may not be willing to discuss in person. That's not cool has an "Adult Allies" section, where clinicians and others can sign up to access free resources related to digital dating and online safety and boundaries. Once in the Allies section, there are numerous areas that can be accessed: "Overview," "Learn," "Teach," "Organize," "Engage," and "Help." Resources can be accessed and downloaded for free within each of these areas. Under the "Help" area, the clinician can explore "Get Help" resources that will help the clinician talk with adolescents about digital safety, in language that makes sense to the adolescent (https://thatsnotcool.com/help/). Also under "Help," there is a "Give Help" section that provides resources on teen dating, talking about

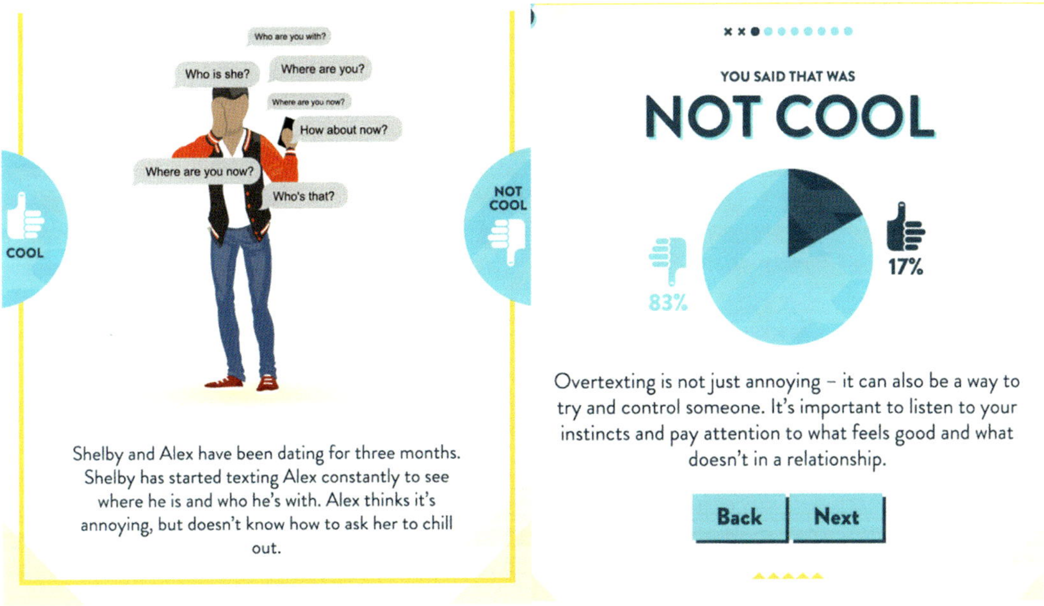

Fig. 19.15 That's Not Cool quiz (Source: http://www.coolnotcoolquiz.org/)

dating violence, and a brochure to address relationship abuse.

The clinician can use the site and resources as prevention or tertiary intervention. From a prevention approach, the clinician could play the PSA videos in their waiting room and place pamphlets and posters in the waiting room. That's not cool could be used as a supplemental intervention to explore with the adolescent or provide as resources. For example, if the clinician assesses that the adolescent is struggling with dating issues and technology or sexting, the clinician can introduce and walk through the website and materials with the adolescent. During follow-up sessions, the clinician can use That's not cool as a way to bring up difficult topics and guide any other conversations.

AnxietyBC™ and AnxietyBC™ Youth

AnxietyBC™ (Anxiety Disorders Association of British Columbia) was established in 1999 as a nonprofit organization in Canada that uses evidence-based tools and technology to help individuals learn more about and address anxiety (https://www.anxietybc.com/about_us.php).

The AnxietyBC Youth page is geared toward adolescents. The site includes fact sheets, quizzes, resources, and videos (Fig. 19.16).

The user can access each of the tabs at the top (Anxiety 101, Facing Fears, Thinking Right, How to Chill, Videos, Health Habits, and Common Problems).

AnxietyBC Youth tabs use a unique approach to present the information in a relatable and graphically pleasing manner. With each highlighted area, the pictures guide the user through different areas he/she may want to explore based on what they want to know or do about anxiety. The Anxiety 101 tab has different types of information on anxiety and includes a self-guided quiz to help the user determine if anxiety is an issue for them (Fig. 19.17).

The Facing Fears tab walks the user through exercises on how to face fears, what does exposure mean, structured activities to help them face their fears, and rewarding themselves when they have overcome fears (Fig. 19.18).

The Thinking Right page includes materials on positive thinking, being kinder to oneself, and exposing thinking traps (Fig. 19.19). The puzzle provides the user with tools for how to think differently including "Challenge your Stinkin' Thinkin"

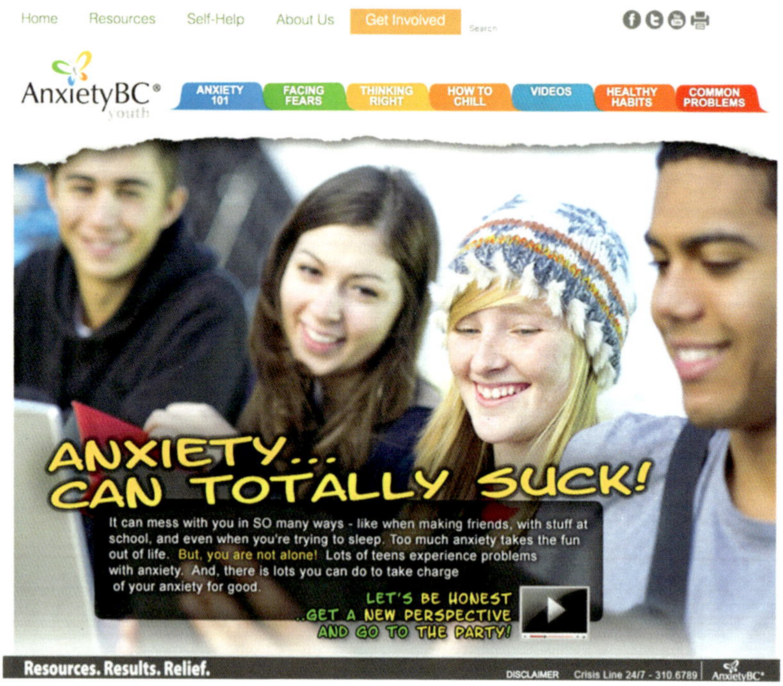
Home
Resources
Self-Help
About Us
Get Involved
AnxietyBC®
youth
ANXIETY 101
FACING FEARS
THINKING RIGHT
HOW TO CHILL
VIDEOS
HEALTHY HABITS
COMMON PROBLEMS
ANXIETY...
CAN TOTALLY SUCK!
It can mess with you in SO many ways - like when making friends, with stuff at school, and even when you're trying to sleep. Too much anxiety takes the fun out of life. But, you are not alone! Lots of teens experience problems with anxiety. And, there is lots you can do to take charge of your anxiety for good.
LET'S BE HONEST
..GET A NEW PERSPECTIVE
AND GO TO THE PARTY!
Resources. Results. Relief.
DISCLAIMER
Crisis Line 24/7 - 310.6789

Fig. 19.16 AnxietyBC Youth home page (Source: http://youth.anxietybc.com/)

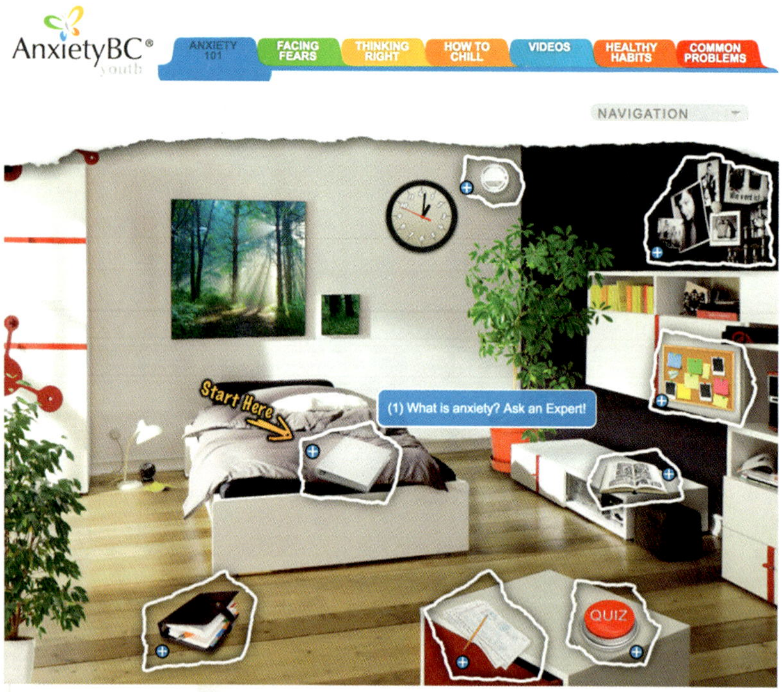
AnxietyBC®
youth
ANXIETY 101
FACING FEARS
THINKING RIGHT
HOW TO CHILL
VIDEOS
HEALTHY HABITS
COMMON PROBLEMS
NAVIGATION
Start Here
(1) What is anxiety? Ask an Expert!
QUIZ

Fig. 19.17 AnxietyBC Youth Anxiety 101 tab (Source: http://youth.anxietybc.com/anxiety-101)

"Telling Yourself Helpful Things," "Letting Thoughts Go," and "Make Uncertainty Your Friend."

How to Chill tab provides the user with different approaches to relaxing (Fig. 19.20). Some of the approaches include visualizations, mindfulness exercises, and other approaches to relaxing.

The AnxietyBC Youth website also includes tabs where users can watch videos and learn other ways to address anxiety.

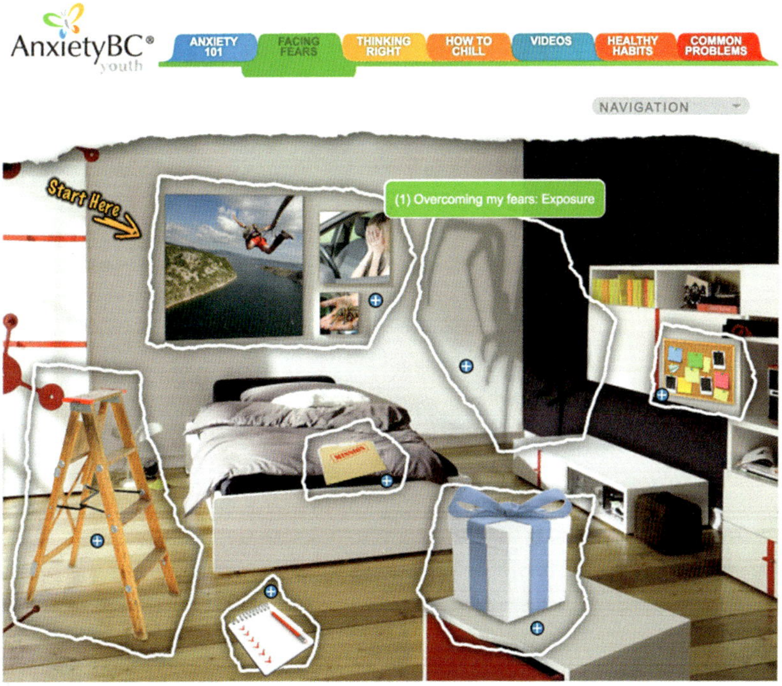

Fig. 19.18 AnxietyBC Youth Facing Fears tab (Source: http://youth.anxietybc.com/facing-fears)

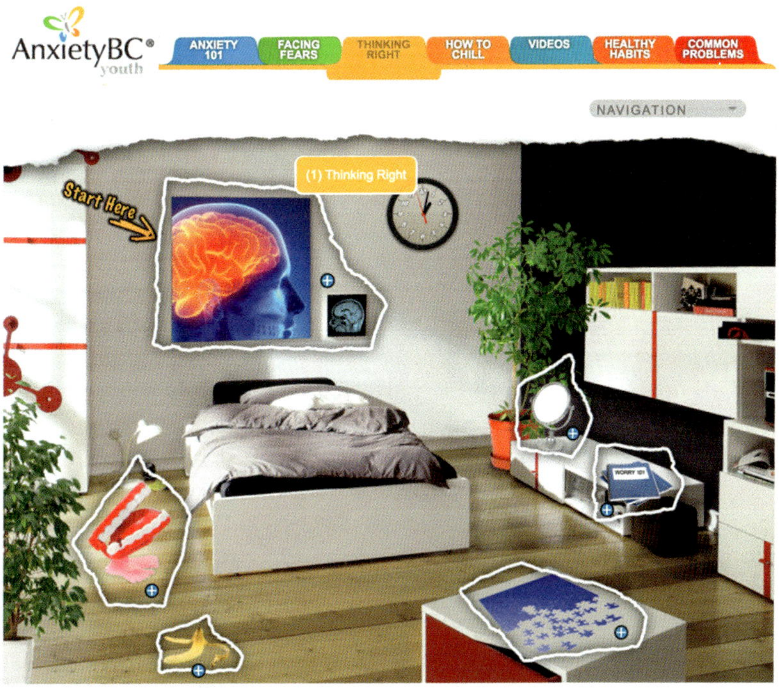

Fig. 19.19 AnxietyBC Youth Thinking Right tab (Source: http://youth.anxietybc.com/right-thinking/)

MindShift App

The MindShift app operates on the same premise as the AnxietyBC app, where there are different domains that the user can explore. Examples from the MindShift app screens are presented in Fig. 19.21. The app helps the user tailor his/her specific experiences and goals around anxiety and download resources to have on-the-go.

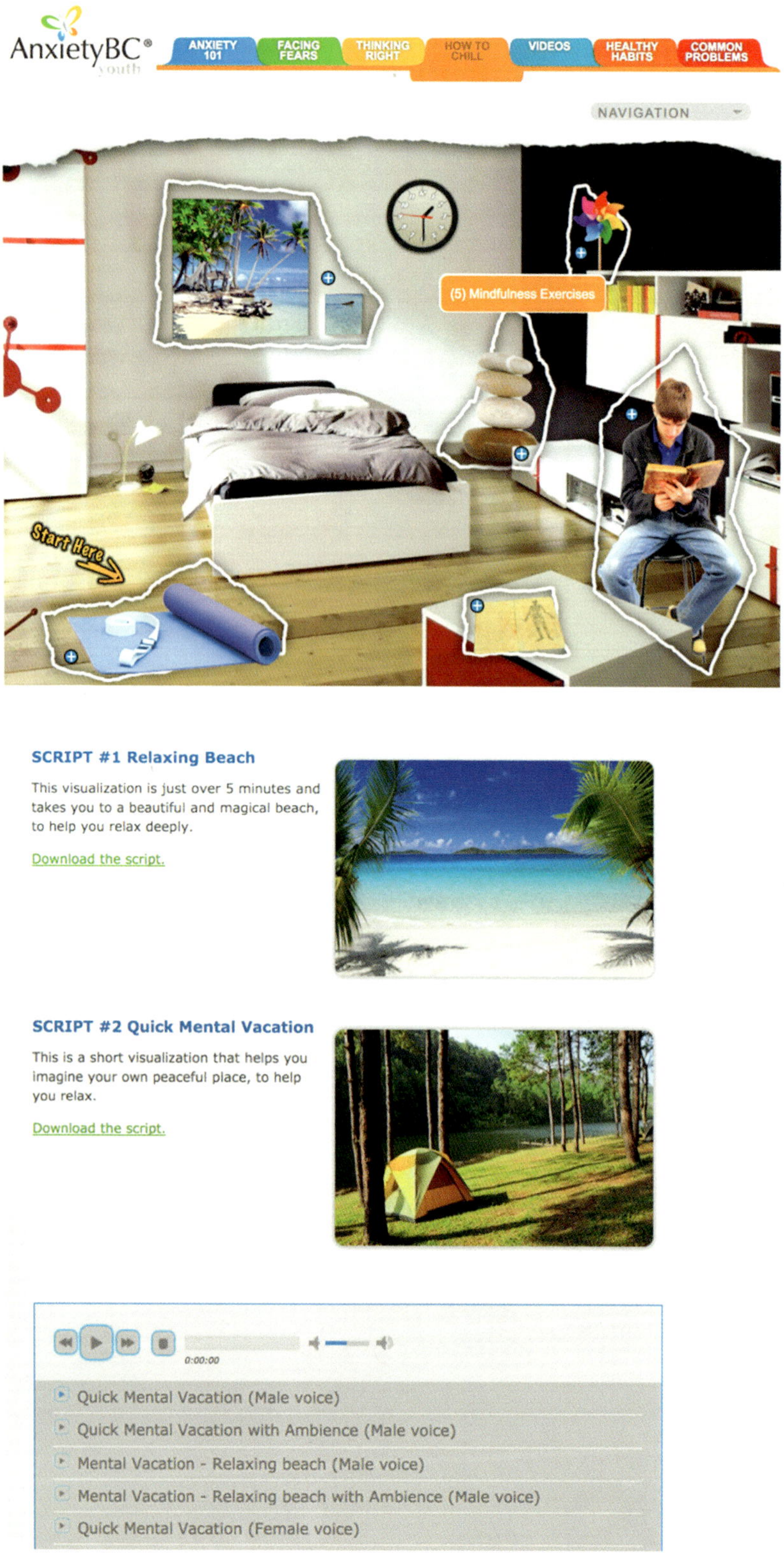
AnxietyBC®
youth
ANXIETY 101
FACING FEARS
THINKING RIGHT
HOW TO CHILL
VIDEOS
HEALTHY HABITS
COMMON PROBLEMS
NAVIGATION
(5) Mindfulness Exercises
Start Here
SCRIPT #1 Relaxing Beach
This visualization is just over 5 minutes and takes you to a beautiful and magical beach, to help you relax deeply.
Download the script.
SCRIPT #2 Quick Mental Vacation
This is a short visualization that helps you imagine your own peaceful place, to help you relax.
Download the script.
0:00:00
Quick Mental Vacation (Male voice)
Quick Mental Vacation with Ambience (Male voice)
Mental Vacation - Relaxing beach (Male voice)
Mental Vacation - Relaxing beach with Ambience (Male voice)
Quick Mental Vacation (Female voice)

Fig. 19.20 AnxietyBC Youth How to Chill tab (Source: http://youth.anxietybc.com/relaxation/)

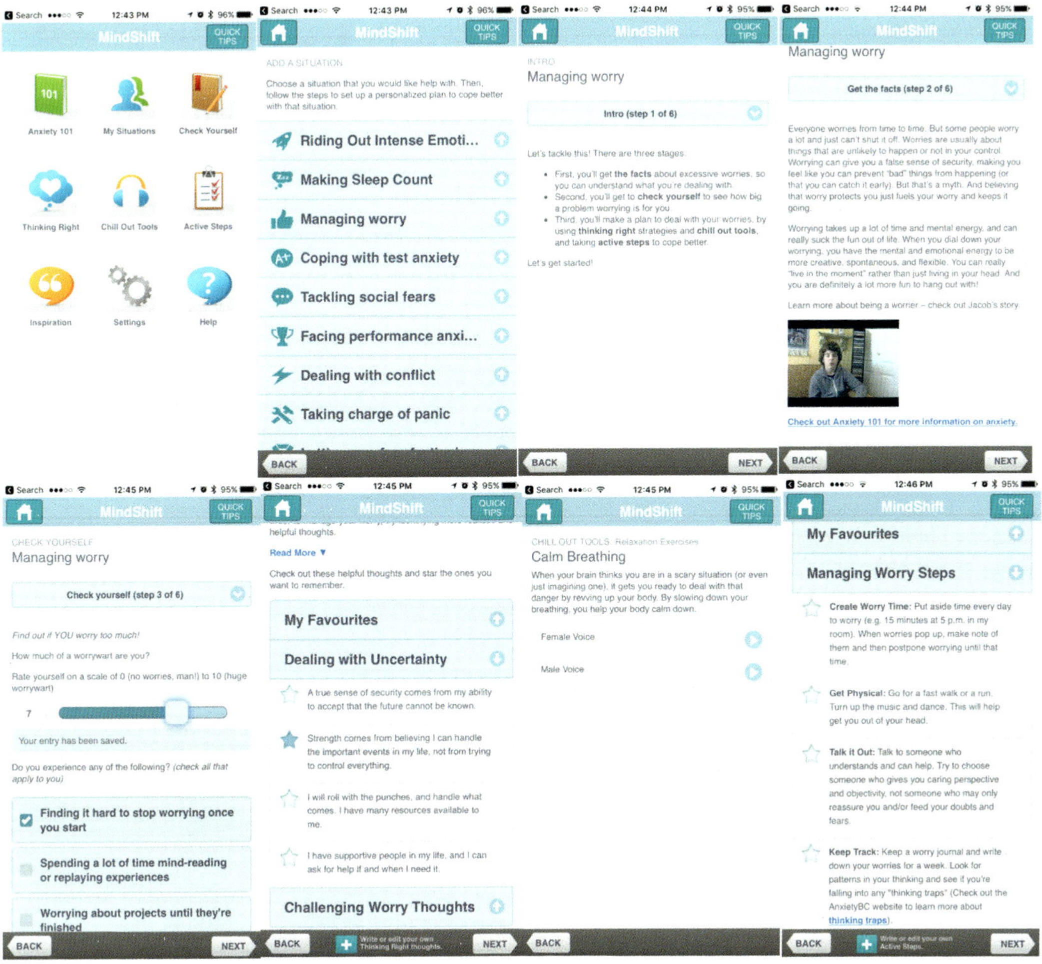

Fig. 19.21 AnxietyBC Youth MindShift app

AnxietyBC also has presence on Facebook, YouTube, and Twitter (Fig. 19.22).

How Clinicians Can Use This Site

Similar to the other resources and initiatives presented in this chapter, the clinician can direct their adolescent patients and parents to the site and website to review and download the resources. With the MindShift app, the clinician could walk through the app with the youth, and they could co-develop a treatment plan with the app's recommendations as the treatment. The clinician could ask the patient to complete a brief anxiety assessment scale prior to introducing the app, and they could monitor progress over time. The clinician could also use the app and website's resources as stand-alone treatments for the adolescent to use in between appointments.

Case Study

Tyler is a 16-year-old boy, who is a junior in high school. He lives with his father in a two-bedroom duplex in a small town outside of Dallas, Texas. Two years ago, Tyler's mother committed suicide after years of struggling with major depression. Tyler always thought that his mother was sad, but never understood that she had been diagnosed with depression. Tyler was often embarrassed

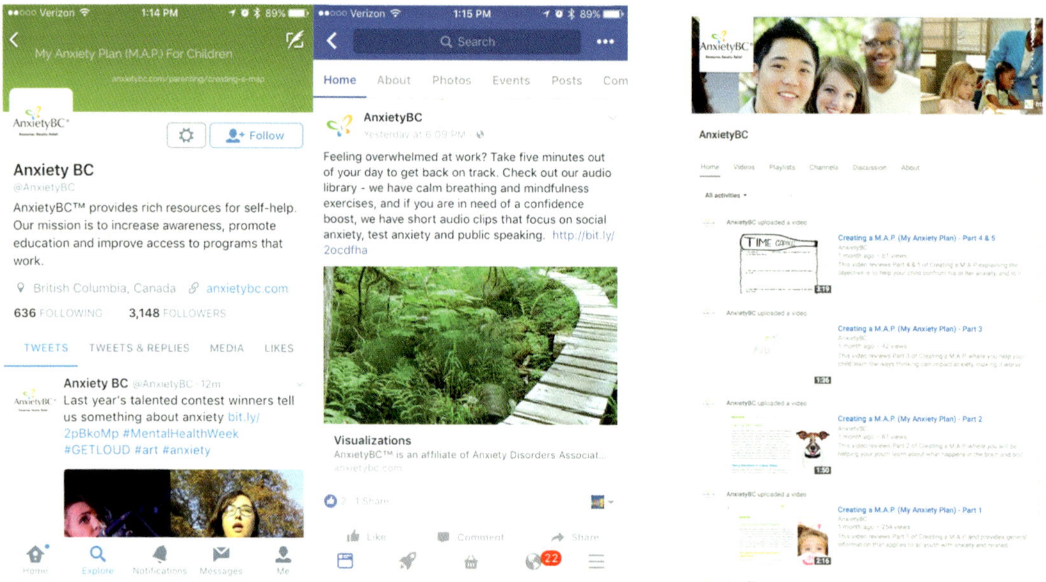

Fig. 19.22 AnxietyBC Youth Twitter, Facebook, and YouTube examples

that his mom didn't seem like the other moms, and he rarely had friends over to his house.

Over the past 2 months, Tyler started skipping school and has not been hanging out with his friends like he used to. One of Tyler's best friends, Alyssa, started worrying about Tyler and decided to look up information on depression. Alyssa struggled to find information on depression and adolescents that wasn't too technical or wasn't written about adult depression. After doing several Google searches, Alyssa found these two sites, ReachOut.com and au.reachout.com websites, and was able to find ways that she could help her friend. She checked out ReachOut.com and was intrigued that there was a specific section for Getting Help when you are worried about a friend (http://us.ReachOut.com/get-help/help-a-friend). She spent time reading through the fact sheets and learned a few ways to start conversations with Tyler about his feelings. She also appreciated that the fact sheets weren't written for a textbook, but were relevant to her and her friends. Alyssa also decided to check out the forum pages, and she read through several posts of users' experiences with depression. When she clicked on the forum page, she saw that there were over 6000 posts on depression and anxiety; however, she noticed that the forum was no longer active. She was still amazed though that she had no idea that there would be so many people out there who would be talking about depression. She decided to check out the Australian site at reachout.com and saw that the forum was still active on this site. She also found that there were similar materials between the US and Australian sites, but the Australian site had a few more features that still were relevant for the US.

Alyssa decided to follow the advice on how to help a friend and she asked Tyler how he was doing; initially he was very hesitant to talk with her. She thought through the website's suggestions about how to talk with someone who is struggling with their feelings and didn't press him on opening up right away. She let him know that she was there if he wanted to talk. She also mentioned to Tyler that she didn't know what Tyler was going through but found two websites, www.ReachOut.com and www.au.reachout.com, and that these two sites provided her with information and resources. She told Tyler that she liked both the US and Australian sites and that the Australian version had a few more features and they had cool accents in the video clips. Tyler thanked her for the information and let her know that he was doing okay. But inside, Tyler knew he was struggling.

The next day, Tyler decided to stay home from school. He told his dad he wasn't feeling well and needed a day to catch up on his homework. After his dad left for work, Tyler decided to first look at the US ReachOut.com website. He was skeptical at first, but when he saw that the website wasn't trying to diagnose him or make him feel like he had to bear his soul, he decided to keep exploring. Tyler clicked on the "Real Stories" (http://us.ReachOut.com/real-stories) page and read about other people's struggles with anxiety, depression, and other mental health issues. There was even one story where the person talked about how they had always been embarrassed about their struggles with mental illness. Before Tyler realized it, he had spent 4 h reading the stories and facts on mental health issues. Tyler thought that he would also check out the Australian version and saw that they had a section "The Toolbox" (http://au.reachout.com/sites/thetoolbox) where he could find and identify what he wanted to work on, and it gave him ideas of websites and apps that he could use to possibly help himself feel better.

The next day Tyler decided to explore the Toolbox feature and picked the goal "Improve General Well-being." Tyler found the app Music eScape, which maps the music on his iPhone to different moods. He downloaded the app and loved that it used his music and that he was able to identify the mood he was currently in and then tell the app how he wanted to feel. He couldn't believe that the app chose his own music to help him feel better, the way he wanted to feel.

Throughout the next week, he continued to use both the US and Australian version of ReachOut.com and decided that the next time he saw Alyssa he would thank her for sharing the information. Tyler realized that he wasn't alone and that there were people just like him, including other guys, who struggled with depression. Tyler decided to write an email to his dad letting him know that he was struggling with depression and sent him the links to the ReachOut.com website. While he was looking around the Australia ReachOut.com site, he also found there was a place for parents to get support. Tyler also sent his dad the link to the Australia ReachOut.com Parent. Tyler was able to have a conversation with his dad, and they made an appointment with a community mental health provider.

When Tyler and his dad met with the mental health provider, the clinician asked Tyler how he was feeling. Tyler indicated that he has been "feeling off" for the past several months. He mentioned that at first he thought it would pass, but then he realized that he was no longer wanting to do anything except be by himself, sleep, and didn't feel like eating. He also told her that he had been embarrassed to talk about his feelings because he didn't want anyone to think he was weird or just being a big baby. Tyler and his dad told the clinician about the support they both found on the US and Australian version of ReachOut.com, and Tyler realized that he wasn't alone in feeling the way he was feeling. Tyler showed the clinician the Music eScape app that he had been using and that he found that it had helped him with his mood, but he knew that he also needed to check with a professional to see if he needed more help.

Conclusion

The age of digital media is upon us, and research has documented that youth have access to and use technology to connect to their world. Australia has led the way in their use of technology to deliver online and youth-based services to support mental health. Mental health issues among youth are prevalent, and many youth have low levels of mental health literacy and high levels of mental health stigma and aren't likely to seek help when they are struggling. Initiatives though need to be dynamic and provided at multiple levels. For example, beyondblue uses different mechanisms to reach the public. Their media campaigns inform the public about mental health issues, specifically depression, anxiety, and suicide. On the beyondblue website, they have mental health promotion material and support for seeking help. The materials include fact sheets, videos, and vetted apps. At a different level, MindMatters is a free program that schools can implement to administrators, staff, and students to promote well-being and identify and support the entire school system to address mental health. ReachOut.com in Australia and the United States provides youth with content and support for mental health issues. Their goal is to increase mental health literacy, reduce stigma, and increase help seeking in the general population. The Australian version also includes quiz components to help guide youth to applications and materials that specifically relate to their needs.

We R Native fills a significant gap in the online resources available that specifically address mental health issues for Native American Youth, the American Indian, and Alaska Native youth (AI/AN). They sought to harness the enormous opportunities the Internet could offer to AI/AN youth in a safe space and method that would support them in culturally specific ways.

The initiatives in this chapter represent only a few of the many approaches to support youth mental health. The opportunities for clinicians to incorporate these resources are endless. Ideally, the resources could be used for prevention and interventions. Clinicians could have lists of evidence-informed websites and apps and could provide these to the patients. Specifically, as a primary prevention approach, clinicians could hang up posters and/or pass out pamphlets in their offices and waiting rooms about these digital resources. If there are video screens in the waiting rooms, the clinicians could upload a series of videos on the different mental health issues (e.g., anxiety, depression, etc.) that could automatically play. During a session, clinicians could introduce the different resources with the patients and walk through how they might be beneficial for supporting the adolescent going through their specific issue. The clinician could also do follow-up with patients to determine if the resources are helpful and gain the patient's perspective on what is most helpful.

The future of supporting mental health will likely include apps and methods to measure and track wellness through biometric approaches combined with other technologies. In order to ensure that interventions are evidence-based and meet youth's specific needs, ongoing research needs to occur. What is difficult, however, is that there may not always be opportunities and funding to assess every intervention with the gold standard of science, randomized controlled trials, to determine if each intervention does lead to positive outcomes, however defined. Optimally, these organizations will have defined outcome measures (ReachOut.com and au.reachout.com, mental health literacy, stigma, and help-seeking behaviors; That's not cool, healthy relationship beliefs; AnxietyBC, anxiety), and the organization will partner with academics to evaluate their processes and outcomes. Clinicians can't provide every service to every person 24 h a day, 7 days a week. Mental health technologies, though, may be one solution for providing patients with support in ways that make sense to them and that are readily accessible even outside the clinician's office.

Acknowledgment *We R Native* is supported, in part, with funds from the Indian Health Service and the Secretary's Minority AIDS Initiative Fund.

References

1. Burns J, Birrell E. Enhancing early engagement with mental health services by young people. Psychol Res Behav Manag. 2014;7:303–12.
2. Eisenberg D, Downs MF, Golberstein E, Zivin K. Stigma and help seeking for mental health among college students. Med Care Res Rev. 2009;66(5):522–41.
3. Hunt J, Eisenberg D. Mental health problems and help-seeking behavior among college students. J Adolesc Health. 2010;46(1):3–10.
4. Nam SK, Choi SI, Lee JH, Lee MK, Kim AR, Lee SM. Psychological factors in college students' attitudes toward seeking professional psychological help: A meta-analysis. Prof Psychol Res Pract. 2013;44(1):37–45.
5. Yap MBH, Reavley NJ, Jorm AF. Associations between stigma and help-seeking intentions and beliefs: Findings from an Australian national survey of young people. Psychiatry Res. 2013;210(3):1154–60.
6. Yap MBH, Wright A, Jorm AF. The influence of stigma on young people's help-seeking intentions and beliefs about the helpfulness of various

sources of help. Soc Psychiatry Psychiatr Epidemiol. 2011;46(12):1257–65.
7. Yap MBH, Reavley N, Jorm AF. Where would young people seek help for mental disorders and what stops them? Findings from an Australian national survey. J Affect Disord. 2013;147(1–3):255–61.
8. Moreno MA, Jelenchick LA, Kota R. Exploring depression symptom references on facebook among college freshmen: a mixed methods approach. Open J Depress. 2013;2(3):35–41.
9. Cash SJ, Bridge JA. Meeting them where they are: An exploration of technology use and help seeking behaviors among adolescents and young adults. San Francisco: American Association of Child and Adolescent Psychiatry; 2012.
10. Keyes S, Cash S. ReachOut.com March 2012 User Survey. Inspire USA Foundation; 2012.
11. Duggan M. Mobile Messaging and Social Media 2015 [Internet]. Pew Research Center: Internet, Science & Tech. 2015 [cited 2017 Mar 10]. http://www.pewinternet.org/2015/08/19/mobile-messaging-and-social-media-2015/
12. Lenhart A. Teens, Social Media & Technology Overview 2015 [Internet]. Pew Research Center: Internet, Science & Tech. 2015 [cited 2017 Mar 10]. http://www.pewinternet.org/2015/04/09/teens-social-media-technology-2015/
13. Our story | About ReachOut Australia [Internet] [cited 2017 Mar 9]. http://about.au.reachout.com/us/story/
14. What we do | About ReachOut Australia [Internet] [cited 2017 Mar 9]. http://about.au.reachout.com/what-we-do/
15. Collin PJ, Metcalf AT, Stephens-Reicher JC, Blanchard ME, Herrman HE, Rahilly K, et al. ReachOut.com: The role of an online service for promoting help-seeking in young people. Adv. Ment Health. 2011;10(1):39–51.
16. Kessler, R.C., Andrews, G., Colpe, LJ, Hiripi, E.Short screening scales to monitor population prevalences and trends in non-specific psychological distress. Psychological Medicine. 2002;32(6):959–76.
17. Metcalf AT, Ivancic L, Blake V, Buhagiar K, Wilson C, Kauer S, et al. ReachOut.com Cohort study: a prospective follow-up study examining the role of online initiatives in promoting mental health literacy and early help-seeking. Montreal: International Association for Youth Mental Health; 2016.
18. Center for Native American Youth. Drawing strength from our cultures: State of Native Youth 2016. In: State of Native Youth Report 2016. The Aspen Institute.
19. Bureau USC. American FactFinder - Results [Internet] [cited 2017 Mar 11]. https://factfinder.census.gov/faces/tableservices/jsf/pages/productview.xhtml?pid=ACS_10_1YR_S0201&prodType=table
20. Evans-Campbell T. Historical trauma in American Indian/Native Alaska communities. J Interpers Violence. 2008;23(3):316–38.
21. Centers for Disease Control and Prevention. High school youth risk behavioral survey data results [Internet]. 2011. http://apps.nccd.cdc.gov/youthonline/App/Default.aspx
22. Centers for Disease Control and Prevention. Suicide 2015 [Internet]. 2015. www.cdc.gov/violenceprevention/pdf/suicide-datasheet-a.pdf
23. Hansen-Mitchell D. Preventing native youth suicide: #WeNeedYouHere Campaign Spreads Love and Help. Verona: Indian Country Media Network.
24. Craig Rushing S, Stephens D. Use of media technologies by Native American teens and young adults in the Pacific Northwest: exploring their utility for designing culturally appropriate technology-based health interventions. J Prim Prev. 2011;32(3):135–45.
25. Rushing S. Using technology to promote health and wellbeing among American Indian and Alaska Native teens and young adults. In: Dyson L, Grant S, Hendriks M, editors. Indigenous people and mobile technologies. New York: Routledge.
26. Bryant C, McCormack Brown KR, McDermott RJ. Community-Based Prevention Marketing: Organizing a Community for Health Behavior Intervention. Health Promot Pract. 2007;8(2):154–63.
27. beyondblue. Who we are and what we do [Internet] [cited 2017 Mar 10]. https://www.beyondblue.org.au/about-us/who-we-are-and-what-we-do
28. beyondblue. Home [Internet] [cited 2017 Mar 10]. https://www.youthbeyondblue.com
29. Dix KL, Slee PT, Lawson MJ, Keeves JP. Implementation quality of whole-school mental health promotion and students' academic performance. Child Adolesc Ment Health. 2012;17(1):45–51.
30. MindMatters. MindMatters Live Stats [Internet]. MindMatters Live Stats [cited 2017 Jun 28]. https://www.mindmatters.edu.au/about-mindmatters/live-stats

Index

M.A. Moreno, A. Radovic (eds.), *Technology and Adolescent Mental Health*,
https://doi.org/10.1007/978-3-319-69638-6

B

Printed by Printforce, the Netherlands